Advances in Veterinary Science
and Comparative Medicine

Volume 34

Domestic Animal Cytogenetics

Advances in Veterinary Science and Comparative Medicine

Edited by

C. E. Cornelius
California Primate Research Center
University of California
Davis, California

R. R. Marshak
School of Veterinary Medicine
University of Pennsylvania
New Bolton Center
Kennett Square, Pennsylvania

E. C. Melby
Animal Health Products Research and Development
Smith, Kline, Beckman
West Chester, Pennsylvania

Advisory Board

Kalman Perk
André Rico
Irwin Arias
Bennie Osburn
W. Jean Dodds

Advances in Veterinary Science
and Comparative Medicine

Volume 34

Domestic Animal Cytogenetics

Edited by

Richard A. McFeely

Department of Clinical Studies
School of Veterinary Medicine
University of Pennsylvania
New Bolton Center
Kennett Square, Pennsylvania

Academic Press, Inc.
Harcourt Brace Jovanovich, Publishers
San Diego   New York   Boston
London   Sydney   Tokyo   Toronto

This book is printed on acid-free paper.

COPYRIGHT © 1990 BY ACADEMIC PRESS, INC.
All Rights Reserved.
No part of this publication may be reproduced or transmitted in any form or by any means, electronic or mechanical, including photocopy, recording, or any information storage and retrieval system, without permission in writing from the publisher.

ACADEMIC PRESS, INC.
San Diego, California 92101

United Kingdom Edition published by
ACADEMIC PRESS LIMITED
24-28 Oval Road, London NW1 7DX

LIBRARY OF CONGRESS CATALOG CARD NUMBER: 53-7098

ISBN 0-12-039234-8 (alk. paper)

PRINTED IN THE UNITED STATES OF AMERICA
90 91 92 93   9 8 7 6 5 4 3 2 1

CONTENTS

Preface ix

Introduction
Richard A. McFeely

I. History	1
II. Chromosomes	4
III. Chromosome Abnormalities	10
IV. Genes	12
V. Molecular Genetics	15
References	16

Chromosome Methodology
Susan E. Long

I. Preparation of Chromosomes	19
II. Chromosome Identification	29
References	37

Chromosomes of the Cow and Bull
Paul C. Popescu

I. Normal Karyotype	41
II. Chromosome Abnormalities	44
III. Y Chromosome Polymorphism	62
IV. The Y Chromosome of Zebu Cattle	62
V. Sexing of Bovine Embryos	64
References	66

Chromosomes of the Pig
Ingemar Gustavsson

I. Introduction	73
II. Evolutionary Aspects on the Pig Karyotype	74
III. The Normal Mitotic and Meiotic Chromosomes	76
IV. Polymorphism	80
V. Spontaneous Chromosome Aberrations and Their Phenotypic Effects	81
VI. Intersexuality and Chimerism	90
VII. Chromosomes of the General Population	92
VIII. Use of the Pig and Pig Chromosomes for Experimental Purposes	93
IX. Future Cytogenetic Research Work in the Pig	97
References	99

Chromosomes of Sheep and Goats
Susan E. Long

I. Normal Chromosome Complement	109
II. Chromosome Abnormalities in Sheep	113
III. Chromosome Abnormalities in Goats	120
IV. Goat–Sheep Hybrids	124
References	125

Chromosomes of the Horse
Monica M. Power

I. Historical Introduction	131
II. Techniques for the Study of Horse Chromosomes	132
III. The Normal Horse Karyotype	143
IV. Clinical Application of Cytogenetics in the Horse	146
V. Horse Breeds and Interspecific Hybrids	157
References	160

Chromosomes of Chickens
N. S. Fechheimer

I. Introduction	170
II. Methodology	172

III.	The Mitotic Karyotype	177
IV.	Meiotic Chromosomes and Synaptonemal Complexes	183
V.	Incidence of Heteroploidy	189
VI.	Origins and Etiology of Heteroploidy	192
VII.	Structural Aberrations	196
VIII.	Effects of Structural Aberrations	198
IX.	Concluding Remarks	201
	References	203

Chromosomes of Fish
C. Larry Chrisman, Kent H. Blacklidge, and Penny K. Riggs

I.	Fish Genetic Research	209
II.	Cytogenetic Tools	218
III.	Summary	222
	References	223

Chromosome Abnormalities and Pregnancy Failure in Domestic Animals
W. Allan King

I.	Introduction	229
II.	Cytogenetic Study of Germ Cells and Embryos	230
III.	Germ Cells	231
IV.	Embryos	235
V.	Effects of Chromosome Abnormalities	243
VI.	Embryonic and Fetal Loss	244
VII.	Conclusions	245
	References	246

Gene Mapping in the Cow
James E. Womack

I.	Introduction	251
II.	Methods of Bovine Gene Mapping	253
III.	Current Status of the Cow Map	257
IV.	Comparative Maps	262
V.	Considerations for the Future	268
	References	270

Gene Mapping in the Pig
R. Fries, P. Vögeli, and G. Stranzinger

I. Gene Mapping and Animal Breeding	273
II. Methods Applied in Gene Mapping	275
III. Status of the Map	281
IV. Conclusions	281
V. Appendix: Gene Loci in the Pig	283
References	292

Glossary of Commonly Used Terms	305
Index	309

PREFACE

My first introduction to the discipline of cytogenetics was in the summer of 1962 when, as a young veterinarian fresh from a farm animal clinical practice, I reported to Professor John Biggers' laboratory at the University of Pennsylvania to begin a postdoctoral training program in reproductive biology. It was an exciting time. Many pioneering efforts in ova and early embryo culture were under way, and a steady stream of scientists, legendary in this emerging field, were either training in the laboratory or visiting for periods of time. As I had no preconceived ideas about which direction my research should take, Professor Biggers suggested looking at the chromosomes of some of the domestic animals because he felt that the discipline of mammalian cytogenetics was about to come into its own.

After a few trips to the library I had learned, among other things, that there were two fewer human chromosomes since I had taken the basic genetics course at my undergraduate university 8 years ago. Since I was sure that evolution did not occur that rapidly, it was apparent that a major breakthrough in technology had taken place, and that it was now possible to study mammalian chromosomes in a great deal more detail. Not only was the normal human chromosome complement now well defined, but certain developmental defects in children had been linked to specific chromosome abnormalities, and the "Philadelphia chromosome" associated with human chronic granulocytic leukemia had been described by colleagues working in the same building in which our laboratory was located. I decided that the time was right for me to learn more about this field and to begin to apply some of the techniques to domestic animals.

Professor Paul Moorhead, who, with his colleagues, had just published a method for displaying chromosomes after short-term culture of cells obtained from peripheral blood, was located across the street in the Wistar Institute, and he was kind enough to take the time to help me get started. My colleague and good friend, W. C. D. Hare, was also getting started in the chromosome business as part of his research on bovine leukemia. He also shared his ideas and knowledge with me, and before long we were able to establish the laboratory which I still occupy today. Doug Hare's interests eventually took him from the University of Pennsylvania and from a direct association with mammalian chromosomes, but his help and encouragement in my formative years as a scientist will never be forgotten. With the encouragement and support of John Biggers and W. C. D. Hare, I embarked on a study of chromosome abnormalities in pig embryos and of developmental defects associated with reproductive failure, a study which continues to this day.

In the mid 1960s, most of those interested in mammalian cytogenetics in the United States assembled in Gatlinburg, Tennessee for the first of what was to become an annual Mammalian Chromosomes and Somatic Cell Genetics Conference. The discussions were informal and lively, and information was exchanged freely. The pioneer spirit which prevailed must have been similar to the feelings of other early explorers. Regardless of the species involved, interest in new developments was keen.

As the number of workers interested in chromosomes of domestic animals increased, it was necessary to create a new forum for the exchange of ideas. The European workers gathered first in Giessen in 1970, and have continued to meet every other year; their most recent meeting, the 9th European Colloquium on Cytogenetics of Domestic Animals, was held in Toulouse, France in July 1990. Several years later, the North American workers began to meet on years alternate to the European meeting. The 7th North American Colloquium on Domestic Animal Chromosomes and Gene Mapping will convene in Philadelphia in July 1991.

When approached by the editorial staff of Academic Press about this volume, I agreed to serve as editor conditional on the recruitment of appropriate authorities to write the individual chapters. All of the contributors are leading authorities in the field, and all agreed to participate with minimal persuasion.

The purpose of the book is to provide a comprehensive review of the status of domestic animal chromosomes and to serve as an introduction to the literature. Two chapters on gene mapping, a relatively new field in cytogenetics, have been included.

A very special acknowledgment is due my wife, Lynne R. Klunder, who has worked as a colleague in the laboratory, and who has supported and enthusiastically encouraged my efforts in this field for the last 15 years.

RICHARD A. MCFEELY

Introduction

RICHARD A. McFEELY

Department of Clinical Studies, School of Veterinary Medicine, University of Pennsylvania, New Bolton Center, Kennett Square, Pennsylvania

I. History
II. Chromosomes
III. Chromosome Abnormalities
IV. Genes
V. Molecular Genetics
   References

I. History

Cytogenetics is defined as the study of the morphology and behavior of chromosomes. Chromosome studies in domestic animals and man have evolved as a modern scientific discipline in the past three decades, although human chromosomes were first observed in dividing cells by Virchow (1857) over 100 years earlier. The significance of their true nature apparently was not appreciated at that time.

The process of cell division called mitosis, in which chromosomes can be visualized, was described by von Török (1874), and detailed descriptions of human chromosomes were made by Arnold (1879). During the next decade several long treatises amplified the knowledge about cell structure and function. Flemming (1882) introduced the term *chromatin* for the darkly staining portions of the nucleus. That chromatin was the physical basis of inheritance was concluded independently by Weismann (1883), Strasburger (1884), and von Kölliker (1885). Waldeyer (1888), after a lengthy review and discussion of the literature, introduced the term *chromosome* for these chromatin structures.

During the middle of the nineteenth century, the Austrian monk, Gregor Mendel (1866), developed his theories about inheritance, which were published in 1866. However, his concepts were so far ahead of his time that it was not until the early part of the twentieth century that his ideas were rediscovered and became widely accepted. In 1903, Sutton and Boveri independently formulated the connection between chromosomes and Mendelian inheritance (Peters, 1959).

Through the first half of the twentieth century, geneticists working primarily with plants and insects began to develop a large body of knowledge about chromosome morphology and behavior during cell division. In contrast, relatively less was known about chromosomes of domestic animals and man. Three events stimulated increased interest in mammalian cytogenetics in the years following World War II. The first was the discovery of a sexual dimorphism in the neurons of cats. In 1948 Dr. Ewart G. Bertram, a postgraduate student, was working with Professor Murray Barr on a project involving stimulation of the hypoglossal nerve of cats and subsequent histologic evaluation of the affected neurons. It was noted that in the neurons of some animals, a darkly staining body, which they called a nucleolar satellite, was present in a large number of cells, but was absent from virtually all cells of other animals subjected to the same treatment. Analysis of the records quickly revealed that the structure was present in nerve cells from female cats, but was absent in similar cells from males. Similar findings were reported for nerve cells in humans. The discovery of the sex chromatin body, as it was subsequently named, was published by Barr and Bertram (1949).

The second event was the result of a fortuitous observation of a laboratory mistake. Techniques for culturing mammalian cells *in vitro* were being developed, and these cell cultures provided the scientist with a source of cells undergoing mitosis. The use of colchicine, an alkaloid derived from the autumn crocus, inhibited mitotic spindle formation and arrested cells in metaphase when the chromosomes were maximally condensed and could be most easily identified. However, when viewed through the microscope, the chromosomes were overlapped and identification of individual chromosomes was not possible. In fact, it was not possible to accurately count the number of chromosomes in a cell. Hsu (1952) observed that the chromosomes were separated and could be visualized and counted without difficulty in cells that had been washed, accidentally, with a hypotonic solution instead of an isotonic solution prior to fixation. Hypotonic treatment opened the door for the mammalian cytogeneticist.

The third event was the report by Tjio and Levan (1956) that the diploid number of chromosomes in man was 46 rather than 48. Shortly thereafter, the discovery of an extra chromosome associated with Down's syndrome (Lejeune *et al.*, 1959) started a massive search for other types of chromosomal anomalies. The technique for the display of chromosomes after short-term culture of cells obtained from peripheral blood hastened the process (Moorhead *et al.,* 1960). In the decade that followed, reports of human chromosome abnormalities associated with congenital defects, reproductive disorders, spontaneous abortions, and neoplasia proliferated at an unprecedented rate.

Although the number of workers interested in chromosomes of domestic animals was quite small, there was general interest in the normal chromosome complement of a wide variety of species, and by 1975 an *Atlas of Mammalian Chromosomes* (Hsu and Benirschke, 1967) containing about 500 entries had been published. Reports of chromosome abnormalities associated with developmental defects and reproductive failure in domestic animals began to appear in the literature in 1964. Until the early part of the 1970s, it was still very difficult to identify individual chromosomes, especially in those species in which the morphology was similar and the only discernible difference was the size of the chromosome. The development of techniques using quinacrine mustard initially, and subsequently, a variety of other treatments that allowed differential staining of individual chromosomes, facilitated their identification. The banding patterns also permitted the cytogeneticist to identify minor structural chromosomal rearrangements, which had previously gone undetected. Today, chromosome analysis is frequently requested as part of breeding soundness examinations of valuable stallions and is one of the requirements for importation of certain species into various countries.

Currently, new technology is permitting scientists to investigate the structure and function of individual chromosomes. Single genes have been isolated, purified, and cloned and their chemical sequence has been identified. They have been introduced into cells in tissue culture to study how genes are regulated and have been introduced as foreign genes into other species, where, in some instances, they function as if in their own species. The possibility of using laboratory-purified genes as therapy for some genetic diseases now seems to be technically feasible.

Determining the exact location of each gene on individual chromosomes is known as gene mapping. Today, a major effort is being made to map the entire human genome. This is an extraordinarily ambitious undertaking and can only be accomplished with the efforts of many cooperating laboratories and the expenditure of vast sums of money. As usual, similar studies in domestic animals lag behind these efforts to study the human genome, but many laboratories have made impressive beginnings and there is considerable worldwide interest in such studies. For gene mapping to proceed, it is necessary to have general acceptance of the standardized karyotype for each species. With this goal in mind, workers on standarization committees for the cow, sheep, goat, and horse met for the Second International Conference for Standardization of Domestic Animal Karyotypes in Jouy en Josas, France in May 1989 to update the standards published as the result of the first standardization meeting held in Reading, England in 1976 (Ford et al., 1980). The standard karyotype for the pig has been published (Gustavsson, 1988) and the results of the Jouy en Josas conference will appear in early 1990.

II. Chromosomes

Although chromosomes have been studied extensively since the beginning of the century, it has only been in recent years that we have gained detailed knowledge of their structure and function. Chromosomes are best visualized during certain stages of cell division, when they are maximally condensed and can be seen through a light microscope.

Mitotic chromosomes have certain fundamental characteristics. First, the number of chromosomes is constant for all normal animals in a given species (Table I). Second, when the chromosomes are photographed, cut out, and arranged in pairs, the resulting karyotype is identical for all members of that species. Third, with one exception, the chromosomes occur in pairs and are called autosomes. The exception is the sex chromosomes, which are paired in females but are unpaired in

TABLE I

DIPLOID CHROMOSOME NUMBERS

Species	Number
Pig	38
Cat	38
Sheep	54
Cow	60
Goat	60
Horse	64
Dog	78
Chicken	78

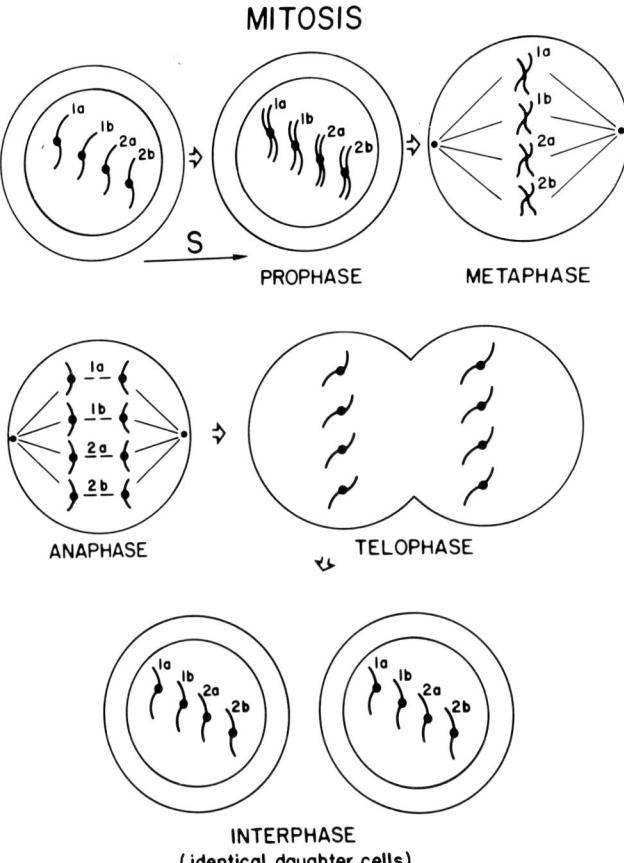

FIG. 1. Mitosis: cell division producing two identical daughter cells, each with an exact duplicate of the nuclear DNA of the parent cell. (From Kelly, T., "Clinical Genetics and Genetic Counseling," 2nd Ed. Year Book Med. Publ., Chicago, Illinois, 1986.)

males. In domestic mammals, the female X chromosome is generally much larger than the male Y chromosome. In birds, the female is the heterogametic sex with ZW sex chromosomes; the male has two Z chromosomes.

Cell division in somatic cells is called mitosis, a process in which two genetically identical cells are produced from a single cell (Fig. 1). The cell cycle can be divided into two phases—interphase and cell division. During interphase, the chromosomes are present as uncoiled molecules of deoxyribonucleic acid (DNA). The interphase portion of the cell cycle is subdivided into three periods. During G1 the cell carries out its normal metabolic functions under the control of its DNA. Following the G1 period, the cell enters the S period, during which the DNA is replicated, producing an exact copy of itself. Each chromosome then consists of two daughter chromatids. After a short G2 period, cell division begins.

Mitosis consists of four stages. During prophase the DNA molecules begin to spiral, forming coils that are recognizable as chromosomes. The nuclear membrane disappears and the mitotic spindle begins to form as the centrioles move to opposite poles of the cell. The second stage of mitosis is metaphase, when the chromosomes are fully condensed and are clearly visible. It is during late prophase or metaphase that the chromosomes are usually analyzed. At this point, the centromere, which unites the two daughter chromatids, attaches to the mitotic spindle and the chromosomes align along the middle of the cell. During anaphase the centromere divides along the longitudinal axis and the sister chromatids of each chromosome migrate toward opposite poles to become a chromosome of the daughter cell. The final phase of mitosis is called telophase. The chromosomes uncoil and return to their interphase state, the nuclear membrane is reestablished, duplication of the centriole occurs, and the cytoplasm divides, completing the formation of two identical daughter cells. The normal chromosome number for a somatic cell is called the diploid number and may be represented as $2n$.

Meiosis is a type of cell division, restricted to germ cells, in which gametes containing one chromosome from each pair are produced (Fig. 2). Thus, the chromosome number of a gamete is one-half the diploid ($2n$) number and is referred to as the haploid number *(n)*. At the moment of fertilization, when a male and female gamete unite to begin the formation of a new individual, the diploid number is restored.

Meiosis is more complex than mitosis and differs in two critical ways. The first involves the exchange of genetic material among homologous chromosomes, a process called *crossing over*. The net effect is that the new chromatids resulting from the exchange now have genes derived from the original maternal and paternal chromosomes. Unlike mitosis, the chromosomes in which crossing over has occurred are not exact copies of the original parental cell, but have new genetic combinations. The second major difference between meiosis and mitosis is that the number of chromosomes in the resulting gametes is reduced from the diploid to the haploid number. Meiosis consists of two cell divisions; meiosis I is a reductional division and meiosis II is an equational division. Both crossing over and the reduction in chromo-

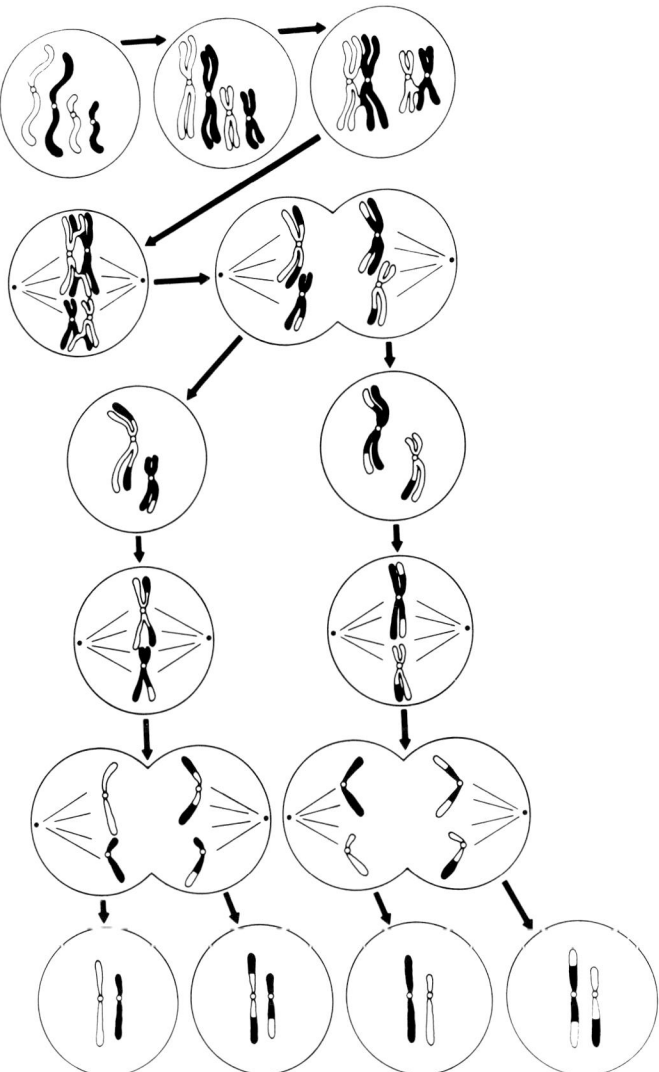

FIG. 2. Meiosis: cell division of germ cells producing haploid gametes. Note that crossing over and reduction of the diploid chromosome number occur in the first meiotic division. (From Kelly, T., "Clinical Genetics and Genetic Counseling," 2nd Ed. Year Book Med. Publ., Chicago, Illinois, 1986.)

some numbers occur in prophase I, which is divided into five stages. Prior to the onset of prophase I, as in mitosis, DNA replication has occurred and the cell contains four times the amount of DNA that the gametes will finally have.

The first stage of prophase I is called the leptotene stage, in which the chromatin condenses into recognizable forms of individual chromosomes. During the zygotene stage, homologous chromosomes come into intimate, side-by-side contact, forming a bivalent. This process is called synapsis. As the X and Y chromosomes are not homologous, they pair in an end-to-end fashion in males. In females, the two X chromosomes form a bivalent in a manner similar to that of the autosomes. In the pachytene stage, the chromosomes are sufficiently condensed so that individual bivalents are visualized as having four chromatids joined at the centromere; these are referred to as tetrads. In the diplotene stage, exchange of identical portions of chromatin between homologous chromosomes occurs. The sites of crossing over are known as chiasmata. Normally, at least one (and frequently more than one) exchange is made for each chromosome pair. The final stage of prophase I is diakinesis, whereby the exchange bridges are broken and the bivalents separate from each other. Prophase I stops with the breakdown of the nuclear membrane.

In metaphase I the bivalents align along the equatorial plate of the meiotic spindle. As the segregation of homologous chromosomes is random, and because the crossing over exchanges have created chromosomes with new gene combinations, the likelihood that the gametes will be different is assured. Anaphase I and telophase I are similar to mitosis except that in meiosis homologous members of a chromosome pair are separated, each containing two chromatids. Metaphase II is similar to mitosis except that there is no S phase, as no DNA replication occurs. The end result is four daughter cells, each with a haploid number of chromosomes. In the case of the mammalian male, the four gametes become spermatozoa, whereas in the female, meiosis is arrested in prophase I, and meiosis I is not completed until around the time of ovulation. Meiosis II is completed around the time of fertilization. In the female only one of the daughter cells becomes the ovum, while one is shed as a diploid polar body at the end of meiosis I and the second is a haploid polar body shed at the completion of meiosis II.

Basically, the techniques used for the display of mammalian chromosomes begin with a source of rapidly dividing cells. These cells can be harvested from cell culture preparations or obtained directly from tissues such as bone marrow, testes, or certain rapidly growing tumors in which cell division is occurring at a high rate. When peripheral

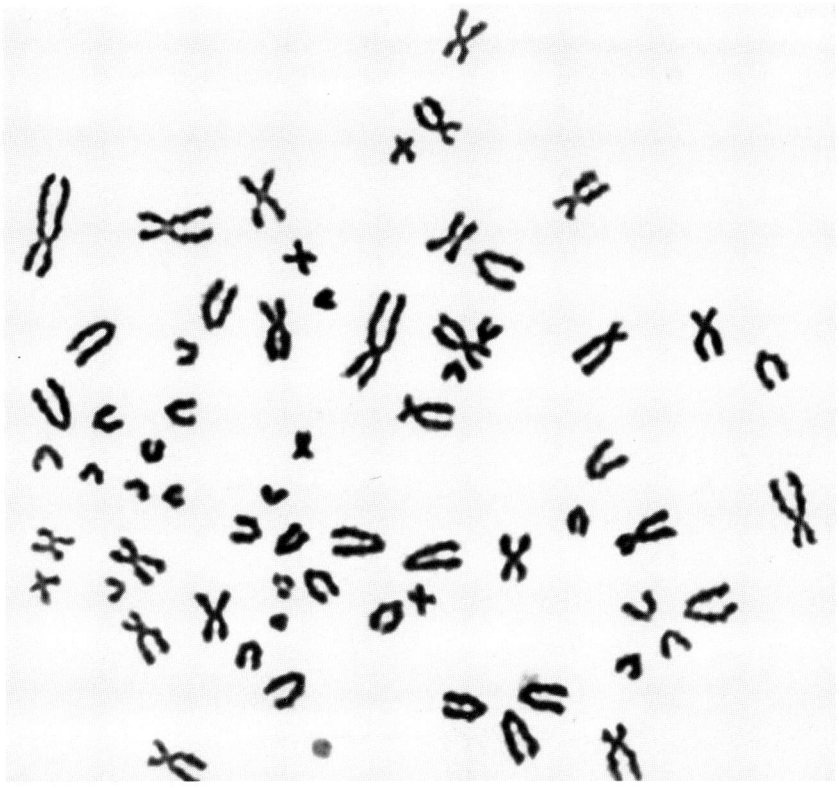

FIG. 3. Equine metaphase chromosomes obtained from a cultured lymphocyte.

blood leukocytes are used in cell culture, they must be stimulated to divide. The most commonly used mitotic stimulators are phytohemagglutinin (PHA), which is derived from the red kidney bean, or pokeweed mitogen (PWM). Normally, for mitotic preparations, colchicine or a related compound is added to the cell medium for a short period of time; this interferes with the formation of the spindle in the dividing cells and arrests cell division in metaphase. The cells are suspended in a hypotonic solution such as potassium chloride or sodium citrate to allow for osmotic swelling, which facilitates subsequent visualization of the chromosomes. The cells are then fixed using a simple methanol:acetic acid fixative and are placed on a glass slide and stained for examination with a conventional light microscope. Figure 3 is a metaphase spread obtained from a peripheral blood culture of cells from a horse. For analysis, the metaphase chromosomes are counted and photographed and each chromosome is cut out, matched with its homologue, and displayed in a standardized manner. The resulting display is called a karyotype.

Mammalian chromosomes obtained from cells in metaphase have three basic shapes, depending upon the location of the centromere. The centromere is the specialized region of the chromosome to which the spindle fibers attach during cell division. During metaphase it is the junction point of the two daughter chromatids. If the centromere is located near the middle of the chromosome, it is referred to as a metacentric chromosome. If the centromere is located at or near the end of the chromosome, the chromosome is called an acrocentric chromosome. Some cytogeneticists refer to chromosomes whose centromere is located at the terminal end of the chromosome as telocentric, although there is controversy on the question of whether short arms to the chromosome are always present even if they are not readily observed. When the centromere lies in an intermediate position, the chromosome is said to be a submetacentric chromosome. By convention, the short arm of the chromosome is referred to as the p arm and the long arm is called the q arm.

III. Chromosome Abnormalities

Chromosome abnormalities are frequently associated with developmental anomalies. Many abnormalities are severe enough to result in embryonic death and are manifested as various levels of infertility. There are two types of chromosome abnormalities. The first type involves chromosome numbers. Abnormalities of chromosome numbers can be subdivided into a group in which individual chromosmes may be either missing or duplicated, and a group in which whole haploid sets of chromosomes may be added or lost. When a single chromosome is missing from a cell, the cell is said to be monosomic for that chromosome. When an extra chromosome is present in a cell, that cell is referred to as a trisomy. The general condition whereby single chromosomes are either missing or present in excess is called aneuploidy. When whole sets of extra chromosomes are present in a cell, the condition is called polyploidy. Triploidy is the condition whereby a cell has one extra set of chromosomes ($3n$); tetraploidy refers to two extra sets of chromosomes ($4n$), etc.

Aneuploidy occurs as the result of nondisjunction when, in mitosis, there is failure of the chromatids to separate during anaphase, result ing in one daughter cell with an extra chromosome and one missing that same chromosome. In meiosis, nondisjunction is the result of failure of a bivalent to separate during the first meiotic division or failure of the sister chromatids to separate during the second meiotic division.

Polyploidy can arise by a number of mechanisms. The most common cause in mammals is probably the fertilization of an ovum by more than one spermatozoon. Aging of the ovum after ovulation may be an important factor in allowing polyspermy to occur. Failure of the ovum to shed the second polar body during meiosis results in a gamete with two haploid sets of chromosomes, which, when fertilized, produces a triploid embryo. Fusion of two diploid cells results in a tetraploid cell, as does nuclear division without subsequent division of the cytoplasm. Endoreduplication occurs when there is DNA replication without nuclear division, resulting in a tetraploid cell. In this condition the sister chromosomes are observed side by side during metaphase.

The second type of chromosome abnormality results from structural rearrangement of a chromosome or chromosomes. A variety of agents can produce chromosome damage, including viruses, drugs, and radiation. A deletion occurs when a chromosome becomes damaged and a fragment of the chromosome breaks off and fails to reunite. As deletions contain no centromere, they become lost at the next cell division. Inversion is a condition in which a chromosome suffers several breaks and a portion of the chromosome is turned end-for-end and is incorporated back into the chromosome. If the inversion incorporates the centromere, it is called a pericentric inversion. A translocation involves a fragment breaking off from one chromosome and attaching to another chromosome. The translocation is spoken of as a reciprocal translocation if fragments are exchanged among two chromosomes. A translocation frequently alters the size and shape of the affected chromosomes. When two acrocentric chromosomes join at the centromeric region to form a metacentric or submetacentric chromosome, it is called a centric fusion or a Robertsonian translocation.

Some animals possess more than one cell line in their bodies. A mosaic is defined as an individual with a mixture of genetically different cells that were derived from a single fertilized egg. A chimera, on the other hand, is an individual with a mixture of genetically different cells that originated from more than one individual. The bovine freemartin, a sterile heifer born co-twin with a bull, is the best example of a chimera. In the freemartin and in the bull twin, there are leukocytes containing XX sex chromosomes derived from the heifer and leukocytes containing XY sex chromosomes derived from the bull. The intermingling of white cells results from the fusion of the vessels in the two placentas early in gestation and the exchange of blood through the conjoined circulation.

IV. Genes

Genes have been considered the basic unit of heredity since the early part of the twentieth century. Knowledge about genes developed in three stages. In the early half of the century, scientists defined genes, using breeding experiments and working primarily with plants and insects, in terms of the traits or characteristics they produced. Traits were determined by one or two alternative expressions of a gene and were said to be either dominant, if expression could be elicited with only one copy of the gene, or recessive, if two copies were necessary for expression. These scientists also confirmed Mendel's conclusion that one copy was inherited from the father and the other from the mother. It was also established that genes were arrayed in a linear fashion along the length of the chromosomes. In species such as *Drosophila*, genes began to be mapped to specific chromosome locations.

In the second stage of gene study, the hypothesis was proved that each gene was responsible for the production of a single protein. In 1909 Archibald Garrod (1909) described a number of metabolic diseases in humans which he characterized as "inborn errors of metabolism." He hypothesized that those diseases were caused by the absence of specific enzymes that were normally synthesized under the direction of certain genes. It was not until 30 years had passed that the hypothesis was shown to be valid, first with mold cells and later on in studies of human sickle-cell anemia. The discovery that genes determined the structure of proteins was a fundamental development in the field of genetics, but it had no immediate importance because very little was known about the molecular structure of chromosomes. In the early part of the 1950s, considerable effort was spent in trying to delineate the structure of deoxyribonucleic acid, which was believed by many to be the prime candidate for the genetic material.

The third stage of knowledge about genes began in 1953, when Watson and Crick (1953) presented their classic description of the spiraled double helix model of the DNA molecule, thus introducing the age of molecular biology. Up to that time it was known that DNA was made up of a series of nucleotides linked end to end. A nucleotide is composed of a phosphate group, a sugar (deoxyribose), and either a purine or a pyrimidine base. The two purines in DNA are adenine (A) and guanine (G). The pyrimidines in DNA are cytosine (C) and thymine (T). It had also been determined that in the DNA of all species studied, the amount of adenine was equal to the amount of thymine and the amount of guanine equalled the amount of cytosine, although the amount of adenine and thymine did not necessarily equal the amount of cytosine and guanine. X-Ray defraction studies had provided a number of structural parameters for the DNA molecule. Watson and Crick took all this information and constructed a model, which time has proved to be amazingly accurate.

The fundamental unit of DNA consists of two strands of nucleotides that are linked end to end by chemical bonds between the 5′ carbon atom of one deoxyribose residue and the 3′ carbon atom of the successive nucleotide, forming the backbone of the molecule. The two strands are linked to each other by hydrogen bonds between a purine base on one strand and a pyrimidine base on the other—adenine is always paired with thymine and cytosine is always paired with guanine. As the base pairs can occur in any order along the backbone, the DNA molecule has a high degree of individuality. Because the bases always pair in the same manner, the two strands have complementary shapes and can be thought of as being a positive and negative template. During replication the helix is unwound and the two strands serve as a pattern to copy two new strands of DNA. Replication takes place simultaneously at many sites along the DNA strand, proceeding in both directions until the entire strand has been reproduced. Thus, replication generates two daughter DNA molecules with sequences identical to the parental molecule (Fig. 4). During the process of replication, mutations can occur as the result of simple copying errors, resulting in nucleotide substitutions.

In addition to DNA, eukaryotic chromosomes contain proteins, which, together with DNA, make up the chromatin. The most prominent proteins associated with metaphase chromosomes are the histones. There are also some nonhistone proteins associated with the DNA molecule. Although the function of the proteins is not entirely clear, they serve as a type of scaffold for the metaphase chromosome.

Once the structure of DNA was determined, it was possible to begin to crack the genetic code. It was clear that the genetic information in DNA was related to the linear sequences of the four bases—adenosine, cytosine, guanine, and thymine. As it was known that a single gene codes for a specific protein, and proteins are made up of some combination of 20 different amino acids, it was hypothesized that some combination of the four bases would be specific for a given amino acid. If only two bases were involved in the code, just 16 permutations would be possible—four too few to code for the 20 amino acids. However, if

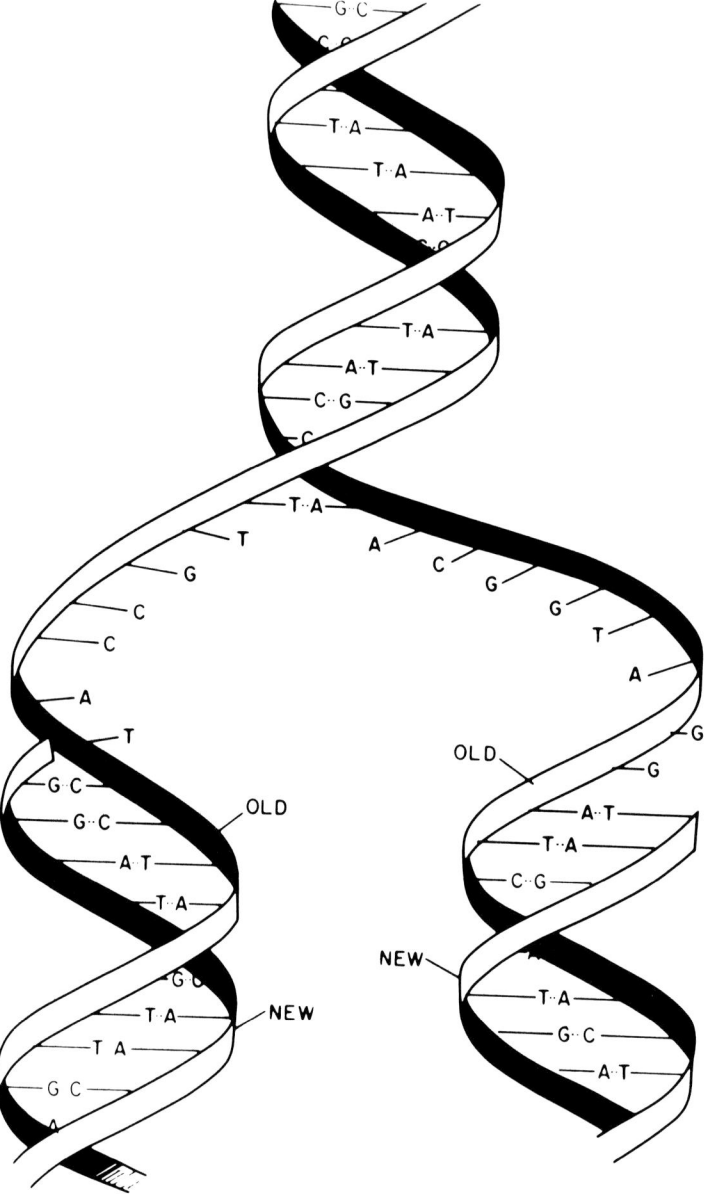

FIG. 4. DNA replication in which the two strands of DNA are used as a template for synthesis of two identical strands. (From Kelly, T., "Clinical Genetics and Genetic Counseling," 2nd Ed. Year Book Med. Publ., Chicago, Illinois, 1986.)

three bases were involved in the code, 64 combinations are possible—more than enough to specify all of the amino acids. It is now well established that groups of three nucleotides, or codons, as they are called, code for a specific amino acid. All but 3 of the 64 possible combinations of bases code for an amino acid. Therefore, some amino acids have more than one codon. With very few exceptions, the codon for a specific amino acid is the same for all known organisms. The codon for the amino acid methionine is also the "start" codon, as methionine is the first amino acid in all protein chains. Three of the codons are the "stop" signal, indicating the end of the protein chain. Within the sequence of codons for a specific protein (exons), there may be codons that play no known role (introns). In addition to the codons that code for amino acid sequences, there are numerous codons that serve as control sequences. There are also very large segments of the DNA molecule that have no known function at this time. A "model" gene might begin with promotor sequences somewhat upstream from the initiation (start) codon, one or more exons interspersed with one or more introns, and a termination (stop) codon.

As DNA resides primarily in the nucleus of eukaryotic cells, and protein syntesis takes place outside the nucleus, there has to be a method for the transfer of genetic information from one part of the cell to the other. Ribonucleic acid (RNA) serves in this role. RNA is chemically very similar to DNA except that ribose is substituted for deoxyribose and uracil replaces thymine as the base that pairs with adenine. There are three types of RNA involved in protein synthesis. Messenger RNA (mRNA) is a linear template of DNA that is transcribed or copied from the DNA in the nucleus. Ribosomal RNA (rRNA) is part of the ribosomal complex, the site of protein synthesis in the cytoplasm. Transfer RNA (tRNA) carries amino acids to the ribosome for incorporation into the newly synthesized proteins. In summary, a single strand of DNA serves as a template for a complementary DNA molecule during the process of cell division or for a complementary RNA molecule during transcription. In turn, the mRNA carries the message to the ribosomes, where rRNA and tRNA translate the genetic language into the proper amino acid sequence for the desired protein.

V. Molecular Genetics

The techniques for the study of genetic material at the molecular level have developed at an extremely rapid pace and our understanding of gene structure and function has expanded greatly in the last decade. It is now possible to isolate a single, discrete segment of DNA from a population of genes, purify this segment, and then amplify it to produce enough material for chemical and biological analysis.

Molecular cloning utilizes well-defined restriction endonuclease enzymes that cleave the DNA molecule at specific sequences of nucleotides. Other enzymes are used to ligate specific fragments into the cleaved DNA of a vector that is either an autonomously replicating circular DNA molecule (plasmid) or a bacterial virus (phage). The vector containing the DNA fragment of interest is introduced into a bacterial cell. After many rounds of replication, the hybrid molecule can be reisolated and purified, providing ample material for further study.

The amino acid sequence of the encoded protein can be predicted by determining the nucleotide sequence of the cloned DNA segment. Using a radioactive label of the purified DNA, complex cell genomes can be probed for copies of related DNA sequences. The cloned DNA segment can be reengineered back into bacteria or yeast, allowing expression of its protein coding sequence and providing an inexpensive or otherwise unobtainable source of protein of biological or medical importance.

Gene cloning will have major medical applications in the future in the diagnosis of genetic diseases. Foreign genes have been successfully introduced into laboratory animals and it is reasonable to expect that engineered genes may be introduced therapeutically into animals suffering from genetic diseases. The potential for further development is enormous.

References

Arnold, J. (1879). Beobachtungen über Kerntheilungen in den Zellen der Geschwülste. *Virchows Arch. Pathol. Anat.* **78**, 279–301.

Barr, M. L., and Bertram, E. G. (1949). A morphologic distinction between neurons of the male and female and the behavior of the nucleolar satellite during accelerated nucleoprotein synthesis. *Nature (London)* **163**, 676–677

Flemming, W. (1882). "Zellsubstanz." Kern & Zelltheilung, Leipzig.

Ford, C. E., Pollock, D. L., and Gustavsson, I. (1980). Proceedings for the First International Conference for the Standardization of Banded Karyotype of Domestic Animals. *Hereditas* **92**, 145–162.

Garrod, A. (1909). "Inborn Errors of Metabolism." Oxford Univ. Press, Oxford.

Gustavsson, I. (1988). Standard karyotype of the domestic pig. *Hereditas* **109**, 151–157.

Hsu, T. C. (1952). Mammalian chromosomes *in vitro*. I. The karyotype of man. *J. Hered.* **43**, 172.

Hsu, T. C., and Benirschke, K. (1967). "An Atlas of Mammalian Chromosomes." Springer-Verlag, New York.

Lejeune, J., Gautier, M., and Turpin, R. (1959). Etude des chromosomes somatiques de neuf enfant mongoliens. *C. R. Hebd. Seances Acad. Sci.* **248,** 1721–1722.

Mendel, G. (1866). Versuche über pflanzen-hybriden. *Verh. Naturforsch. Ver. Bruenn* **4,** 3–47.

Moorhead, P. S., Nowell, P. C., Mellman, W. J., Battips, D. M., and Hungerford, D. A. (1960). Chromosome preparations of leucocytes cultured from human peripheral blood. *Exp. Cell Res.* **20,** 613–616.

Peters, J. A. (1959). "Classic Papers in Genetics." Prentice-Hall, Englewood Cliffs, New Jersey.

Strasburger, E. (1884). "Neue Untersuchungen über den Befruchtungsvorgang bei den Phanerogamen als Grundlage für eine Theorie der Zeugung." Fischer, Jena.

Tjio, J. H., and Levan, A. (1956). The chromosome number of man. *Hereditas* **42,** 1–6.

Virchow, R. (1857). Ueber die Theilung der Zellenkerne. *Virchows Arch. Pathol. Anat.* **11,** 89–92.

von Kölliker, A. (1885). Die Bedeutung der Zellenkerne für die Vorgänge der Vererbung. *Z. Wiss. Zool.* **42,** 1–46.

von Török, A. (1874). Die formative Rolle der Dotterplättchen beim Aufbau der Gewebestructur. *Centralbl. Med. Wiss.* **12,** 257–261.

Waldeyer, W. (1888). Über Karyokinese und ihre Beziehung zu den Befruchtungsvorgängen. *Arch. Mikrosk. Anat.* **32,** 1–181.

Watson, J. D., and Crick, F. H. C. (1953). Molecular structure of nucleic acids: A structure for deoxyribose nucleic acid. *Nature (London)* **171,** 737–738.

Weismann, A. (1883). "Über der Verabung." Fischer, Jena.

Chromosome Methodology

SUSAN E. LONG

Department of Animal Husbandry, School of Veterinary Science, University of Bristol, Bristol, England

I. Preparation of Chromosomes
   A. Interphase Cells
   B. Mitotic Metaphase Chromosomes
   C. Meiotic Chromosomes
II. Chromosome Identification
   A. Chromosome Morphology and Chromosome Markers
   B. Autoradiography
   C. Differential Staining Techniques
   References

I. Preparation of Chromosomes

It is now possible to examine the chromosomes of domestic animals in a number of very different ways. For example, although in the interphase cell the chromatin is usually dispersed throughout the nucleus so that individual chromosomes cannot be identified, in some tissues there is a sex dimorphism in the chromatin arrangement, facilitating deduction of the chromosomal sex of the animal. More usefully, cells at mitotic metaphase have chromosomes that are condensed and easily visible, allowing examination of the whole chromosome complement. Examination of chromosomes during meiotic divisions will often reveal small exchanges that are difficult, if not impossible, to detect in mitotic chromosomes. Differential staining techniques can now help to reveal not only structural variations in chromosomes, but also differences in the dynamics of how each chromosome divides. The science and art of cytogentics lie in obtaining the most suitable cells, at the correct stage of division, and treating them appropriately so that the chromosomes can be clearly seen and identified.

A. INTERPHASE CELLS

1. Sex Chromatin (Barr Body)

Interphase cells are not very informative as regards chromosome complement because the chromatin is dispersed throughout the nucleus and individual chromosomes are not visible. However, in the late 1940s, a postgraduate student, during the process of examining some histological slides of spinal cords of cats, noticed that some samples had nuclei with a mass of chromatin next to the nucleolus, whereas others did not. To his infinite credit he checked through his material and discovered that all of the samples with the chromatin mass came from female specimens and those without the mass were from males (Barr and Bertram, 1949). This was the first description of the Barr body, or sex chromatin body, which was to be used for a number of years in the determination of chromosomal sex in humans as well as domestic animals. It was originally designated the nucleolar satellite but was renamed when it was realized that its position was different in cells of nonnervous origin. It is visible in a wide variety of tissue, but its presence may be masked by other chromocenters. This is particularly true of the epithelial cells of most of the domestic animals. Only in the dog and cat is there a recognizable sex dimorphism in cells from a buccal smear, for example (Moore, 1962).

The sex chromatin is visible only in the interphase cell, is approximately 0.7×1.2 μm, and stains darkly with nuclear stains (Fig. 1). We now know that it is a condensed, facultative heterochromatic X chromosome. It can be of either paternal or maternal origin and this condensation is believed to be a mechanism whereby females, who have two X chromosomes, can compensate for the extra genes compared to the male, with only one X chromosome. The current theory is that proposed by Lyon (1961) and has become known as the "Lyon hypothesis of X inactivation." This hypothesis is based on the following statements:

1. Genes on the sex chromatin-forming X chromosome are inactive.
2. The decision as to which of a pair of X chromosomes is to be inactivated is made early in embryonic life.
3. Once the decision is made, the descendants of each X chromosome will be like the parent chromosome (i.e., either active or inactive).
4. The original inactivation in each embryonic cell occurs at random, so that in some cells a paternal and in others a maternal X chromosome will be inactivated. Therefore, the mammalian female is a mosaic with two populations of somatic cells, one with

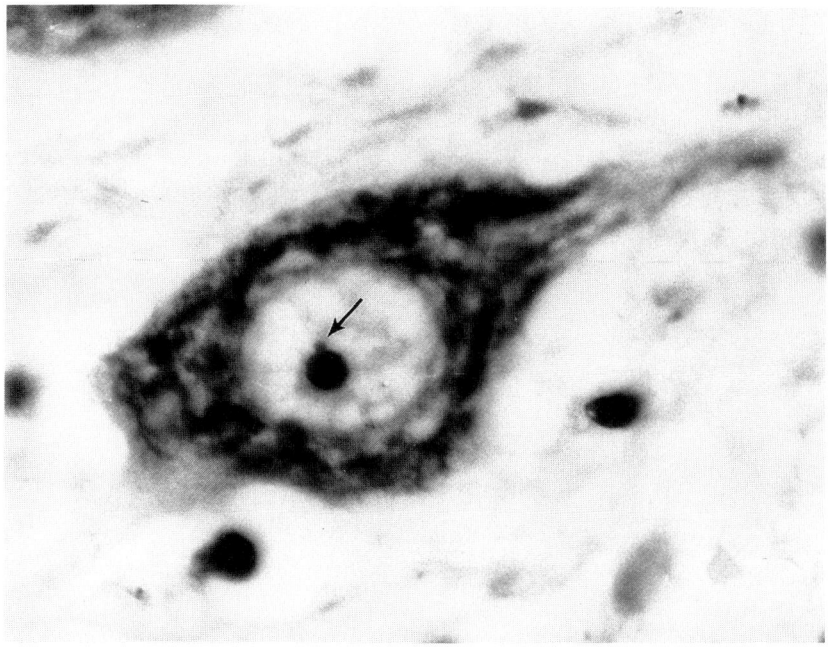

FIG. 1. Spinal cord neurone from a female lamb showing the sex chromatin or Barr body (arrow). Stain: hematoxylin and eosin.

a functional, paternally derived X chromosome and the other with a functional, maternally derived X chromosome.

The result of the inactivation of one of the two X chromosomes is that animals of both sexes receive a single dose of X-linked genes. This is the basis of the gene dosage compensation theory. Inactivation occurs very early in embryonic development. In the pig, dog, and cat it is at about the late blastocyst stage (Lyon, 1972).

This hypothesis is somewhat over simplified, because some genes on the "inactive" X chromosome may be functional at some stage in the cell cycle. For example, during the meiotic divisions of the gamete in the female, which take place during early fetal life, the inactivated X chromosome is reactivated and both X chromosomes are functional (Gartler et al., 1973).

2. Drumstick Appendages (Accessory Nuclear Lobules)

The inactivated X chromosome can also be seen as a small lobule on the nucleus of polymorphonucleocytes in routine blood smears. These

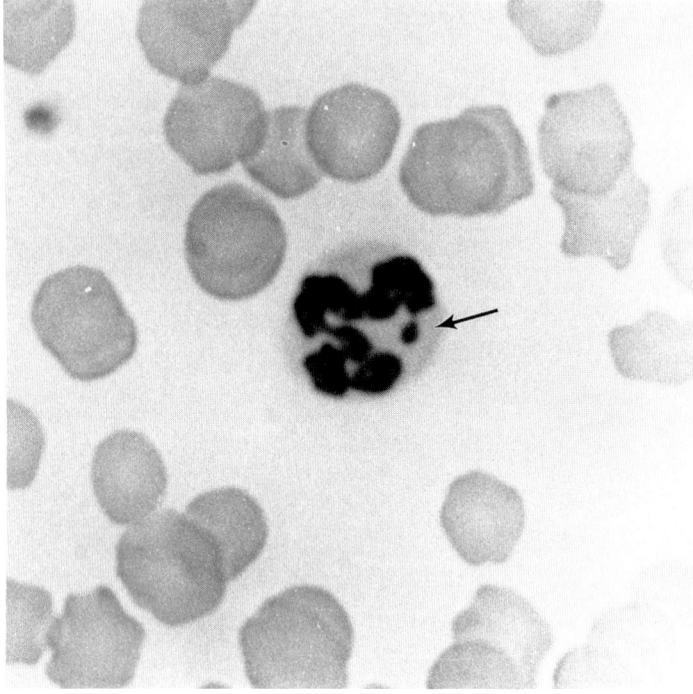

FIG. 2. Polymorphonucleocyte showing a drumstick appendage (arrow) from a male tortoiseshell cat with a 39, XXY chromosome complement. Stain: Wright's.

lobules were first recognized in the human (Davidson and Smith, 1954) but have been investigated in a variety of domestic animals by Colby and Calhoun (1963) (Fig. 2). Recognition of the drumstick appendage requires good preparation of the blood smear, which should be made and stained as soon as the blood sample is collected. Care has to be taken not to confuse the drumstick appendages with other nuclear appendages. The distinctive drumstick appendage is approximately 1.2 × 1.6 μm in size. In poor preparations the nucleus is not well spread and the drumstick appendage becomes obscured. Six lobules in 500 cells were considered to be diagnostic of a female in the dog, cat, sheep, goat, and horse (Colby and Calhoun, 1963). In the pig it was recommended that more than 500 cells should be counted before a male was diagnosed, but the technique was considered to be unsuitable for cattle because of the nuclear morphology.

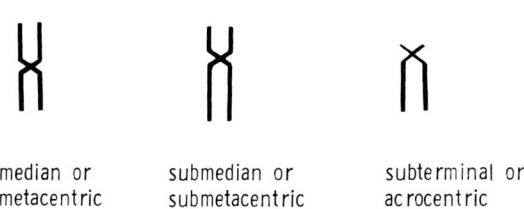

FIG. 3. Diagrammatic representation of chromosome morphology based on centromeric position.

B. Mitotic Metaphase Chromosomes

For chromosome examination, a stage much more useful than interphase is mitotic metaphase. At this stage, the chromatin is condensed and individual chromosomes are visible under the light microscope as two chromatids held together at the centromere. The centromere may be at one end of the chromosome or at some point along its length. The different positions of the centromere give the chromosomes different morphologies at metaphase. These have been classified by Levan *et al.* (1964) and are shown in Fig. 3.

Dividing cells can be obtained directly from certain tissues, for example, from bone marrow. However, most tissues require the establishment of *in vitro* cultures before a supply of dividing cells can be obtained. Tissue biopsy and *in vitro* culture is time consuming and invasive. A major breakthrough for clinical cytogenetics came with the development of short-term (2–3 days) peripheral blood lymphocyte cultures.

1. Lymphocyte Cultures

Blood is an easily obtainable source of cells. However, peripheral blood leukocytes do not normally divide *in vitro*. Nevertheless, during the course of work on human leukemia it was noted that there was a dramatic rise in the number of mitoses in the *in vitro* cells on the third day of culture (Nowell, 1960b). It was shown that this rise was due to the lymphocytes, primarily the small lymphocytes, undergoing transformation and active mitosis (MacKinney *et al.*, 1962). The transformation occurred only in cultures where phytohemagglutinin (PHA) had been used to separate the white cells from whole blood (Nowell, 1960a). Following this discovery, Nowell and his co-workers developed a method of lymphocyte culture for chromosome analysis that combined the use of PHA to stimulate cell division, the use of a hypotonic solution to swell the cells (Hsu, 1952), and the air-drying technique of Rothfels and Siminovitch (1958). This became the basic technique for chromosome preparations from blood samples from humans (Moorhead *et al.*, 1960) and it was adapted for use in cattle by Basrur and Gillman (1964). This basic lymphocyte culture technique, with minor modifications, is now used for all domestic animals. Either whole blood or buffy coat samples are cultured for 2 or 3 days, the cells are harvested, and slide preparations are made for chromosome examination. Because this is such an important technique, a detailed explaination is appropriate.

a. Mitogens. Phytohemagglutinin is the generic name given to aqueous extracts of certain plants, most notably those of the *Phaseolus* sp. The PHA used by Nowell was a partially purified mucoprotein extract prepared from the red kidney bean, *Phaseolus vulgaris*. Nowell had used the PHA for separating leukocytes from whole blood because of its powerful erythroagglutinating property. It has since been shown that as well as having mitogenic and hemagglutinating properties, PHA also stimulates the production of interferon and lymphotoxin (Haber *et al.*, 1972). The multivalent activity of PHA can present problems and it is often advisable to test each batch for its mitogenic potency before purchasing large quantities. PHA stimulates a population of lymphocytes dependent on or influenced by the thymus (T-lymphocytes).

Although PHA is the most commonly used mitogen, others are available. Many plant substances, known collectively as lectins or phytomitogens, induce blast cell transformation and mitosis. For example, saline extracts of the roots of pokeweed *(Phytolacca americana)* contain five different types of mitogens. Four of these stimulate only T-lymphocytes, but the fifth also produces proliferation in B-lymphocytes. Pokeweed mitogen (PWM) seems to be more successful than PHA in stimulating cat lymphocytes in culture and is the mitogen of choice in this species. There is now good evidence of species specificity in the mitogenic lectins as a group (Sharon, 1976). Another commonly used mitogen is concanavalin A (Con A), which is also a T-lymphocyte stimulator. Lymphocyte activation requires macromolecules in the culture medium (Forsdyke, 1973) and so most systems entail the supplementation with 20% fetal calf serum that has been heated to 56°C for 30 minutes to destroy the complement activity.

b. Blockage of Cell Division at Mitotic Metaphase. Once the blood culture has been established and the mitoses induced, cell division is blocked by the use of colchicine, a plant alkaloid, or its synthetic analog, deacetymethylcolchicine (Colcemid). These compounds act by

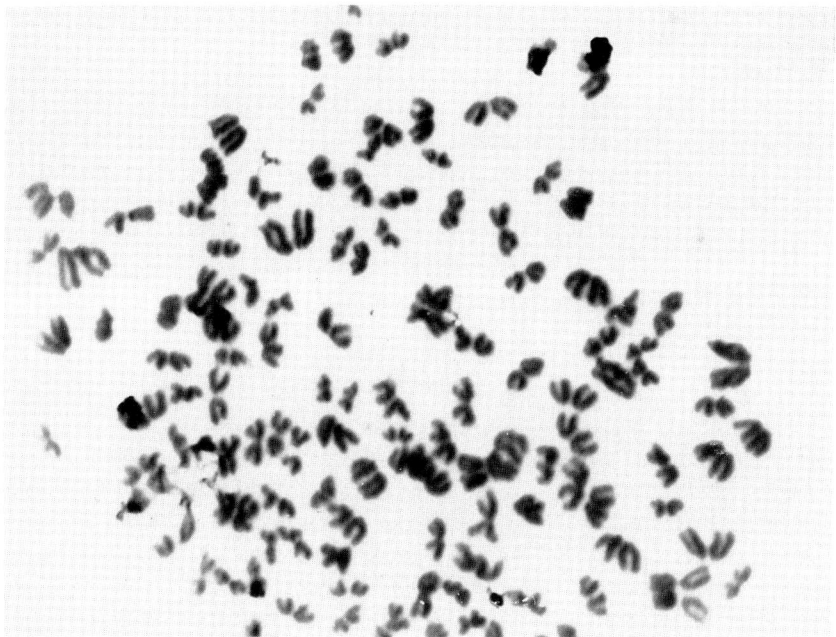

FIG. 4. Metaphase chromosomes from a dog fibroblast cell showing endoreduplication. Stain: Giemsa.

binding to the protein subunits in the microtubles of the mitotic spindle (Borisy and Taylor, 1967). Above a critical level this binding prevents the assembly of the subunits into microtubules and the cell is unable to form a functional mitotic spindle. Dividing cells thus stop at metaphase because they are unable to progress to anaphase. Too low a concentration of Colcemid results in incomplete blocking and may lead to endoreduplication, wherein the chromosomes divide but the cytoplasm does not (Fig. 4).

 c. *Hypotonic Treatment.* The arrested lymphocytes in culture are subjected to a hypotonic solution before fixation. This has the double effect of hemolyzing the red blood cells if a whole blood culture has been used and also of swelling the lymphocytes and enhancing chromosome separation. A hypotonic treatment was first reported by Hsu (1952) in an addendum. The discovery was in fact the result of an accident whereby a hypotonic Tyrode solution was used as a wash instead of an isotonic saline solution. This resulted in better separation of the chromosomes. A hypotonic potassium chloride solution, first recommended by Hungerford (1965), is now most commonly used.

d. *Fixation.* The final fixation procedure is an important step, because this can affect not only the morphology of the chromosomes but also their ability to stick to the slide and their receptivity to the stain. The standard fixative is a 3 : 1 mixture of methanol : acetic acid, which must be freshly made before each use. Better results are obtained if the fixative is chilled to 4°C or lower before use. Slide preparations are made by dropping a cell suspension in fixative onto the slide. The alcohol in the fixative evaporates and the chromosomes are spread and flattened on the slide.

2. Fibroblast Cultures

Examination of tissue other than blood is carried out either when blood samples are unobtainable, for example, from a specimen post mortem, or when a mosaic or chimera is suspected. Fibroblast cultures can be established from most tissue and dividing cells can be harvested after a suitable period of time. Initiation of *in vitro* division requires that the fibroblasts remain undisturbed on the surface of the culture vessel for a "lag period," during which time they adapt to the artificial conditions. For attachment to take place the flasks must be clean and free of detergent; there are a number of special disposable culture flasks that are commonly used now in preference to glass flasks that have to be washed and reused.

There are three basic methods for the establishment of primary cultures. When the tissue to be examined is rapidly dividing, e.g., fetal tissue, fibroblast growth can be obtained simply by chopping the tissue into small fragments (1 mm^3) and allowing them to settle on to the bottom of the flask with enough medium just to cover them. Each flask should be gassed with 5% CO_2 in air before use (Basrur *et al.*, 1963).

Alternatively, a single cell suspension may be obtained from tissue by trypsinization. The material is finely chopped as for the previous method and then treated with a 0.04% trypsin solution at 37°C for 30 minutes. The suspension is centrifuged and the deposit inoculated into culture flasks. If this method is used for anything other than rapidly dividing tissue, results are often disappointing, because attachment of the cells to the culture flask is poor. For more consistent results the tissue has to be fixed to the flask surface using a plasma clot. With the plasma clot method, small fragments of tissue are attached to the flask surface by means of small clots of chicken plasma. This keeps the tissue fragments immobile and closely adhered to the flask surface. Fibroblasts then grow out, attaching themselves to the flask surface.

a. Subculturing. Once growth has begun cell division is usually quite rapid. When half to two-thirds of the flask is covered by a monolayer of cells, the tissue should be subcultured. The cells are removed from the flask surface by means of a weak trypsin solution (0.15%). They are then spun down, resuspended in fresh culture medium, and distributed to fresh culture flasks. Two or more subcultures are derived from the initial primary culture, which will also continue to provide further fibroblast growth in most cases.

b. Harvesting. After subculturing, the cells rapidly attach and begin to divide. There is also the added advantage that this cell division is fairly synchronous. During mitosis, fibroblasts change from being spindly to being round. This gives a good indication of the mitotic index. Peak mitotic activity occurs 18–24 hours after subculturing but even greater synchrony of mitoses can be achieved by cold-shock treatment. That is, the cultures are placed in the refrigerator at 4°C for 30 minutes and are then allowed to regain a temperature of 37°C before further treatment. Further mitoses can also be accumulated by the use of Colcemid. The cells are then treated with a hypotonic solution followed by fixation in a manner similar to the lymphocyte culture procedure.

3. Direct Preparations from Bone Marrow Cells

This method utilizes a source of actively dividing cells and has the advantage that results can be obtained in a matter of hours. In addition, it avoids the possibility of cultural artifacts. It has the disadvantage that the cells are relatively difficult to obtain, unless post mortem, and for this reason is now not frequently used.

The technique was first described by Tjio and Wang (1962), who recommended the aspiration of approximately 0.5 ml of bone marrow; the aspirated marrow should be placed immediately into a 1 µg/ml Colcemid solution. The bone marrow cells are washed in this solution to remove blood clots and to break up cell clumps. They are incubated for 1–2 hours to accumulate cells in metaphase and are then centrifuged and treated with a 1% sodium citrate hypotonic solution. Fixation and slide preparation are as for lymphocyte cultures.

4. Amniotic Fluid Cells

Interest in obtaining chromosome preparations from amniotic fluid cells stemmed from the desire for the prenatal diagnosis of gender in cattle. Bongso and Basrur (1975) described a method for amniocentesis in cows between 70 and 100 days of gestation. Access to the amniotic cavity was by means of a 12-inch, 18-gauge needle that was inserted into the pelvic cavity via the dorsal fornix of the cervix. Between 15 and 20 ml of amniotic fluid was aspirated and centrifuged to obtain a cell button. These cells were then cultured at 37°C in Leighton tubes in tissue culture medium for 4–7 days. Another approach is via the sacrosciatic ligament or ischiorectal fossa.

Timing and route of amniocentesis is important because some techniques have a high risk to the embryo (Mitchell and Eaglesome, 1975). The best results have been obtained when aspiration was attempted between 70 and 90 days of gestation (Eaglesome and Mitchell, 1977).

C. MEIOTIC CHROMOSOMES

Meiosis is much more easily studied in the male than in the female. In the male, meiotic divisions begin at puberty and continue well into old age. By contrast, in the female, meiotic divisions begin during fetal life but are arrested until there is oocyte maturation initiated by the luteinizing hormone (LH) surge just before ovulation in adult life. Therefore, whereas male meiosis can be examined using direct preparations, study of female meiosis requires *in vitro* culture systems.

The examination of meiotic chromosomes provides information on a number of important questions. Before differential staining techniques for mitotic chromosomes were developed, meiotic studies were the only method of detecting inversions and interchanges that did not alter chromosome morphology. Even now, it is a very useful method of confirming that small rearrangements have taken place, because differences in apparent homologous chromosomes are highlighted.

During meiotic prophase the chromosomes condense (leptotene) and pair closely, forming a synaptonemal complex (zygotene). Crossing-over takes place (pachytene) and the chromosomes begin to pull apart and the chiasmata become visible (diplotene). As the chromosomes continue to contract (diakinesis), the chiasmata terminalize. Meiotic prophase is followed by metaphase I and anaphase I. In the latter stage there is separation of chromosomes but no centromeric division. Anaphase I is followed by a short interphase during which there is no replication of chromosomal material, and then the cells go into the second meiotic division, which is identical to a mitotic division.

During pachytene the synaptonemal complex can be studied to assess the pairing of homologous chromosomes (Hulten *et al.*, 1986). At diplotene and diakinesis, chiasmata counts can be made to assess crossing-over frequencies, and at second metaphase, nondisjunction (ND) can be assessed. Nondisjunction can be calculated in two ways.

$$\%\text{ND} = \frac{2 \times \text{no. of hyperhaploid cells}}{\text{total no. of cells counted}} \times 100 \qquad (1)$$

This method assumes that the number of hyperhaploid cells is real and not a technical artifact and that the number of hypohaploid cells equals the number of hyperhaploid cells. It is the calculation used when there is a great excess of hypohaploid cells due to technical artifacts.

$$\%\text{ND} = \frac{(n-1) + (n+1)\,\text{cells}}{(n-1) + n + (n+1)\,\text{cells}} \times 100 \qquad (2)$$

where n is the haploid number. This calculation is used when the number of technical artifacts is believed to be low.

1. Male Meiosis

Samples from any species can be obtained at slaughter, castration (Long, 1978), or biopsy (Eaglesome et al., 1979; Hare et al., 1979). Single cell suspensions are made in a hypotonic solution; these are fixed and microscope preparations are made in a manner similar to that for lymphocyte preparations. Such preparations produce a predominance of cells at pachytene, but other stages can also be found in numbers sufficient to be informative (Fig. 5).

2. Female Meiosis

Until recently, very little work was carried out on female meiosis. However, with the commercial interest in in vitro culture and in vitro fertilization of bovine embryos, techniques have been developed that allow the analysis of both the later stages of meiotic prophase and of metaphase II (Greve et al., 1983; Farver Koenig et al., 1983; Suss et al., 1988). Similar, although much less extensive, work has been carried out on lambs (Logue et al., 1978) and pigs (McGaughey and Polge, 1971).

Techniques for the study of female meiosis require a period of in vitro culture of the arrested oocyte to simulate resumption of the meiotic division. Careful timing of harvesting will then result in the recovery of oocytes at diakinesis or second metaphase.

II. Chromosome Identification

Once techniques were available for the visualization of well-spread chromosomes, methods were developed to identify the individual chro-

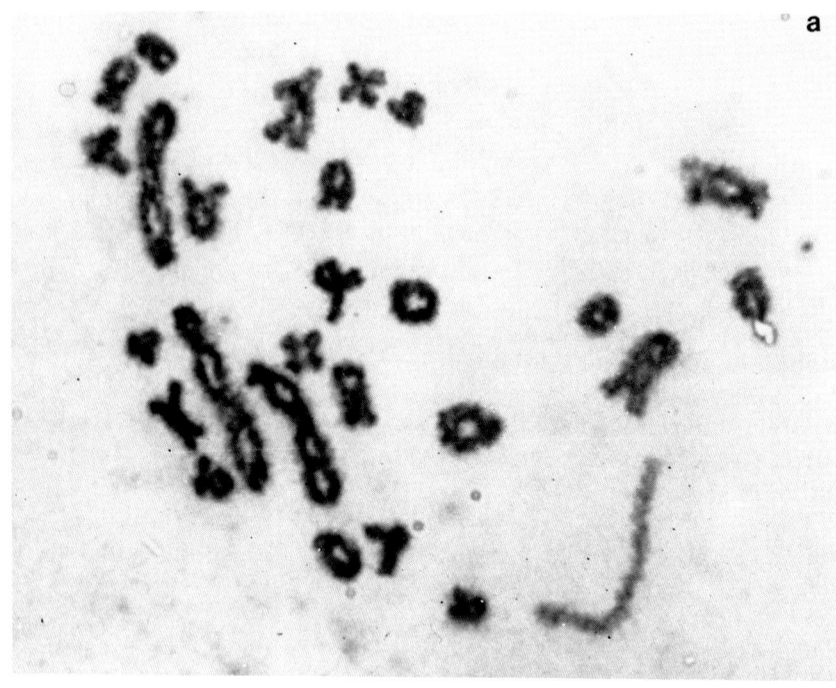

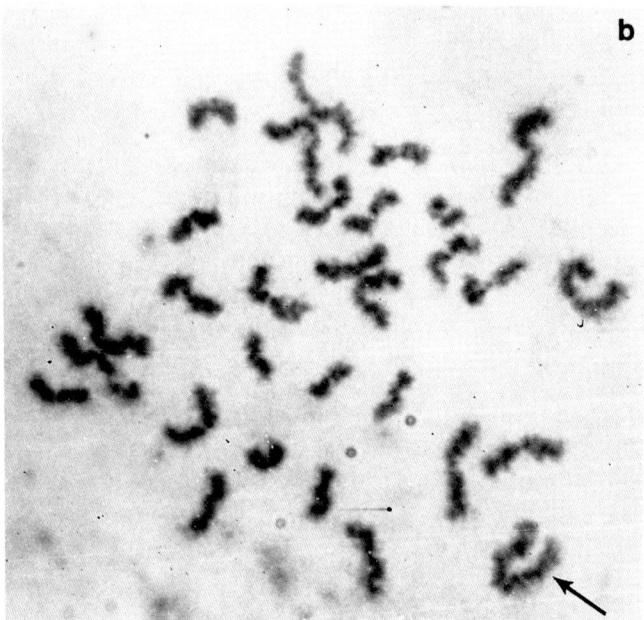

FIG. 5. (a) Ram cell at late diplotene/early diakinesis. Stain: Giemsa. (b) Ram cell at second metaphase. The arrow indicates the X chromosome. Stain: Giemsa.

mosomes and even specific parts of chromosomes. Most of these techniques are used on mitotic metaphase chromosomes, but many are applicable to meiotic chromosomes as well.

A. CHROMOSOME MORPHOLOGY AND CHROMOSOME MARKERS

One of the simplest ways of identifying homologous chromosomes is on the basis of centromeric position (Fig. 3). However, none of the domestic animals has a chromosome complement wherein each homologue is morphologically distinct. Indeed, in species such as the goat, cattle, and dog, the autosomes are morphologically the same and vary only in size. Identification of homologues in these species requires careful measurement and the construction of an idiogram. One can either measure the length of the chromosome arms or the arm ratio relative to the total chromosome length, from a photographic print. However, because of the practical difficulties of measuring chromosomes, regarding deciding where the arms really end and at what point the centromere is situated, the errors involved can be quite high. Some early workers tried weighing cut out photographs of each chromosome but again this was subject to considerable error.

Chromosome markers such as satellites or secondary constrictions can be used for identification. For example, chromosome E_1 in the cat has satellites on the short arms and chromosomes 10 in the pig is identifiable by means of a large secondary constriction on the short arm. However, for the most part, chromosomes of domestic animals do not carry specific markers. Even "markers" may be inconsistent. For example, secondary constrictions can vary with the specific cultural conditions, such as the concentration of colchicine (Palmer and Funderburk, 1965), the type of medium (Sasaki and Makino, 1963), the type of hypotonic solution (Bruere and McLaren, 1967), and the fixative (Sasksela and Moorhead, 1962).

B. AUTORADIOGRAPHY

Chromosomes can be identified to a certain extent on the basis of the dynamics of cell division, because some chromosomes replicate later than others during the S phase of the cell cycle. If a radiolabeled substance is added to the culture system for a short time before harvesting, only the late-replicating chromosomes will be labeled and thus identified. This technique is called autoradiography and was first described by Doniach and Pelc (1950) but was modified by Taylor et al. (1957). Labeled thymidine, in the form of tritium incorporated into the pyrimidine ring, is added to the culture medium. This is then taken up and incorporated into any chromosome that is replicating at the time. Tritium is a β-particle emitter and β particles have a relatively low energy. Thus, if the chromosome preparations are overlayed with photographic emulsion, only the emulsion over the chromosomes that have incorporated the labeled thymidine will be fogged.

This procedure is particularly useful for identifying the inactivated X chromosome, because it is one of the last to replicate in the cell. However, the disadvantage is that the procedure is somewhat prolonged and it still does not identify every chromosome individually.

C. Differential Staining Techniques

Real progress in chromosome identification was not made until the development of differential staining techniques that resulted in unique patterns of bands on homologous chromosomes. This not only enabled individual chromosomes to be identified but also allowed recognition of specific parts of chromosomes.

1. Q-Bands

The first technique for differential staining of chromosomes was described by Caspersson et al. (1968). They stained chromosomes with quinacrine mustard and produced distinctive bands (Q-bands) of high- and low-intensity fluorescence, because the quinacrine was preferentially staining areas of heterochromatin (Caspersson et al., 1969). One useful advantage of this technique in human cytogenetics was that the human Y chromosome fluoresced brightly and could even be identified in interphase cells, including spermatozoa (Pearson et al., 1970; Sumner et al., 1971). Unfortunately, the Y chromosomes of the domestic species do not have this property (Pearson et al., 1971).

Since this original work, a number of other fluorochromes have been used, e.g., quinacrine dihydrochloride (Pearson et al., 1970), acroflavine and proflavine (Caspersson et al., 1969), chlorinetine (Salamanca et al., 1972), and Hoechst 33258 (Raposa and Natarajan, 1974). All have the disadvantage that the fluorescence fades under illumination so that preparations have to be kept in the dark and photographs must be taken immediately.

2. G-Bands

Another type of band is similar to Q-bands in that where there are bright Q-bands there are dark (positive) Giemsa bands (G-bands). These bands were originally produced by incubating the chromosome preparations in various salt solutions and then staining with Giemsa. The major example of this method is the acid/saline/Giemsa (ASG) technique of Sumner et al. (1971). However, the most common method currently used depends on partial enzyme digestion followed by staining with Giemsa. This is the trypsin G-band technique described by Seabright, (1971, 1972a,b, 1973), which each laboratory has modified slightly to fit its own requirements.

3. R-Bands

These bands are produced in a reverse fashion compared to the Q-bands. There are basically two methods. The first involves the incubation of the preparations in a phosphate buffer at pH 6.8 at 87°C followed by staining with Giemsa (Dutrillaux and Lejeune, 1971). The second method involves the incorporation of 5-bromodeoxyuridine (5BrdU) into the culture for the last 6–10 hours of incubation. The BrdU causes differential contraction along the chromosome and subsequent staining with acridine orange results in fluorescent bands (Dutrillaux et al., 1973). A modification of this staining technique is the fluorescent-plus-Giemsa (FPG) technique of Perry and Wolff (1974). This involves staining with 33258 Hoechst, exposing the preparation to exciting light, and then counterstaining with Giemsa. Bands of light and dark Giemsa staining are produced, correlating to the positive and negative fluorescence of the fluorochrome.

As well as Q-, G-, and R-band staining, which produce bands along the whole length of the chromosome, there are special staining techniques that stain specific sites on the chromosome.

4. C-Bands

The C-band techniques result in preferential staining of highly repetitive DNA that is found in constitutive heterochromatin. The process involves the denaturation and renaturation of the DNA by sequential treatment with acid and alkali. The highly repetitive sequences renature rapidly and stain darkly with Giemsa (Pardue and Gall, 1970; Britten and Kohne, 1968; Arrighi and Hsu, 1971). The method most commonly used in domestic animals involves the treatment of cells with 0.1 N HCl at room temperature for 1 hour, immersion in a barium hydroxide solution at 60°C for 3 minutes, and incubation in 2× saline sodium citrate (SSC) at 60°C for 15 minutes. This is a modification of the technique described by Sumner (1972). The technique is particularly useful in the identification of the X chromosome in the horse. In this species all the autosomes (except the number 11) and the X chromosome have centromeric heterochromatin, which stains positively with C-banding, but in addition the X chromosome has a band of constitutive heterochromatin on the long arm that is also C-band positive and which distinguishes it from the autosomes.

5. T-Bands

These bands are produced by a variation of the phosphate buffer R-band technique (Dutrillaux, 1973). If the pH of the buffer is maintained at pH 5.1–5.3 instead of pH 6.5, most of the R-bands fail to appear. Those remaining are located on the terminal region of the chromosome.

6. Centromeric Staining

Centromeric (Cd) staining is a modification of the C-band technique and results in specific staining of the centromeric region (Eiberg, 1974). Preparations are treated at high temperature (85°C) at high pH (8.5–9.0) and are then stained with Giemsa. The process produces two identical dots at the centromere, one on each chromatid. The technique is particularly useful in assessing whether there are one or two centromeres in a centric fusion translocation.

7. Nucleolar Organizer Regions

The original method used to identify the nucleolar organizer regions (NORs) involved extraction of DNA and RNA with appropriate enzymes and removal of histone proteins with acid (Matsui and Sasaki, 1973). When the chromosomes were stained with Giemsa, the NORs appeared as purplish spots. Later, a silver staining technique was developed that resulted in black spots at the site of the NORs (Goodpasture and Bloom, 1975; Bloom and Goodpasture, 1976). This was further modified by Howell and Black (1980) to provide more rapid and reliable results. In their method a colloidal developer consisting of gelatin in water plus formic acid is mixed with silver nitrate on the slide. The slide is then heated on a 70°C hotplate until the staining mixture turns dark brown.

8. Sister Chromatid Staining

Latt (1973) was the first to describe a technique for the differential staining of sister chromatids. After two rounds of replication in the presence of 5BrdU followed by staining with acridine orange or 33258 Hoechst, the unifilarily substituted chromatid fluoresces more brightly than the bifilarily substituted sister chromatid (Fig. 6). This technique therefore allows the identification of sister chromatid exchanges (SCEs) (Fig. 7). The FPG staining method of Perry and Wolff (1974)

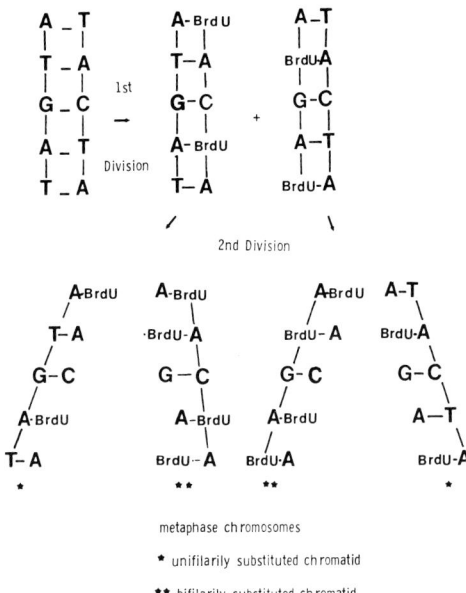

FIG. 6. Diagrammatic representation of sister chromatid staining with 5-bromodeoxyuridine incorporation.

can also be used to produce Giemsa-stained preparations and this can be combined with G-band staining (Fonatsch, 1979) so that the exact point of exchange can be identified. Sister chromatid exchanges are very sensitive indices of chromosome damage. The technique is of particular use in identifying mutagenic or toxic agents. Although it has been extensively used in man (Evans, 1982), it is rarely used in domestic animals.

9. High-Resolution Banding

Whereas the differential staining of midmetaphase chromosomes permits the identification of individual homologues, it does not allow the detection of minute deletions or rearrangements. In addition, gene mapping requires much more elongated chromosomes so that the loci of closely linked genes can be differentiated. For these reasons techniques were developed to increase the number of prometaphase and prophase chromosomes in the culture. The G-banding of these chromosomes showed that the major bands at metaphase result from the progressive coalescence of numerous small bands.

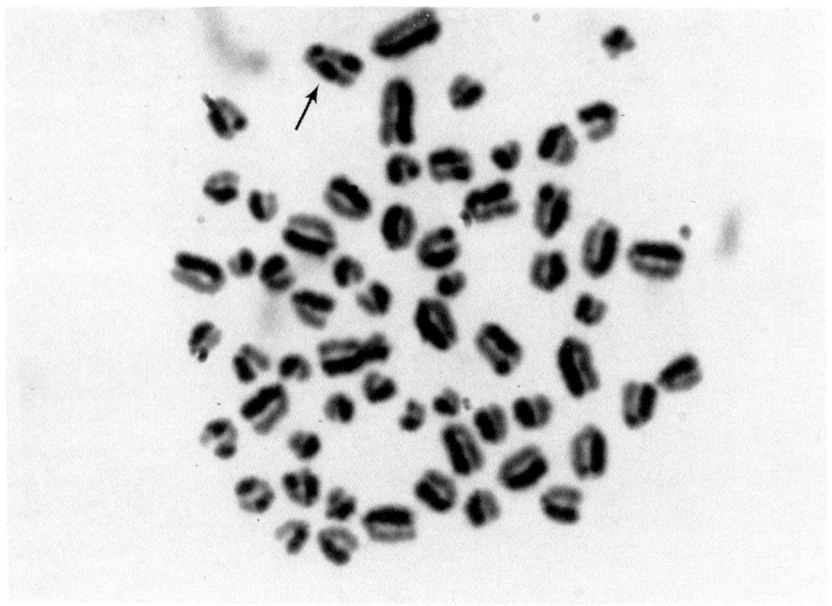

FIG. 7. Metaphase chromosomes from a bull showing sister chromatid exchanges (arrow). Stain: fluorescent-plus-Giemsa (Perry and Wolff, 1974).

Many techniques are now available that either synchronize the cultures so that the cells can be harvested while still in late prophase or inhibit the contraction of the chromosomes so that they are blocked in prophase. The two main substances used are methotrexate, which blocks cell division (Yunis, 1976), and ethidium bromide, which inhibits coiling of the chromatin fibers (Ikeuchi, 1984). High-resolution banding has been carried out in cattle (Di Berardino et al., 1985), pigs (Rønne et al., 1988a), and cats (Rønne et al., 1988b).

Other methods for the production of elongated chromosomes include treatment with thymidine (Viegas-Pequignot and Dutrillaux, 1978), acridine orange (Matsubara and Nakagome, 1983), distamycin A, Hoechst 33258 (Rønne, 1983), and methotrexate plus leucovorin synchronization (Rønne et al., 1985). With so many different staining methods a system of nomenclature is required. That used in domestic animal cytogenetics is the one adopted for human nomenclature (ISCN, 1978). The system is based upon one, two, or three code letters. The first decribes the type of banding; the second, the general technique; and the third, the stain. Examples of the code system are shown in Table 1.

TABLE I

Chromosome Banding Nomenclature

Code	Description
Q	Q-bands
QFQ	Q-bands by fluorescence using quinacrine
G	G-bands
GAG	G-bands by acetic saline using Giemsa
GTG	G-bands by trypsin using Giemsa
C	C-bands
CBG	C-bands by barium hydroxide using Giemsa
R	R-bands
RFA	R-bands by fluorescence using acridine orange
RHG	R-bands by heating using Giemsa
RBG	R-bands by 5BrdU[a] using Giemsa
RBA	R-bands by 5BrdU using acridine orange

[a]5BrdU, 5-Bromodeoxyuridine.

References

Arrighi, F. E., and Hsu, T. C. (1971). Localization of heterochromatin in human chromosomes. *Cytogenetics* **10**, 81–86.

Barr, M. L., and Bertram, E. G. (1949). A morphological distinction between neurones of the male and female, and the behavior of the nucleolar satellite during accelerated nucleoprotein synthesis. *Nature (London)* **163**, 676–677.

Basrur, P. K., and Gilman, J. P. W. (1964). Blood culture method for the study of bovine chromosomes. *Nature (London)* **204**, 1335–1337.

Basrur, P. K., Basrur, V. R., and Gilman, J. P. W. (1963). A simple method for short term cultures from small biopsies. *Exp. Cell Res.* **30**, 229–232.

Bloom, S. E., and Goodpasture, C. (1976). An improved technique for selective silver staining of nucleolar organizer regions in human chromosomes. *Hum. Genet.* **34**, 199–206.

Bongso, T. A., and Basrur, P. K. (1975). Prenatal diagnosis of sex in cattle by amniocentesis. *Vet. Rec.* **96**, 124–127.

Borisy, G. G., and Taylor, E. W. (1967). The mechanism of action of colchicine. Colchicine binding to sea urchin eggs and the mitotic apparatus. *J. Cell Biol.* **34**, 535–548.

Britten, R. J., and Kohne, D. E. (1968). Repeated sequences in DNA. *Science* **161**, 529–540.

Bruere, A. N., and McLaren, R. D. (1967). The idiogram of the sheep with particular reference to secondary constrictions. *Can. J. Genet. Cytol.* **9**, 543–553.

Caspersson, T., Faber, S., Foley, G. E., Kudynowski, J., Modest, E. J., Simonsson, E., Wagh, U., and Zech, L. (1968). Chemical differentiation along metaphase chromosomes *Exp. Cell Res.* **49**, 219–222.

Caspersson, T., Zech, L., Modest, E. J., Foley, G. E., Wagh, W., and Simonsson, E. (1969). Chemical differentiation with fluorescent alkylating agents in *Vicia faba* metaphase chromosomes. *Exp. Cell Res.* **58**, 128–140.

Colby, E. B., and Calhoun, L. (1963). Accessory nuclear lobule on the polymorphonuclear neutrophil of domestic animals. *Acta Cytol.* **7,** 346–350.

Davidson, W. M., and Smith, D. R. (1954). A morphological sex difference in the polymorphonuclear neutrophil leucocytes. *Br. Med. J.* **ii,** 6–7.

Di Berardino, D., Iannuzzi, L., and Lioi, M. B. (1985). The high-resolution RBA-banding pattern of bovine chromosomes. *Cytogenet. Cell Genet.* **39,** 136–139.

Doniach, I., and Pelc, S. R. (1950). Autoradiographic technique. *Br. J. Radiol.* **23,** 184–192.

Dutrillaux, B. (1973). Nouveau système de marquage chromosomique: les bandes T. *Chromosoma* **41,** 395–402.

Dutrillaux, B., and Lejeune, J. (1971). Sur une nouvelle technique d'analyse du caryotype humain. *C. R. Hebd. Seances Acad. Sci., Ser. D* **272,** 2638–2640.

Dutrillaux, B., Laurent, C., Couturier, J., and Lejeune, J. (1973). Coloration des chromosomes humains par l'acridine orange après traitement par le 5-Bromodeoxyuridine. *C. R. Hebd. Seances Acad. Sci.* **276,** 3179–3181.

Eaglesome, M. D., and Mitchell, D. (1977). Collection and cytogenetics of fetal fluids from heifers during the third month of pregnancy. 1. Collection. *Theriogenology* **7,** 195–201.

Eaglesome, M. D., Hare, W. C. D., and Singh, E. L. (1979). Studies on obtaining meiotic chromosomes for analysis in the bull. 1. Testicular biopsy. *Theriogenology* **12,** 263–270.

Eiberg, H. (1974). New selective giemsa technique for human chromosomes, Cd staining. *Nature (London)* **248,** 55.

Evans, H. J. (1982). Sister chromatid exchanges and disease states in man. *In* "Sister Chromatid Exchange" (S. Wolff, ed.), pp. 183–228. Wiley, New York.

Farver Koenig, J. L., Eldridge, F. E., and Harris, N. (1983). A cytogenetic analysis of bovine oocytes cultured *in vitro. Proc. A.D.S.A., Annu. Meet., 78th* p. 253.

Fonatsch, C. (1979). A technique for simultaneous demonstration of G bands and sister chromatid exchanges. *Cytogenet. Cell Genet.* **23,** 144–146.

Forsdyke, D. R. (1973). Serum and lymphocyte activation by phytohemagglutinin (PHA). *Exp. Cell Res.* **77,** 216–222.

Gartler, S. M., Liskay, R. M., and Gant, N. (1973). Two functional X chromosomes in human fetal oocytes. *Exp. Cell Res.* **82,** 464–466.

Goodpasture, C., and Bloom, S. E. (1975). Visualization of nucleolar organizer regions in mammalian chromosomes using silver staining. *Chromosoma* **53,** 37–50.

Greve, T., King, W. A., Bousquet, D., and Betteridge, K. J. (1983). Chromosomes of the bovine oocyte in culture. *Proc. A.D.S.A., Annu. Meet., 78th* p. 245.

Haber, J., Rosenau, W., and Goldberg, M. (1972). Separate factors in phytohemagglutinin induced lymphotoxin, interferon and nucleic acid synthesis. *Nature (London), New Biol.* **238,** 60–61.

Hare, W. C. D., Singh, E. L., and Eaglesome, M. D. (1979). Studies on obtaining meiotic chromosomes for analysis in the bull. II. Direct and culture methods. *Theriogenology* **12,** 271–281.

Howell, W. M., and Black, D. A. (1980). Controlled silver staining of nucleolus organizer regions with a protective colloidal developer: A 1-step method. *Experientia* **36,** 1014–1015.

Hsu, T. C. (1952). Mammalian chromosomes *in vitro.* 1. The karyotype of man. *J. Hered.* **43,** 167–172.

Hulten, M. A., Saadallah, N., Wallace, B. M. N., and Creasy, M. R. (1986). Meiotic studies in man. *In* "Human Cytogenetics: A Practical Approach" (D. E. Rooney and B. H. Czepulkowski, eds.). IRL Press, Oxford.

Hungerford, D. A. (1965). Leucocytes cultured from small inocula of whole blood and the preparation of metaphase chromosomes by treatment with hypotonic KCl. *Stain Technol.* **40**, 333–338.

Ikeuchi, T. (1984). Inhibitory effect of ethidium bromide on mitotic chromosome condensation and its application to high-resolution chromosome banding. *Cytogenet. Cell Genet.* **38**, 56–61.

ISCN (1978). An international system for human cytogenetic nomenclature. *Cytogenet. Cell Genet.* **21**, 309–404.

Latt, S. A. (1973). Microfluorometric detection of deoxyribonucleic acid replication in human metaphase chromosomes (33258 Hoechst/BrdU-dependent fluorescence). *Proc. Natl. Acad. Sci. U.S.A.* **70**, 3395–3399.

Levan, A., Fredga, K., and Sandberg, A. A. (1964). Nomenclature for centromeric position on chromosomes. *Hereditas* **52**, 201–220.

Logue, D. N., Berry, J. E., and Bruere, A. N. (1978). In vitro culture and karyotyping of oocytes from 4 to 6 week old lambs. *Anim. Reprod. Sci.* **1**, 25–30.

Long, S. E. (1978). Chiasma counts and non-disjunction frequencies in a normal ram and in rams carrying the Massey I (t_1) Robertsonian translocation. *J. Reprod. Fertil.* **53**, 353–356.

Lyon, M. F. (1961). Gene action in the X chromosome of the mouse. *Nature (London)* **190**, 372–373.

Lyon, M. F. (1972). X-Chromosome inactivation and developmental patterns in mammals. *Biol. Rev.* **47**, 1–35.

McGaughey, R. W., and Polge, C. (1971). Cytogenetic analysis of pig oocytes matured *in vitro*. *J. Exp. Zool.* **176**, 383–396.

MacKinney, A. A., Stohlman, F., and Brecher, G. (1962). The kinetics of cell proliferation in culture of human peripheral blood. *Blood* **19**, 349–358.

Matsubara, T., and Nakagome, Y. (1983). High-resolution banding by treating cells with acridine orange before fixation. *Cytogenet. Cell Genet.* **35**, 148–151.

Matsui, S., and Sasaki, M. (1973). Differential staining of nuleolus organizers in mammalian chromosomes. *Nature (London)* **246**, 148–150.

Mitchell, D., and Eaglesome, M. D. (1975). Amniocentesis in cattle. *Vet. Rec.* **96**, 365.

Moore, K. L. (1962). Symposium on sex chromatin: The sex chromatin: Its discovery and variation in the animal kingdom. *Acta Cytol.* **6**, 1–12.

Moorhead, P. S., Nowell, P. C., Mellman, W. J., Batipps, D. M., and Hungerford, D. A. (1960). Chromosome preparations of leucocytes cultured from peripheral blood. *Exp. Cell Res.* **20**, 613–616.

Nowell, P. C. (1960a). Differentiation of human leukemic leucocytes in tissue culture. *Exp. Cell Res.* **19**, 267–277.

Nowell, P. C. (1960b). Phytohemagglutinin: An initiator of mitosis in cultures of normal human leukocytes. *Cancer Res.* **20**, 462–466.

Palmer, C. G., and Funderburk, S. (1965). Secondary constrictions in human chromosomes. *Cytogenetics* **4**, 261–276.

Pardue, M. L., and Gall, J. G. (1970). Chromosomal localization of mouse satellite DNA. *Science* **168**, 1356–1358.

Pearson, P. L., Bobrow, M., and Vosa, C. G. (1970). Technique for identifying Y chromosomes in human interphase nuclei. *Nature (London)* **226**, 78–80.

Pearson, P. L., Bobrow, M., Vosa, C. G., and Barlow, P. W. (1971). Quinacrine fluorescence in mammalian chromosomes. *Nature* **231** 326–329.

Perry, P., and Wolff, S. (1974). New giemsa method for the differential staining of sister chromatids. *Nature (London)* **251**, 156–158.

Raposa, T., and Natarajan, A. T. (1974). Fluorescence banding pattern of human and mouse chromosomes with a benzimidazole derivative (Hoechst 33258). *Humangenetik* **21,** 221–226.

Rønne, M. (1983). Simultaneous R-banding and localization of dA–dT clusters in human chromosomes. *Hereditas* **98,** 241–248.

Rønne, M., Andersen, O., and Hansen, S. O. (1985). Methotrexate–leucovorin synchronization of human lymphocyte cultures. Induction of high resolution R- and G-banding. *Anticancer Res.* **4,** 357–360.

Rønne, M., Poulsen, B. S., and Shibasaki, Y. (1988a). The high resolution R-banded karyotype of *Sus scrofa domestica* L. *Proc. Colloq. Cytogenet. Domest. Anim., 8th, Bristol, Eng.* pp. 106–114.

Rønne, M., Shibasaki, Y., and Poulsen, B. S. (1988b). The high resolution R-banded karyotype of *Feli catus. Proc. Colloq. Cytogenet. Domest. Anim., 8th, Bristol, Eng.* pp. 78–82.

Rothfels, K. H., and Siminovitch, L. (1958). An air drying technique for flattening chromosomes in mammalian cells grown *in vitro*. *Stain Technol.* **33,** 607–609.

Salamanca, F., Guzzman, M., Barbosa, E., and Martinez, I. (1972). A new fluorescent compound for cytogenetic studies. *Ann. Genet.* **15,** 127–129.

Sasaki, M. S., and Makino, S. (1963). The demonstration of secondary constrictions in human chromosomes by means of a new technique. *Am. J. Hum. Genet.* **15,** 24–33.

Sasksela, E., and Moorhead, P. S. (1962). Enhancement of secondary constrictions and the heterochromatic X in human cells. *Cytogenetics* **1,** 225–244.

Seabright, M. (1971). A rapid banding technique for human chromosomes. *Lancet* **ii,** 971–972.

Seabright, M. (1972a). The use of proteolytic enzymes for the mapping of structural rearrangements in the chromosomes of man. *Chromosoma* **36,** 204–210.

Seabright, M. (1972b). Human chromosome banding. *Lancet* **1,** 967.

Seabright, M. (1973). Improvement of trypsin method for banding chromosomes. *Lancet* **1,** 1249–1250.

Sharon, N. (1976). Lectins as mitogens. *In* "Mitogens in Immunology" (J. J. Oppenheim and D. L. Rosenstreich, eds.), pp. 31–41. Academic Press, New York.

Sumner, A. T. (1972). A simple technique for demonstrating centromeric heterochromatin. *Exp. Cell Res.* **75,** 304–306.

Sumner, A. T., Robinson, J. A., and Evans, H. J. (1971). Distinguishing between X, Y and YY-bearing human spermatozoa by fluorescence and DNA content. *Nature (London) New Biol.* **229,** 231–233.

Suss, U., Wuthrich, K., and Stranzinger, G. (1988). Chromosome configurations and time sequence of the first meiotic division in bovine oocytes matured *in vitro*. *Biol. Reprod.* **38,** 871–880.

Taylor, H. J., Woods, P. S., and Hughes, W. L. (1957). The organization and duplication of chromosomes as revealed by autoradiographic studies using tritium-labelled thymidine. *Proc. Natl. Acad. Sci. U.S.A.* **43,** 122–128.

Tjio, J. H., and Wang, J. (1962). Chromosome preparations of bone marrow cells without prior *in vitro* culture or *in vivo* colchicine administration. *Stain Technol.* **37,** 17–21.

Viegas-Péquignot, E., and Dutrillaux, B. (1978). Une méthode simple pour obtenir des prophases et les prométaphases. *Ann. Genet.* **21,** 122–125.

Yunis, J. J. (1976). High resolution of human chromosomes. *Science* **191,** 1268–1270.

Chromosomes of the Cow and Bull

PAUL C. POPESCU

Cytogenetics Laboratory, National Institute for Agricultural Research, Jouy-en-Josas, France

I. Normal Karyotype
II. Chromosome Abnormalities
   A. The 1/29 Robertsonian Translocation
   B. Other Autosomal Structural Abnormalities
   C. Structural Abnormalities of Sex Chromosomes
   D. Numerical Abnormalities
   E. Intersexuality
   F. Freemartinism
III. Y Chromosome Polymorphism
IV. The Y Chromosome of Zebu Cattle
V. Sexing of Bovine Embryos
   References

I. Normal Karyotype

The normal karyotype of domestic cattle (*Bos taurus* L.) follows the pattern of the members of the Bovidae family: 60 chromosomes, including 58 autosomes and 2 sex chromosomes. All autosomes are acrocentric, their centromeres are terminal, and they differ only in length (Fig. 1). The bovine karyotype is therefore arranged according to the latter criterion. The karyotype of bovine cells stained with the usual dyes (for example, Giemsa) is presented as a declining series divided arbitrarily into a few groups. The use of one or more banding methods permits the identification and pairing of homologous chromosomes.

Sex chromosomes are easily identifiable because their centromeres are situated in the median region. The X chromosome is similar in length to the longest autosome, whereas the Y chromosome is one of the shortest chromosomes in the bovine karyotype.

Before the use of banding methods for chromosome identification,

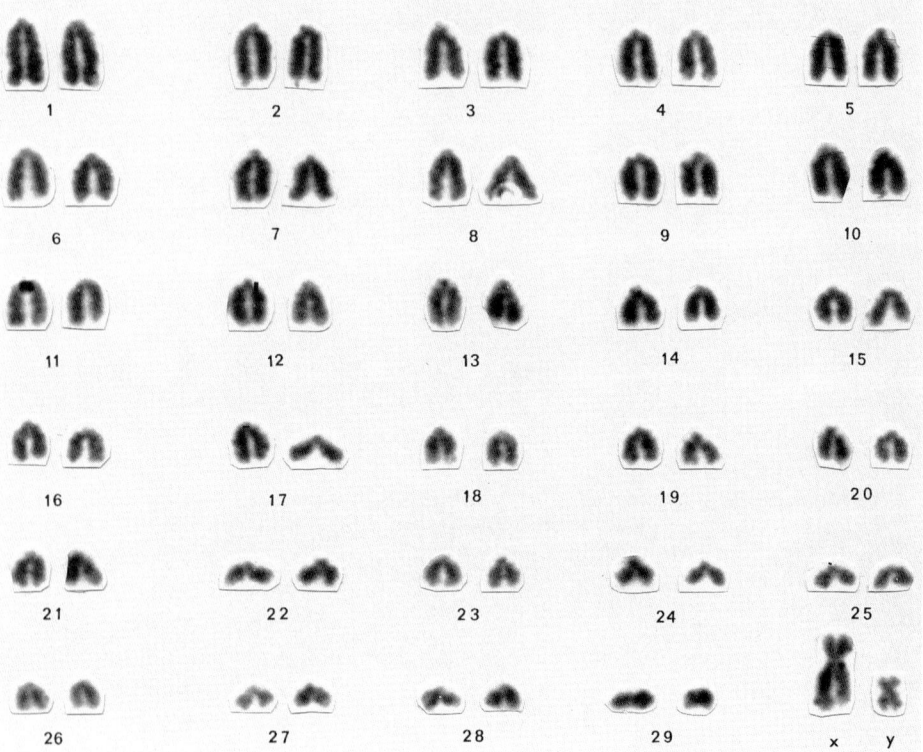

FIG. 1. A karyotype of a normal bull. Giemsa stained.

the only criterion for the identification of abnormal chromosomes was the relative length of each chromosome (per thousand of the total haploid length). This is how the 1/29 translocation was identified (Gustavsson, 1969; Popescu, 1971). However, identification of chromosomes other than the longest and the shortest ones was uncertain, because there are only minor differences in two proximal pairs in decreasing order. Therefore, idiograms established before the era of banding (Gustavsson, 1969; Popescu, 1969, 1971) have shown that, with the exception of the first two easily identifiable pairs, the difference between two proximal pairs does not exceed 1 per 1,000.

Some investigators have applied the usual banding methods for the identification of bovine chromosomes. At present, for this species, G-, R-, and C-banding methods are routinely used. For G bands, the recognized standard for pairing and classification of the 30 chromosomal pairs is that of the Reading Conference (Ford et al., 1980). The pattern of G bands is evident, regardless of the method used (trypsin or saline denaturation). However, the last pairs cannot be easily identified in cells with only low or medium despiralization, whereas they are readily identified in cells with chromosomes showing a high degree of despiralization (Popescu, 1975a).

The R-banding method, using the incorporation of bromodeoxyuridine (BrdU) followed by staining with acridine orange (RBA, Fig. 2) or with Giemsa (RBG, Fig. 2), has been adapted for bovine chromosomes (Popescu, 1975a; Gustavsson and Hageltorn, 1976). Under fluorescent light, the chromosomes appear as intermittent areas emitting a strong fluorescent green light and areas showing red light of lower intensity. The former correspond to the R-bands whereas the latter are situated at the locations of G-bands. In black and white pictures, light bands correspond to green areas and dark bands to red areas. The identification and pairing of homologous chromosomes are therefore possible, in particular on elongated chromosomes. Sex chromosomes are also well delineated. The X chromosome has a large light band in the middle of the long arm, and the short arm of the Y chromosome is very bright.

The intensity of the image obtained after R-banding is strong and durable, contrary to that obtained after Q-banding, and the metaphase spreads, after being photographed, can be decolorized and retreated for another type of banding. All of these advantages contribute to the worldwide routine use of this method for the detection of chromosome anomalies. A translation of the Reading classification system for G-bands into one for R-bands and a standardized bovine karyotype for R-bands have been proposed in the Second Conference for Standardization of Domestic Animal Karyotypes held in Jouy-en-Josas, France this year.

Constitutive heterochromatin that is colored preferentially by the C-banding method appears to be localized to the centromeric region of all bovine autosomes (Popescu, 1973) (Fig. 3). On the Y chromosome, it is situated on the median part of the short arm, and on the X chromosome, it is detected faintly on the proximal part of the short arm. Because the disposition of C-bands is uniform in bovine chromosomes, this technique is not useful for the identification of chromosomes. However, constitutive heterochromatin polymorphism has been detected and involves a quantitative difference between the two homologous chromosomes of the first two autosomal pairs (Popescu, 1974a; Moraes et al., 1979). This polymorphism has also been detected by the T-banding method (Gustavsson, 1980).

These polymorphisms and variants detected by different banding methods constitute a useful instrument for gene mapping. One good

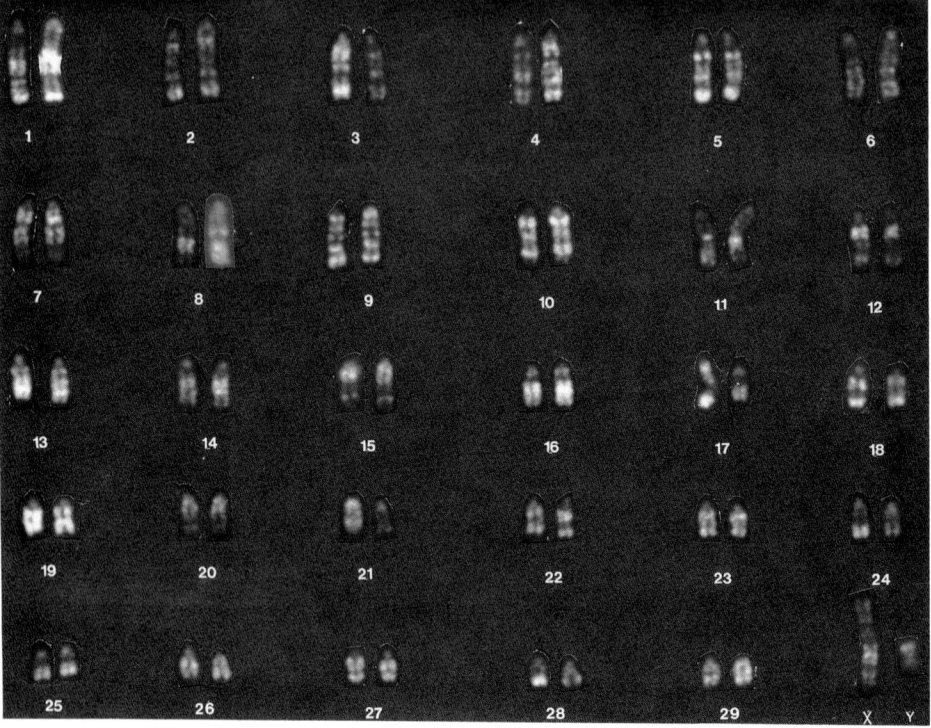

FIG. 2. Above: RBA karyotype of a normal bull. Opposite: RBG karyotype of a normal cow. (Photographs courtesy of H. Hayes, Cytogenetics Laboratory, National Institute for Agricultural Research, Jouy-en-Josas, France.)

example is the C-band polymorphism on chromosome 15 in the pig; this polymorphism has been used as a marker for the localization of the G locus for blood typing (Fries and Ruddle, 1986).

Silver nitrate staining has also been applied to bovine chromosomes for the detection of chromosomes carrying the nucleolar organizer regions (NORs) (Henderson and Bruere, 1979; Di Berardino et al., 1979). Five chromosome pairs have been found to carry NORs: 2, 3, 4, 11, and 28. Again, a great heterogeneity in the expression of nucleolar organizers has been noted in homologous chromosomes of the same pair and in similar chromosomes from different spreads (Di Berardino et al., 1979).

II. Chromosome Abnormalities

In 1977, during the Third Colloquium on Domestic Animal Cytogenetics, the total number of animals examined for karyotyping in cattle

CATTLE CHROMOSOMES

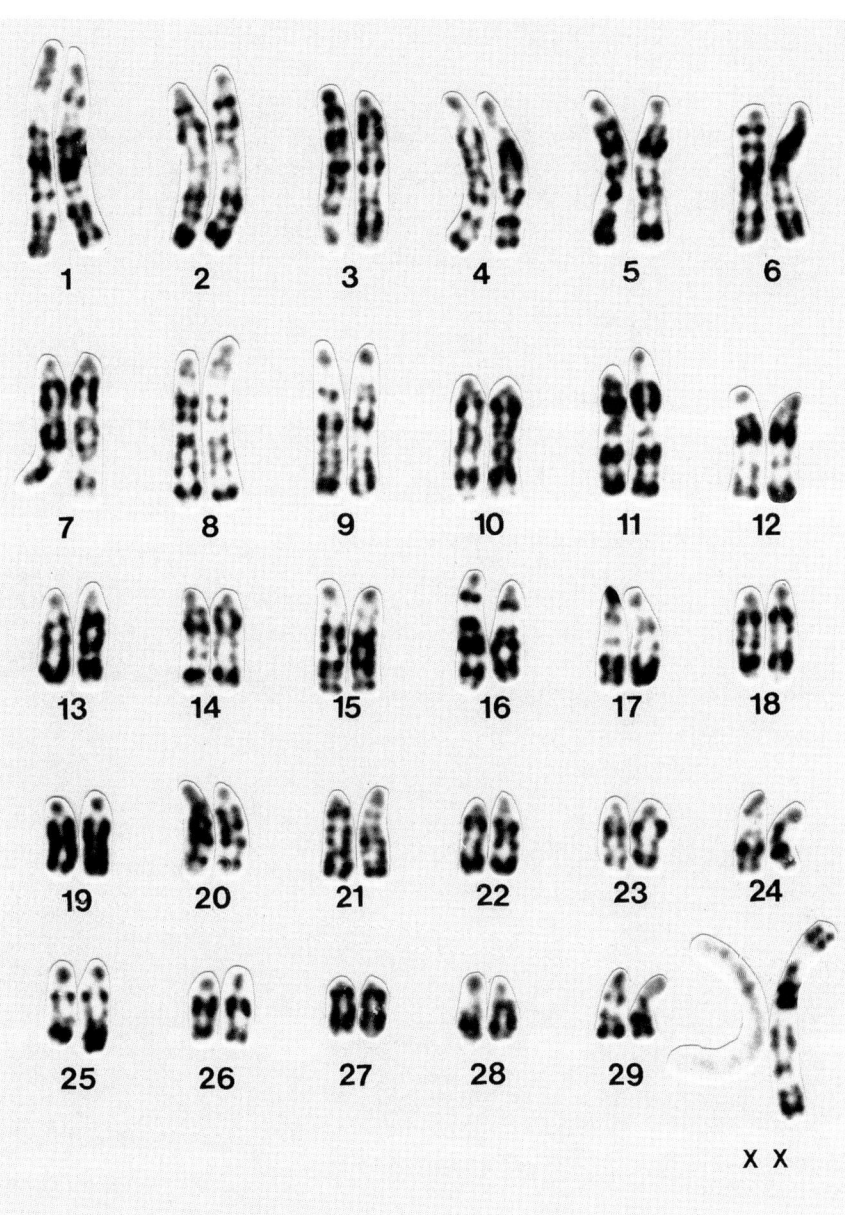

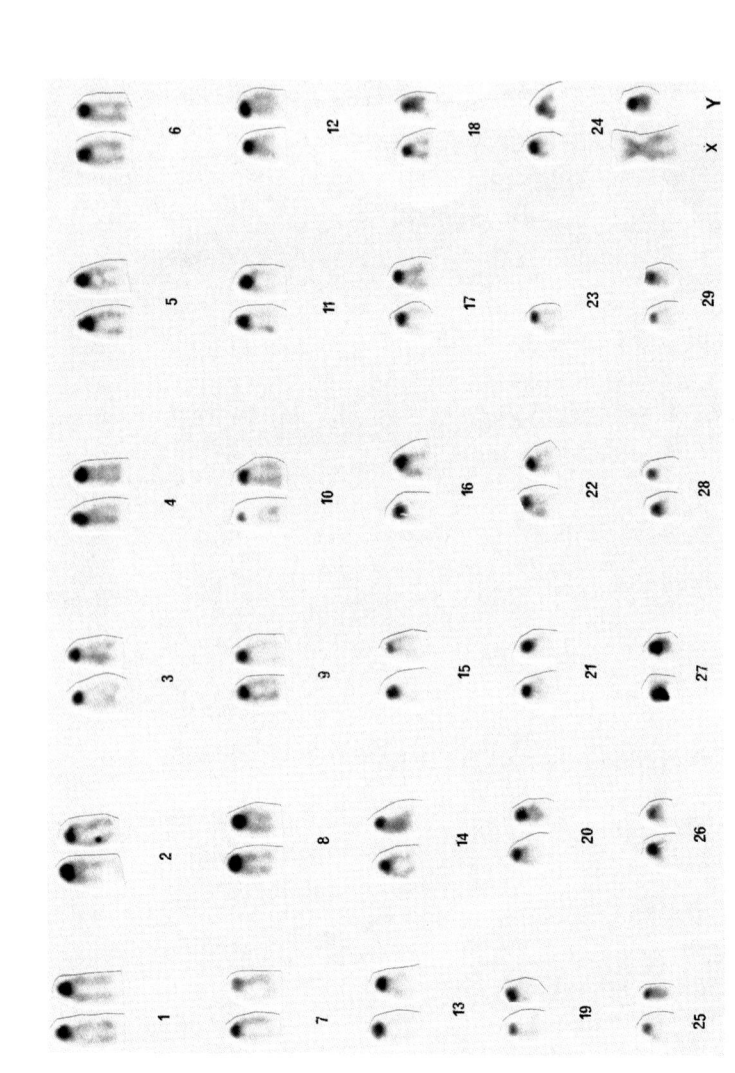

FIG. 3. C-band karyotype of a normal bull.

was estimated at 13,000 animals from 80 different bovine breeds (Popescu, 1977). At present, this number is estimated to be 25,000 animals, which puts cattle, after man and mouse, as the mammalian species most studied from the cytogenetic aspect.

The number of animals examined varies greatly from one breed to the other and among geographical areas. For example, the Swedish Red Pied breed, with almost 6,000 animals examined (I. Gustavsson, personal communication), represents almost a quarter of all cases.

In France, up to the present, about 5,000 animals have been examined; 3,000 in Switzerland (Tschudi, 1984) and 3,000 in Hungary (Kovacs, 1984). In the United States, 2,000 animals have been studied by Fechheimer (1973) and Eldridge et al. (1984); in Australia 1,100 animals have been studied by Halnan (1976), whereas in Africa only 500 animals have been examined (Popescu et al., 1979; Nel et al., 1985). In South America, roughly the same number has been studied (Moraes et al., 1980; Pinheiro et al., 1981).

Chromosome translocations of the Roberstonian type are by far the most frequently reported in cattle. In fact, Gustavsson (1984) and coworkers reviewed 19 different reported types, including 12 detected by banding methods and 7 by classical staining with Giemsa. Interestingly, among the 29 autosomal pairs of the bovine species, only pairs 10, 15, 17, 19, 22, and 26 have not been implicated in Robertsonian type translocations.

A. The 1/29 Robertsonian Translocation

Following the initial description by Gustavsson and Rockborn (1964) in Sweden, the 1/29 translocation was reported in Norway (Amrud, 1969), the United States (Herschler and Fechheimer, 1966), Italy (Rugiati and Fedrigo, 1967), Germany (Rieck et al., 1968), France (Popescu, 1971), and Great Britain (Harvey, 1971) (Figs. 4 and 5).

In 1977 the compilation done during the Third Colloquium on Domestic Animal Cytogenetics showed the presence of the 1/29 translocation in 28 breeds disseminated in Europe, North and Central America, Asia, and Africa (Popescu, 1977). Since that time, that translocation has been identified in South America, including Brazil (Pinheiro et al., 1979; Moraes et al., 1980), Venezuela (G. Munoz, personal communication), and Argentina (Igartua et al., 1985), in Japan (Masuda et al., 1975), in the French West Indies (Popescu et al., 1987), in a Zebu breed in the Ivory Coast (Popescu et al., 1979), in South Africa (Nel et al., 1985), and in a dozen European breeds. Worldwide, the translocation has been reported in approximately 50 breeds.

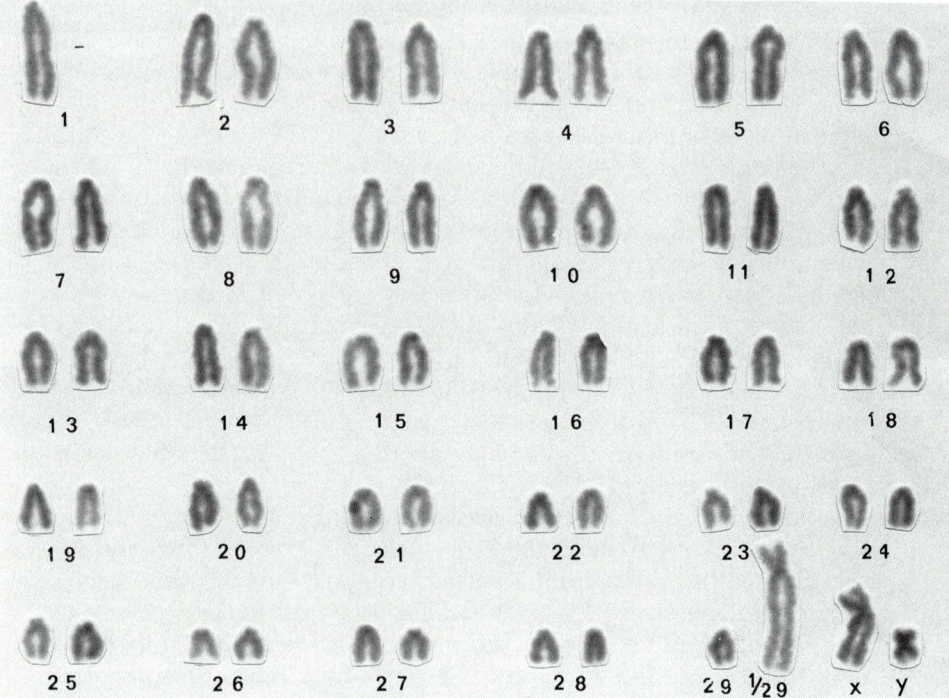

FIG. 4. Karyotype of a bull heterozygous for the 1/29 translocation.

The frequency of heterozygous carriers of this translocation varies greatly depending on breed or size of the population studied. In rare breeds such as the British White (Eldridge, 1975) or the Corsican breed (Hari *et al.*, 1984), high frequencies of 60 and 40%, respectively, are noted.

In France, a survey on the frequency of the translocation in the Blonde d'Aquitaine breed has been completed recently. Among a representative sample of more than 2,000 heifers, the overall frequency of carriers has been estimated at 14.2%. This study has also shown that among the various factors investigated, the geographic location and the type of breeding, artificial insemination or natural breeding, play a major role in the variation of the frequency of the abnormality (Frebling *et al.*, 1987).

1. Origin of the 1/29 Translocation

There are two hypotheses for the worldwide distribution of the anomaly: a recurrent mutation or a common origin. At present, there

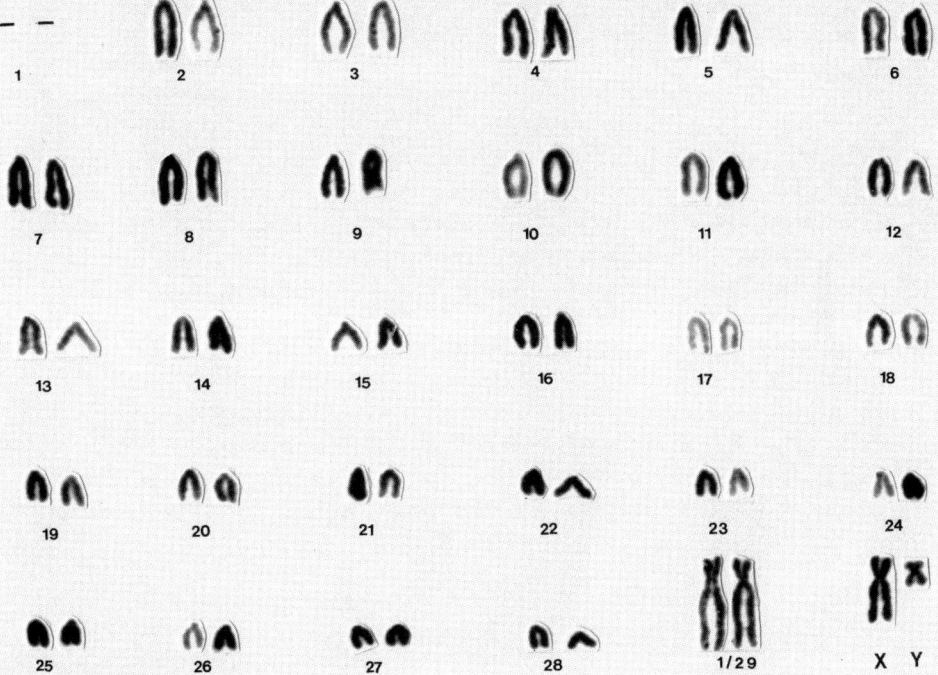

FIG. 5. Karyotype of a bull homozygous for the 1/29 translocation.

is no evidence to support the recurrent mutation hypothesis. Despite the significant number of animals studied and the detected carriers of this anomaly, not a single case of *de novo* appearance of the translocation has been reported. On the other hand, it is well known that chromosomes containing nucleolar organizers remain attached to the nucleolus during the meiotic prophase and, due to their proximity, they are more prone to translocations. If the two chromosomes implicated in this translocation were carriers of nucleolar organizers, one could suggest the possibility of recurrence. However, this circumstance, which would favor repeated fusions, is not confirmed, because chromosome 1 does not carry a nucleolar organizer. In cattle, only chromosomes 2, 3, 4, 11, and 28 carry nucleolar organizers (Henderson and Bruere, 1979; Di Berardino *et al.*, 1979).

Finally, similarities in DNA repetitive sequence patterns in the centromeric area of the two chromosomes, which could favor fusion, has not yet been established (Maio, 1975, cited in Gustavsson, 1979).

On the contrary, many observations support the hypothesis of a common and ancient origin of this anomaly and of a subsequent diffusion among numerous breeds. A monocentric fused chromosome possesses only one block of constitutive heterochromatin at the centromeric level, which suggests an ancient origin for this fusion (Niebuhr, 1972). Two blocks of constitutive heterochromatin in the region of the centromere of the fused chromosome, and therefore termed dicentric, would suggest a recent origin for this fusion, similar to the metacentric chromosomes reported in *Mus poschiavinus* (Forejt, 1982) or in the metacentric neochromosome reported in the goat (Evans *et al.*, 1973). However, the fused 1/29 chromosome has always been described as monocentric when C-banding methods were used; a single block of constitutive heterochromatin has always been detected at the level of the centromere (Popescu, 1973, 1975b; Blazak and Eldridge, 1977).

At a more general level, Hsu and Mead (1969) stated that the probability of a chromosome rearrangement involving the same chromosomes occurring more than once is very low and Taylor *et al.* (1969) considered each translocation of the Robertsonian type to be a unique event.

2. Effects of the 1/29 Translocation

The presence of the 1/29 translocation in a chromosomally balanced karyotype, like other structural anomalies, does not have any visible effect on the phenotype in carriers. Gustavsson (1969) reported that the libido and the sperm characteristics, such as motility or volume, were normal in heterozygous bulls. Only the concentration of spermatozoa appeared slightly reduced. No other physiological parameter seems to be influenced by this anomaly. In France, Darre *et al.* (1972) reported that heterozygous bulls showed better meat production, which was attributed to a growth rate superior to that of normal bulls, but this observation was later retracted (Queinnec *et al.*, 1974).

The only reported impact of this anomaly is a reduction in the fertility of heterozygous carriers. Gustavsson (1969) observed in Swedish Red and White cattle a reduction in fertility at first calving in daughters of heterozygous bulls, compared to that of daughters of normal bulls. The difference was 2.85% on nonreturn rates up to 56 days and 5.8% at 273 days (Gustavsson, 1969). Refsdal (1976) confirmed the decline in fertility and the progressive decrease from 30 to 60 days, in a study involving 20,000 daughters of carrier bulls and 600,000 daughters of normal bulls of the Norwegian Red breed.

Initially, the fertility of heterozygous males appeared to be normal (Gustavsson, 1969), but the study involved only bulls selected for fertility based on the nonreturn rate. Redoing the study, with 12 hetero-

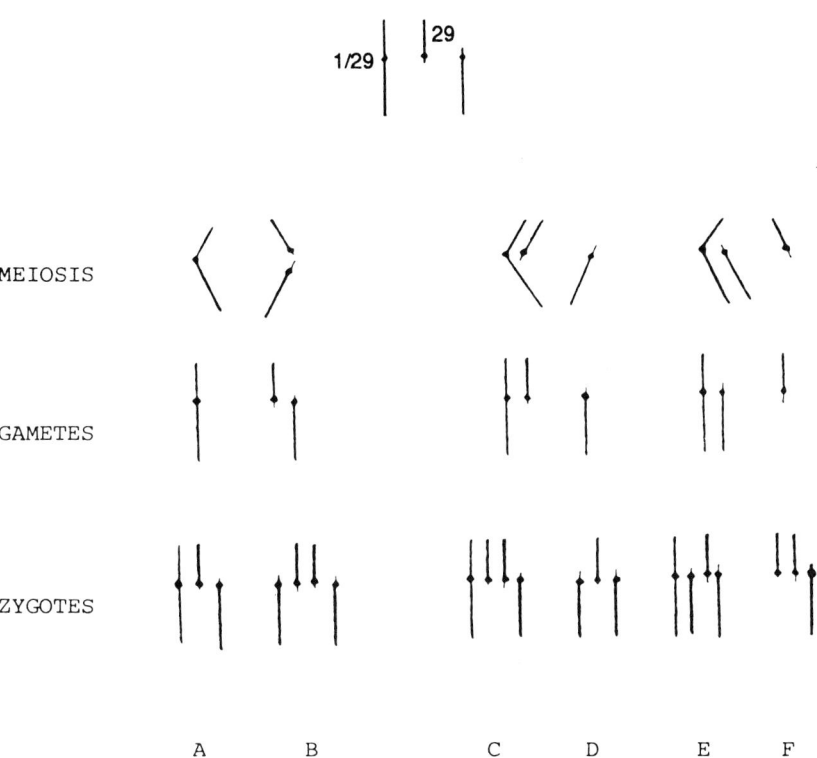

FIG. 6. Different types of gametes and zygotes produced by a bull heterozygous for the 1/29 translocation. (A) Balanced carrier; (B) normal; (C) trisomy 29; (D) monosomy 29; (E) trisomy 1; (F) monosomy 1. [From Gustavsson (1969).]

zygous bulls unselected for fertility, and 45 normal bulls, observations showed in the first group a reduction in the nonreturn rate, at 28 and 56 days, of 4.85 and 7.02%, respectively, compared to the normal group (Dyrendahl and Gustavsson, 1979). Other parameters, such as libido and sperm characteristics, were normal except for a slight diminution in the concentration of spermatozoa, which confirmed the first study.

The reduction in fertility in males and females heterozygous for the 1/29 translocation is explained by Gustavsson (1969) as an increase in early embryonic mortality. To support this proposal, Gustavsson developed a schematic illustration of the meiotic process in an animal heterozygous for the 1/29 translocation and of the formation of zygotes after fertilization with a normal gamete (Fig. 6).

It is apparent that the gametogenesis in an animal carrying the

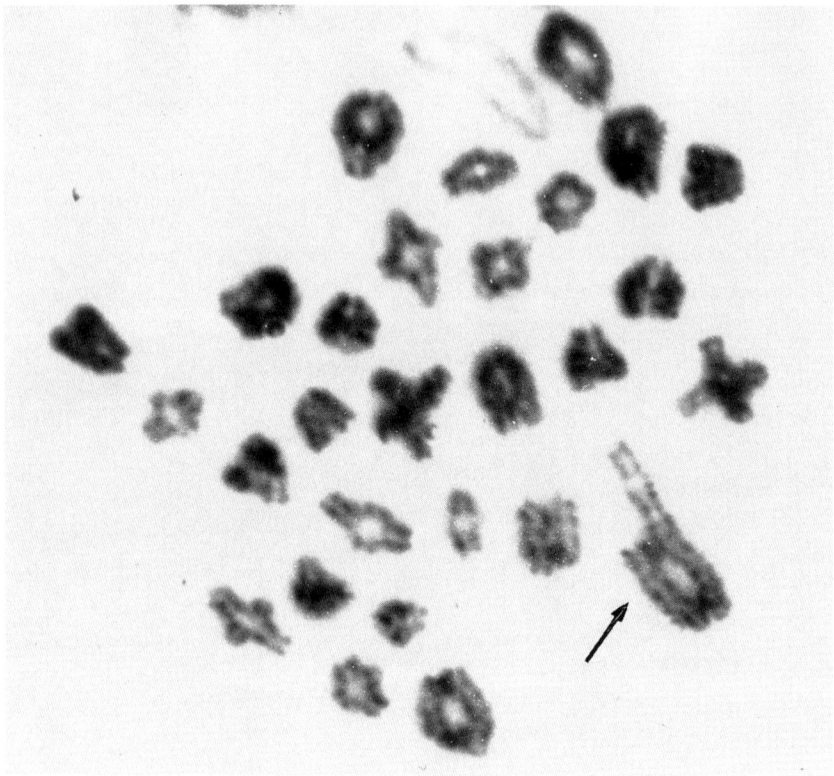

FIG. 7. Diakinesis in a bull carrying the 1/29 translocation.

1/29 translocation is abnormal. For example, the two chromosomes involved in the translocation associate with their free homologues and form a trivalent at diakinesis (Fig. 7). If segregation occured normally, the two free chromosomes would go to one pole and the recombined chromosome, to the other. Gametes from this division would be balanced, because the genetic material would be intact, although one would carry the centric fusion. In some cases, one of the free chromosomes migrates with the recombined chromosome to the same pole. This type of segregation leads to the formation of disomic gametes, carrying a chromosome in two doses and a nullisomic gamete, lacking one chromosome. After fusion with a normal gamete, monosomic or trisomic zygotes are created, with one or three copies of the same chromosome, 1 or 29, respectively. These unbalanced embryos, with an ex-

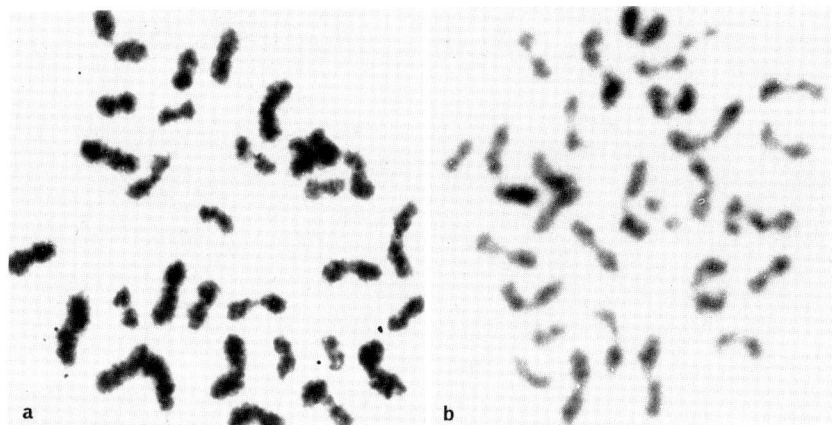

FIG. 8. Metaphase II with unbalanced karyotype: (a) missing one chromosome (29,X); (b) having one extra chromosome (30,t,Y).

cess or a lack of genetic material, are not viable and are rejected at a more or less precocious stage. The embryonic mortality due to unbalanced gametes produced by heterozygous animals would explain the drop in fertility noted in nonreturn rates. The lethality of unbalanced karyotypes for embryos would be confirmed by the fact that although a considerable number of living animals have been karyotyped, not a single case of monosomy of trisomy for the chromosomes implicated in the translocation has been reported.

The theoretical explanation by Gustavsson has been confirmed by meiotic studies and by studies on embryos per se. Studies on meiotic chromosomes in animals heterozygous for the 1/29 translocation have shown that a certain percentage of unbalanced gametes exists (Gustavsson, 1969; Logue, 1977; Logue and Harvey, 1978; Popescu, 1978) (Fig. 8). Therefore, the detection of karyotypes showing monosomy for chromosome 1 in 13-day-old embryos from a heterozygous sire (Popescu, 1980) (Fig. 9) and those showing trisomy for the same chromosome in younger embryos (day 7) (King *et al.*, 1981) confirmed that the theory of Gustavsson is valid and firmly establishes the role of embryonic mortality in the reduction of fertility in heterozygotes.

The 1/29 translocation in a balanced state is transmitted like a simple, dominant Mendelian factor in a 1:1 ratio (Gustavsson, 1969; Popescu, 1974b). The prevalance of the translocation in numerous breeds, sometimes very high despite its negative impact on fertility,

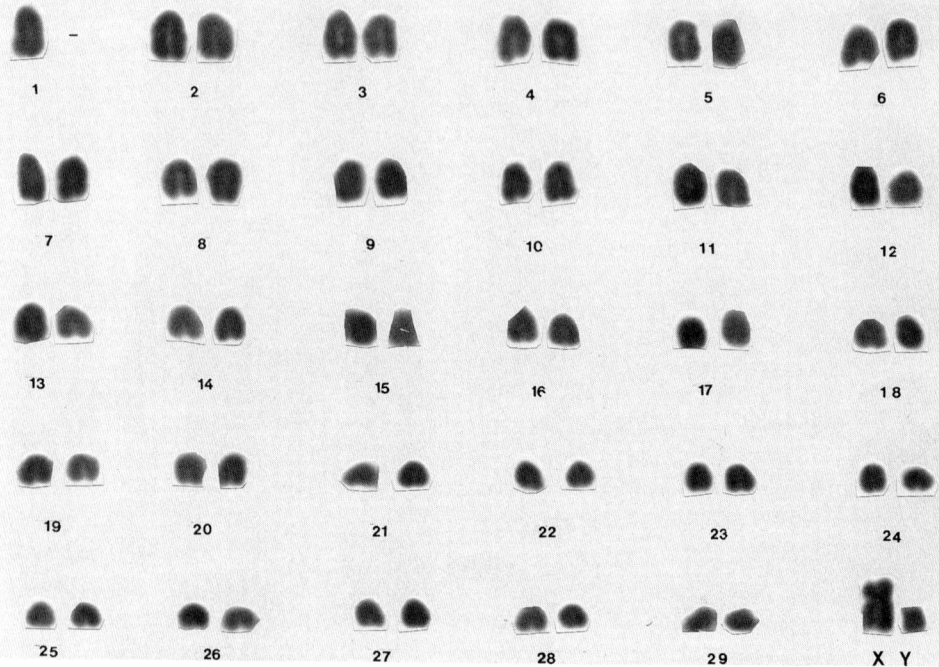

FIG. 9. Karyotype with monosomy 1 from a 13-day-old embryo sired by a bull carrying the 1/29 translocation.

would suggest that there is a selection advantage associated with its presence. In studies using mice, to explain the presence of such an anomaly in a wild-type population, the formation of "coadaptive gene complexes" has been suggested. In the absence of crossing over in the regions near the centromere, due to the translocation, these neoformed gene complexes would have selective advantages, particularly under specific environmental conditions (Cattanach, 1978).

In the case of the 1/29 translocation in cattle, there is no argument in favor of a selective advantage. Gustavsson (1979) and Ford (1982) suggested that there should have been an advantage shortly after its appearance, when selection pressure was different from what it is today. This could explain the high frequency, roughly 10%, of this anomaly in a relatively unselected breed such as the N'Guni (Nel et al., 1985), in which only natural mating is used.

For highly selected breeds, the introduction of artificial insemination has considerably modified the population dynamics. The intensive use of certain sires could be the basis of high frequencies of the translocation in certain breeds. The migration and export of cattle from one country to the other, and sometimes from one continent to the other, could have played a certain role in the dissemination of the anomaly. For example, the 1/29 translocation was introduced in Africa in the Brune d'Atlas breed, through French breeds (Marx, 1979), and in Brazil, in the Pitangueras breed by Red Poll sires (Pinheiro et al., 1981).

3. Eradication Policy

The Swedish Department of Agriculture has estimated that the reduction in fertility attributed to the 1/29 translocation is responsible for an annual loss of 2,000,000 crowns (1 dollar = 6 Swedish crowns). At the same time, it has been noted that for the period 1966–1969, there was an average of a 1% reduction in fertility among the Swedish Red Pied breed. The Swedish government decided at the end of 1969 to carry out a serious and costly program of eradication by eliminating from reproduction all bulls carrying the translocation and to have every young bull karyotyped before entering the testing program (Gustavsson, 1970).

Within 3 years from the beginning of the eradication program, the average fertility of the breed was up by 0.5%, and this has been maintained ever since. The frequency, which had been estimated in 1969 at 14%, is now 3–4% in bulls used for artificial insemination (I. Gustavsson, personal communication).

The application of the eradication policy in Sweden had consequences in other countries. For example, since the beginning of the 1970s, routine cytogenetic evaluations have been conducted in animals used for breeding in France, Germany, Italy, Hungary, Switzerland, and Great Britain. At the same time, Australia and Great Britain decided that all imported cattle should be karyotyped and declared normal before being granted permission to enter the country. In 1985, the French Department of Agriculture adopted a new regulation concerning the 1/29 translocation, which prohibits the certification of carriers and their use for breeding.

After 15 years, the eradication program, although costly at the beginning, because bulls already tested and in use in artificial insemination centers had to be replaced, has proved to be judicious and economically advantageous. On a more general level, the discovery of the 1/29 translocation has had a considerable impact on bovine cytogenetics. There are roughly 200 scientific papers on the subject and, in fact, it is because of the study of its distribution and frequency that large cattle populations have been examined. The translocation's impact on fertility has contributed to the awareness of the danger of breeding animals that are phenotypically normal but carry chromosomal anomalies.

B. Other Autosomal Structural Abnormalities

Very few cases of other chromosomal structural abnormalities, such as tandem or reciprocal translocation, are described in cattle (for review see Popescu, 1989). The paucity of reported cases and the fact that usually they are isolated incidents could be explained by the technical difficulty of detecting the small chromosomal fragment that is involved in these rearrangements, in karyotypes where all autosomes are similar in shape. It is possible that other structural anomalies, such as paracentric inversions, which do not modify the chromosomal structure, totally escape detection.

C. Structural Abnormalies of Sex Chromosomes

1. X/Autosome Translocations

Only two cases of X/autosome translocations have been described in cattle (Gustavsson et al., 1968; Eldridge, 1980). In both cases, the females were phenotypically normal but were repeat breeders. In Canada, a third case of X/autosome translocation has been identified in a cow and her female offspring, an albino. The abnormal X chromosome is active in all cells examined, whereas the normal X chromosome appears inactive (Basrur et al., 1988) The autosome translocated to the X chromosome has been identified by R-banding to be chromosome 18 (Fig. 10).

2. Deletions of the X Chromosome

Chromosomal breaks on the X chromosome have always been reported in females with fertility problems, and all animals examined were mosaics with normal cells (Genest and Guay, 1979; Hanada and Muramatsu, 1980).

D. Numerical Abnormalities

Numerical anomalies, or heteroploidies, are rarely seen after birth, as conceptuses are usually eliminated during pregnancy, due to the deleterious nature of the anomalies. In all cattle cells studied, euploid heteroploidies have never been observed. Only $2n/4n$ or $2n/6n$ mosaics have been detected in cattle with muscular hypertrophy (Culard phe-

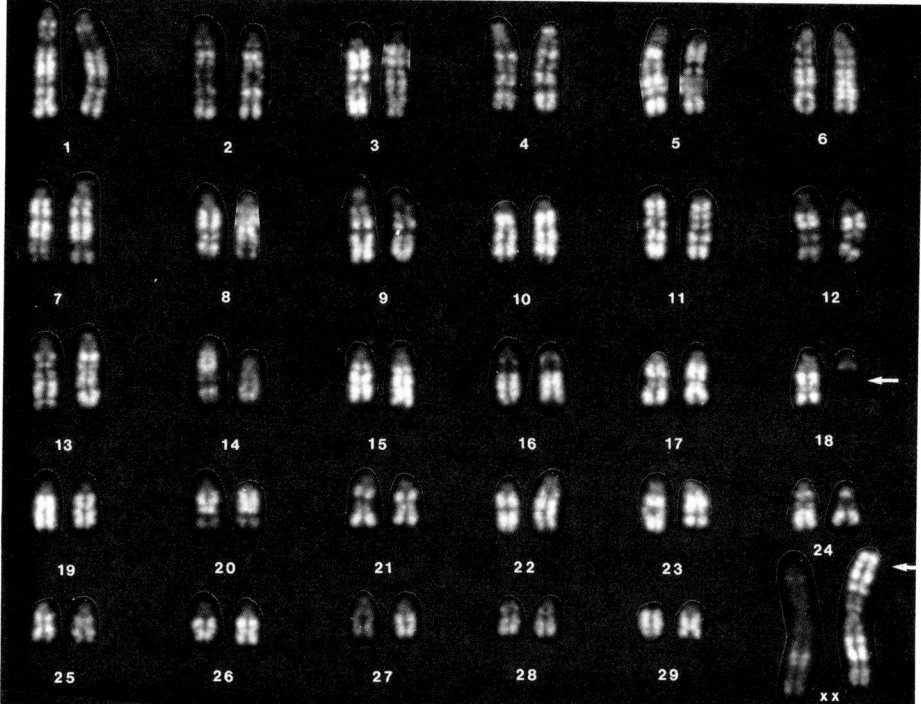

FIG. 10. RBA karyotype of a cow carrying the X/autosome translocation

notype, Popescu, 1968) or in lines selected for meat production (Zartman and Fechheimer, 1967).

1. Autosomal Heteroploidies

Aneuploid heteroploidies are monosomics or trisomies resulting from nondisjunction at mitosis or meiosis. Trisomies are usually tolerated more easily and more frequently than monosomies. Some cases of autosomal trisomies are known in cattle. The oldest, trisomie 18 (Herzog and Hohn, 1968), is always associated with brachygnathia. After the initial German report describing this trisomy, it was detected in Japan (Mori et al., 1979) and in Switzerland (Tschudi et al., 1975). Two other autosomal trisomies, involving chromosome 17 (Herzog et al., 1982) and chromosome 22 (Mayr et al., 1985), have been identified precisely with banding methods. Other trisomies, usually isolated cases, have been reported, but the chromosomes involved were not identified precisely (Dunn and Johnson, 1972; Long, 1984).

Herzog and Hohn (1984) described a novel type of trisomy in cattle, "trisomy with centric fusion." This is a trisomy in which two of the involved chromosomes are fused and the third one is free. Herzog and Hohn suggested that this anomaly occurred after nondisjunction at meiosis or after fertilization, by a normal spermatozoon, of a disomic ovum carrying two associated homologous chromosomes. The two calves described by Herzog and Hohn had similar anomalies, but the chromosomes involved were different: chromosome 12, in the first case, and chromosome 20, in the second animal. Both calves had lower brachygnathia but the second calf, with trisomy 20, also showed scoliosis and microcephaly.

Regardless of the chromosome implicated and the clinical signs, of which lower brachygnathia is the only constant factor, autosomal trisomies are all lethal, and all calves carrying the anomaly die at birth or a few days later.

2. Sex Chromosome Abnormalities

Aneuploidies of sex chromosomes are frequently seen in animals surviving birth because these abnormalities are more easily tolerated due to the mechanism of gene dosage compensation.

In the mammalian female, one of the X chromosomes, either of maternal or paternal origin, is genetically inactivated early in embryonic life (Lyon, 1961). Gene dosage compensation acts as a regulator in cases of X chromosome anomalies. Therefore, in XO females, the only existing X is not inactivated, and in females with one or more extra X chromosomes, only one X chromosome remains active.

Three types of sex chromosomal aneuploidies have been described: an excess of X or Y chromosomes in males and XXX in females. The XO type, well known in horses, has not been reported in cattle.

a. XXY Condition. In humans, this anomaly is associated with the Klinefelter syndrome. Rieck (1984) reported three cases of pure XXY animals and two cases of XY/XX/XXY mosaics in cattle. The anomaly is always associated with bilateral testicular hypoplasia and oligospermia or even azoospermia, resulting from the degradation of seminiferous tubules, which worsens after puberty. The animals affected are therefore sterile and easy to detect.

The anomaly is due to an error in meiotic or mitotic division. Rieck (1984) noted that all cases of hypogonadism could not be attributed to the XXY condition. This investigator suggested that certain types of hypogonadism and an inherited predisposition to nondisjunction of sex chromosomes could be the result of the pleiotropic effect of certain genes.

b. XYY Condition. In cattle, the pure XYY condition has never been observed. Only three cases of XY/XYY mosaics have been reported (Miyake *et al.*, 1984). This anomaly could be explained by the implantation of two male zygotes (one XY and one XYY), followed by the exchange of cells between the two zygotes, and the elimination of the abnormal embryo, or by a nondisjunction in a normal zygote, during the first embryonic divisions. In contrast to what has been observed in man, Miyake *et al.* (1984) showed that the frequency of XYY cells diminished with age in a mosaic bull. Despite poor semen quality, this animal had a normal fertility. Because of its rarity in cattle, this syndrome does not have great importance for reproduction.

c. XXX Condition. Five cases of trisomy for the X chromosomes have been described. Clinical signs are various: irregular cycles, primary anestrus, and repeat breeding. Like the XYY condition, the X trisomy occurs only sporadically and does not have a great impact on reproduction.

E. INTERSEXUALITY

There are three steps in the mammalian sexual development: the chromosomal sex, which is determined at fertilization, the gonadal sex, and the phenotypic sex. Alterations in the normal process can result in three types of intersexuality: true intersexuality or hermaphroditism, male or female pseudohermaphroditism, and freemartinism.

Usually, intersexuality is defined by a mixture in the same individual of characteristics of both sexes. Two types of hermaphroditism can be defined based only on the gonadal characteristics. True hermaphroditism is defined as the presence of both male and female tissues in gonads. Pseudohermaphroditism is characterized by the presence of one type of gonadal tissue. Male pseudohermaphroditism is defined by the presence of male gonadal tissue only, whereas female pseudohermaphroditism occurs when only female gonadal tissue is present.

1. True Hermaphroditism

In humans a wide variety of ambiguous genital organs exists, but usually the organs are of the male type. Clinical signs are very different from one case to the other. Gonads can consist of an ovary on one side and a testis on the other (alternate hermaphroditism), an ovotestis on each side (bilateral), or one ovary or a testis on one side and an ovotestis on the other (unilateral). The bilateral type is rare, comprising only 20% of cases, whereas the other types occur in equal proportions. The karyotypes of true hermaphroditism are usually XX, but

XX/XY mosaics are described in the literature. There has not been a single report of true hermaphroditism in cattle.

2. Female Pseudohermaphroditism

Following a secondary virilization of the female fetus, female pseudohermaphroditism is rare in humans and unknown in cattle.

3. Male Pseudohermaphroditism

There are various forms of male pseudohermaphroditism known in humans and they are usually the result of a genetic mutation with an autosomal recessive or sex-linked recessive mode of inheritance.

4. Testicular Feminization Syndrome

Testicular feminization syndrome (Tfm) is a well-known syndrome in humans and mice. The karyotype of affected individuals is always XY. The primary defect, an absence of the tissue receptor for androgens, is due to a sex-linked genetic mutation. The phenotype is feminine but the gonads are intraabdominal testes.

Nes (1966) reported the first case of testicular feminization in cattle, and subsequent reports came from Germany (Rieck, 1971) and England (Long and David, 1981). In Sweden, Linares et al. (1981) reported four related cases in the Swedish Red Pied breed. Affected animals are sterile but the anomaly, due to genetic mutation, can be transmitted and can have negative effects on certain families.

5. Gonadal Dysgenesis

Gonadal dysgenesis is an extreme case of male pseudohermaphroditism. In humans, affected individuals have a female phenotype, but the secondary sexual characteristics are not accentuated. The karyotype is usually XY, but gonads are reduced to fibrous streaks and usually become malignant.

A few isolated cases have been reported in cattle in France (Bastien et al., 1973), in Roumania (Gluhovschi et al., 1972), and more recently in New Zealand (Chapman et al., 1978) and India (Sharma et al., 1980).

F. FREEMARTINISM

The phenomenon of freemartinism has been known to occur in cattle for centuries. A freemartin is a female, usually sterile, born co-twin to a male. This anomaly is present in 90% of all twin births involving at least one male and one female; the female co-twin, in rare occasions, can be fertile.

The freemartin heifer usually shows masculinization of the internal genitalia, gonads, and genital tract, whereas the external genitalia are not obviously modified. Placental membranes from the male and female twins fuse in the uterus and the differentiation of the gonads and the Müllerian duct is inhibited around day 50 of pregnancy. Later, around day 90, masculinization of the gonads and development of the Wolffian duct occur (Vigier et al., 1976).

Cytogenetically, the freemartin shows a mixture of male and female cells, called chimerism, in blood and hematopoietic organs. The male co-twin is not grossly affected. There is blood chimerism, XX/XY, but the genital organs are normal. However, some investigators consider that these animals should not be used for breeding, because they have poor-quality semen and a nonreturn rate inferior to that of normal bulls (Stafford, 1972).

Different hypotheses have been suggested to explain the freemartin condition. The oldest theory was suggested by Lillie (1916) and is called the hormonal theory, because it considers that the masculinization of the genital tract and the gonads is provoked by androgens that are secreted by the gonads of the male co-twin, and later by the masculinized gonad of the female fetus. The experiments done by Jost (1947) on rabbit fetuses concluded that there is an action of testicular factors toward the masculinization of the female gonad, but did not show any evidence of direct action on the gonad.

The discovery of chromosomal chimerism, XX/XY, in blood and hematopoietic organs in male and female co-twins (Ohno et al., 1962) triggered the cellular origin theory. Fechheimer suggested that the phenomenon is not a result of the transfer of male hormones to the female fetus, but rather is the result of the transfer of male cells and their action on sexual differentiation. The cellular origin hypothesis was formed following numerous experiments by Wachtel and Ohno on the H-Y antigen. The H-Y antigen, a histocompatibility antigen coded on the Y chromosome, could be the initial factor responsible for testicular differentiation (Wachtel et al., 1975; Ohno et al., 1976). Therefore, testicular differentiation could require the presence of the H-Y antigen, and the formation of ovarian structure, on the contrary, would occur in its absence.

Ohno et al. (1976) have looked for the presence of the H-Y antigen in freemartins. At day 150 of pregnancy, they have shown the presence of the antigen on the gonads of three freemartins at a concentration similar to that found on a fetal testis of similar age. They concluded that the male cells migrate to the female gonad and release H-Y antigen; the antigen is taken up by the XX cells and induces the masculinization of the gonad. Later, Wachtel *et al.* (1980) showed the presence of H-Y antigen in sera from male and freemartin fetuses, whereas it was absent in sera from normal female fetuses. The presence of H-Y antigen is explained by the transmission of the circulating form of H-Y antigen secreted by the male fetus, through vascular anastomoses established during the fusion of placental membranes. The time lapse between the masculinization of the male gonad, which started around 40, and that of the freemartin, around day 100, is explained by the requirement for a certain concentration of the antigen, which takes longer to build up in the freemartin, to trigger its action (Carlon, 1982).

III. Y Chromosome Polymorphism

Cases of abnormally long Y chromosomes in bulls were reported in the Ayrshire breed (Fechheimer, 1973) and the Charolais breed (Cribiu and Popescu, 1974). The Y chromosome of the Charolais bull has a G-banding pattern similar to that of the normal Y chromosome, which excludes the hypothesis of a rearrangement. The abnormally long chromosome is explained by a higher degree of despiralization of the chromatin. In both cases, the elongated Y chromosome does not appear to affect reproduction or phenotypic characteristics.

In subsequent studies on five French breeds, Cribiu (1975) found a breed difference for the length of the Y chromosome. Therefore, Maine–Anjou and Normandy bulls would have a smaller Y chromosome than is found in Charolais or Montbeliard bulls, whereas the Y chromosomes of the Black and White French Friesian bulls are mid-sized. The length of the Y chromosome in Charolais bulls has been confirmed by Hansen and Elleby (1975), who found comparable measurements in the Danish Red and Danish Black Pied breeds. The interest in Y chromosome polymorphism in these species pertains to the usefulness of this feature as a genetic marker.

IV. The Y Chromosome of Zebu Cattle

In an old study, Kieffer and Cartwright (1968) were the first to show that the Y chromosomes of Zebu bulls were not identical to those of European cattle. Bulls of the Brahman and Santa Gertrudis breeds, which originated from Zebus imported from India, have an acrocentric

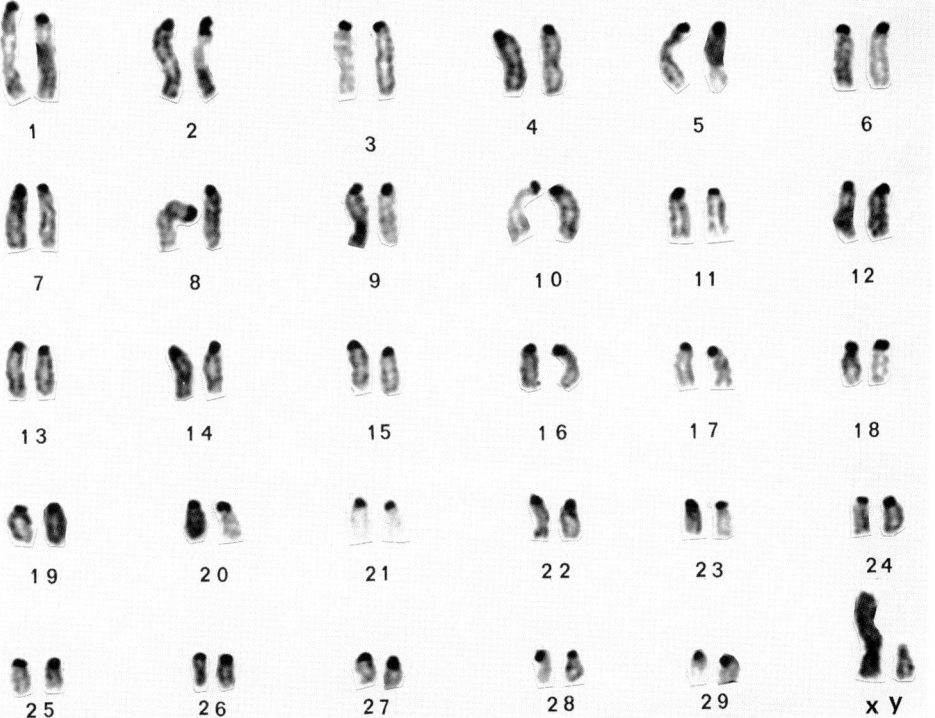

FIG. 11. Karyotype of a Zebu bull.

Y chromosome. This acrocentric morphology (Fig. 11) has been confirmed in numerous Zebu breeds in Asia and in Africa. However, Halnan (1976), studying South African Zebus of the Afrikaaner breed, found a submetacentric Y chromosome similar to that of European cattle. This shape of Y chromosome has been detected by Meyer et al. (1980) in other Zebu breeds in South Africa, i.e., Bonsmara, Drakensberger, Nguni, and Pedi. In the Brazilian Ibage breed, created from Nellore Zebus and Angus, Pinheiro et al. (1980) found the two types of Y chromosomes, acrocentric and submetacentric.

If an acrocentric chromosome is considered more ancient phylogenetically, it is possible that a pericentric inversion occurred in the Y chromosome during the evolution of European cattle. Therefore, the terminal portion of the long arm of the Y chromosome of Zebus shows adjacent bright and dark bands by R- and C-banding methods. Using the same techniques, the same banding pattern is found on the distal part of the short arm of the Y chromosome of European cattle. Only a pericentric inversion involving the proximal half of the long arm, including the centromere, could explain the transformation of an acrocentric to a submetacentric chromosome. This morphological difference in the Y chromosome has been used by Eldridge and Blazak (1977) in the study of evolution and parentage among different breeds.

However, the practical consequence of Y polymorphism seems to be negative in the Zebu × European crosses. It has been reported that in crosses between a Zebu breed with an acrocentric Y chromosome and a European breed with a submetacentric chromosome the F_2 generation shows a calving rate significantly reduced compared to both parental breeds (Rendel, 1980; Rao, 1982). This reduction in the calving rate does not occur if the Zebu breed used for crossing has a submetacentric Y chromosome, as in the Afrikaaner breed (Rendel, 1980). Because the Y chromosome is the only element of the karyotype that differs in the two subspecies, it has been considered responsible for the reduction of fertility in crosses. Different hypotheses have been proposed to elucidate the intimate mechanism of fertility reduction and the role of the Y chromosome. Rendel (1980) thinks that there is a Y/autosome or Y/X translocation, but this is not visible in meiotic chromosomes of Zebus (Sharma and Popescu, 1986). C. R. E. Halnan (personal communication) suggests that the infertility derives from slight differences in the X chromosomes of the two subspecies, and even in certain autosomes responsible for sexual differentiation. These morphological differences could explain modifications in the expression of these genes, which in crossbred animals could not maintain an optimal fertility level.

Because these hypotheses have not been verified, the problem of crossbreeding remains. Crosses of Zebu and European cattle are practiced in various regions of the world to improve the reproductive characteristics of local breeds, which are otherwise well adapted and usually resistant to diseases and parasites.

V. Sexing of Bovine Embryos

The advances in cytogenetic techniques during the last few years have permitted not only the study of large populations of wild and domestic animals, but also the detection of chromosome anomalies before birth, in embryos, and in particular in progeny wherein one parent is heterozygous for a structural anomaly. In that regard, the investigation of the chromosome complement in embryos from a parent heterozygous for the 1/29 translocation has permitted the development of karyotyping techniques from young morulae or blastocysts.

The rapid development of bovine embryo transfer techniques has enabled cytogeneticists to determine the sex of an unborn calf, by chromosomal analysis. The bovine karyotype, difficult to study because of the uniformity of autosomes, nevertheless affords a great advantage: the sex chromosomes are different from the autosomes and are thus easily identifiable. The limiting factor for this technique is the reduced number of dividing cells available at the time, before transfer, that the embryo is biopsied.

The first experiments on sexing were conducted on fragments biopsied from day-13 and day-14 embryos and had a 50% success rate (Hare et al., 1976; Wintenberger-Torres and Popescu, 1980). Because day-13 embryos are too old for transfer and for freezing, methods to sex younger embryos (at day 6 or 7) had to be developed. At this stage, the total number of cells is 40–60 and the mitotic index is around 10%. If 10 cells are removed with a micromanipulator, the probability of getting dividing cells is limited. By the direct method, using whole or half embryos at day 7, there was 74 and 46% success, respectively (Popescu and Cribiu, 1982). To improve the percentage of cells in division, a method was devised to culture blastomeres on a collagen layer (Popescu et al., 1982). However, this method necessitates a lot of equipment and the results are too low to be of practical use in embryo transfer.

Sexing by cytogenetic methods permits not only determination of the sex of the embryo, but also detection of chromosomal anomalies transmitted by the parents or induced during superovulation. Because there are problems with the cytogenetic approach, other approaches have been investigated. In that regard, Brunner et al. (1983) devised a sexing technique based on the fluorescence of the monoclonal antibody for H-Y antigen. Preliminary results showed that the antibody recognized the H-Y antigen at days 6–7 in the bovine embryo, which indicated a practical method for sexing if the success rate could be improved.

The last technique to be tested for sexing involves the identification of the bovine Y chromosome by hybridization with DNA probes; the probes are obtained after cloning DNA specific for the Y chromosome. One of these probe was developed at the National Institute for Agricultural Research in Jouy-en-Josas, France, (Leonard et al., 1987) and has proved to be specific for the bovine Y chromosome (Popescu et al., 1988). Using a bound biochemical marker, this probe will be used for identification of the Y chromosome, on half embryos, or on a few cells biopsied from day-7 embryos, using a micromanipulator.

Ackowledgement

All figures (except for Fig. 6) are reproduced by permission of the Institut National de la Recherche Agronomique.

References

Amrud, J. (1969). Centric fusion of chromosomes in norwegian red cattle. *Hereditas* **62**, 293–302.
Basrur, P. K., Popescu, C. P., Pinheiro, L. E. L., Berepubo, N. A., and Reyes, E. R. (1988). Non-random pattern of X-chromosome inactivation in X-autosome translocation carrier cows. *Int. Congr. Genet., 16th, Toronto* Genome 30, Suppl., p. 1 (Abstr.)
Bastien, G., Dalbiez, J. M., and Nain, M. C. (1973). A propos d'un cas d'intersexualité constaté chez une génisse. *Bull. Soc. Sci. Vet. Med. Comp., Lyon* **75**, 145–146.
Blazak, W. F., and Eldridge, F. E. (1977). A Robertsonian translocation and its effect upon fertility in Brown Swiss cattle. *J. Dairy Sci.* **60**, 1133–1142.
Brunner, M., Moreira-Filho, C., Selden, J. R., Koo, G. C., and Wachtel, S. S. (1983). H-Y antigen in the early embryo. *Symp. Adv. Top. Anim. Reprod., 2nd, Jaboticabal, Bras.* pp. 97–111.
Carlon, N. (1982). Role de l'antigène H-Y dans l'organagénèse des gonades chez l'homme et les mammifères. *Pathol. Biol.* **30**, 49–60.
Cattanach, B. M. (1978). Crossover suppression in mice heterozygous for tobacco mouse metacentrics. *Cytogenet. Cell Genet.* **20**, 264–281.
Chapman, H. M., Bruere, A. N., and Jaine, P. M. (1978). XY gonadal dysgenesis in a Charolais heifer. *Anim. Reprod. Sci.* **1**, 9–18.
Cribiu, E. P. (1975). Variation interraciale de la taille du chromosome Y chez *Bos taurus* L. *Ann. Genet. Sel. Anim.* **7**, 139–144.
Cribiu, E. P., and Popescu, C. P. (1974). Un cas de chromosomes Y anormalement long chez *Bos taurus* L. *Ann. Genet. Sel. Anim.* **6**, 387–390.
Darre, R., Queinnec, G., and Berland, H. M. (1972). La translocation 1/29 des bovins. Etude générale et importance du phénomène dans le Sud-Ouest. *Rev. Med. Vet.* **123**, 477–494.
Di Berardino, D., Arrighi, F. E., and Kieffer, M. N. (1979). Nucleolus organizer regions in two species of Bovidae. *J. Hered.* **70**, 47–50.
Dunn, H. O., and Johnson, R. H. (1972). A 61 XY cell line in a calf with extreme brachygnathia. *J. Dairy Sci.* **55**, 524–526.
Dyrendahl, I., and Gustavsson, I. (1979). Sexual functions, semen characteristics and fertility of bulls carrying the 1/29 chromosome translocation. *Hereditas* **90**, 281–289.
Eldridge, F. E. (1975). High frequency of a Robertsonian translocation in a herd of British White cattle. *Vet. Rec.* **96**, 71–72.
Eldridge, F. E. (1980). X-autosome translocation in cattle. *Eur. Colloq. Cytogenet. Domest. Anim., 4th, Uppsala* pp. 23–30.
Eldridge, F. E., and Blazak, W. F. (1977). Comparison between by the Y chromosome of Chianina and Brahma crossbred steers. *Cytogenet. Cell Genet.* **18**, 57–60.
Eldridge, F. E., Harris, N. B., and Koenig, J. L. F. (1984). Chromosomes of young AI bulls. *Eur. Colloq. Cytogenet. Domest. Anim., 6th, Zurich* pp. 59–67.
Evans, H. J., Buckland, R. A., and Sumner, A. T. (1973). Chromosome homology and heterochromatin in goat, sheep and ox studied by banding techniques. *Chromosoma* **42**, 383–402.

Fechheimer, N. S. (1973). A cytogenetic survey of young bulls in the U.S.A. *Vet. Rec.* **93**, 535–536.
Ford, C. E., (1982). Structural rearrangements and infertility in mammals. *Eur. Colloq. Cytogenet. Domest. Anim., 5th, Milan* pp. 17–41.
Ford, C. E., Pollock, D. L., and Gustavsson, I. (1980). Proceedings of the First International Conference for the Standardization of Banded Karyotype of Domestic Animals, University of Reading, Reading, England, 2–6 August, 1976. *Hereditas* **92**, 145–162.
Forejt, J. (1982). XY involvement in male sterility caused by autosome translocations: A hypothesis. *Serono Clin. Colloq Reprod.* **3**, 135–151.
Frebling, J., Foulley, J. L., Berland, H. M., Popescu, C. P., Cribiu, E. P., and Darre, R. (1987). Resultats de l'enquete sur la frequence de la translocation 1/29 en race bovine Blonde d'Aquitaine. *Bull. Tech. CRZV INRA* No. 67, 49–58.
Fries, R., and Ruddle, F. H. (1986). Gene maping in domestic animals. In "Genetic Engineering of Animals. An Agricultural Perspective" (J. W. Evans and A. Hollaender, eds.), pp. 39–57. Plenum, New York.
Genest, P., and Guay, P. (1979). Structural abnormalities of the X chromosome in a heifer. *Can. J. Comp. Med.* **43**, 110–111.
Gluhovschi, N., Bistriceanu, M., Bilcea, P., and Majina, C. (1972). Klinische histopathologische und zytogenetische Untersuchungen uber die angeborene Ovarienhypoplasie. *Monatsh. Vet. Med.* **27**, 176–179.
Gustavsson, I. (1969). Cytogenetics distribution and phenotypic effects of a translocation in Swedish cattle. *Hereditas* **63**, 68–169.
Gustavsson, I. (1970). Economic importance of a translocation in Swedish cattle. *Eur. Kolloq. Zytogenet. (Chromosomenpathol.) Veterinarmed. Tierzucht Saugetierkd., Giessen* pp. 34–42.
Gustavsson, I. (1979). Distribution and effects of the 1/29 Robertsonian translocation in cattle. *J. Dairy Sci.* **62**, 825–835.
Gustavsson, I. (1980). Banding techniques in chromosome analysis of domestic animals. *Adv. Vet. Sci. Comp. Med.* **24**, 245–290.
Gustavsson, I. (1984). Chromosome evaluation and fertility. *Int. Congr. Anim. Reprod. Artif. Insemin., 10th, Univ. Ill.* **6**, 1–7.
Gustavsson, I., and Hageltorn, M. (1976). Staining technique for definite identification of individual cattle chromosomes in routine analysis. *J. Hered.* **67**, 175–178.
Gustavsson, I., and Rockborn, G. (1964). Chromosome abnormality in three cases of lymphatic leukaemia in cattle. *Nature (London)* **203**, 990.
Gustavsson, I., Franccaro, M., Tiepolo, L., and Lindstcin, J. (1968). Presumptive X-autosome translocation in a cow: Preferential inactivation of the normal X chromosome. *Nature (London)* **218**, 185–184.
Halnan, C. R. E. (1976). A cytogenetic survey of 1101 Australian cattle of 25 differents breeds. *Ann. Genet. Sel. Anim.* **8**, 131–139.
Hanada, H., and Muramatsu, S. (1980). A case of subfertile cow with structural abnormalities of the X chromosome. *Ann. Genet. Sel. Anim.* **12**, 209–213.
Hansen, K. M., and Elleby, F. (1975). Chromosome investigation of danish. A. I. beef bulls. *Nord. Veterinaermed.* **27**, 102–106.
Hare, W. C. D., Mitchell, D., Betteridge, K. J., Eaglesome, M. D., and Randall, G. C. B. (1976). Sexing two-week old bovine embryos by chromosomal analysis prior to surgical transfer: Preliminary methods and results. *Theriogenology* **5**, 243–253.
Hari, J. J., Franceschi, P., Casabianca, F., Boscher, J., and Popescu, C. P. (1984). Etude cytogénétique d'une population de bovins corses. *C. R. Acad. Agric. Fr.* **70**, 191–199.

Harvey, M. J. A., (1971). An autosomal translocation in the Charolais breed of cattle. *Vet. Rec.* **89,** 110–111.
Henderson, L. M., and Bruere, A. N. (1979). Conservation of nucleolus organizer regions during evolution in sheep, goat, cattle and aoudad. *Can. J. Genet. Cytol.* **21,** 1–8.
Herschler, M. S., and Fechheimer, N. S. (1966). Centric fusion of chromosomes in a set of bovine triplets. *Cytogenetics* **5,** 307–312.
Herzog, A., and Hohn, H. (1968). Autosomale Trisomie bei einem kalb mit Brachygnatia inferior und Ascites congenitus. *Den. Tieraerzt. Nochenschr.* **75,** 604–606.
Herzog, A., and Hohn, H. (1984). Two new translocation type trisomies in calves, 60 XX, t(12;12), +12 and 60 XX, t(20;20), +20. *Eur. Colloq. Cytogenet. Domest. Anim., 6th, Zurich* pp. 313–317.
Herzog, A., Hohn, H., and Olyschlager, F. (1982). Autosomal trisomy in calves with dwarfism. *Dtsch. Tieraerztl. Wochenschr.* **89,** 400–403.
Hsu, T. C., and Mead, R. A. (1969). Mechanisms of chromosomal changes in mammalian speciation. *In* "Comparative Mammalian Cytogenetics" (K. Bernischke, ed.), pp. 8–15. Springer-Verlag, Berlin.
Igartua, D. V., Roldan, E. R. S., and Vitullo, A. D. (1985). Cytogenetic studies in beef cattle females with reproductive problems. *Rev. Argent. Prod. Anim.* **5.** (In Span.)
Jost, A. (1947). Recherches sur la différenciation sexuelle de l'embryon de Lapin. III. Role des gonades foetales dans la différenciation sexuelle sematique. *Arch. Anat. Microsc. Morphol. Exp.* **36,** 271–315.
Kieffer, M. N., and Cartwright, T. C. (1968). Sex chromosome polymorphism in domestic cattle. *J. Hered.* **59,** 35–36.
King, W. A., Linares, T., and Gustavsson, I. (1981). Cytogenetics of preimplantation embryos sired by bulls heterozygous for the 1/29 translocation. *Hereditas* **94,** 219–224.
Kovacs, A. (1984). Progress in eradication of the 1/29 translocation of cattle in Hungary. *Eur. Colloq. Cytogenet. Domest. Anim., 6th, Zurich* pp. 52–58.
Leonard, H., Kirszenbaum, M., Cotinot, C., Chesne, P., Heyman, Y., Stinnakre, M. G., Bishop, C., Delouis, C., Vaiman, M., and Fellous, M. (1987). Sexing bovine embryos using Y chromosome specific DNA probe. *Theriogenology* **27,** 248.
Lillie, F. R. (1916). The freemartin: A study of the action of sex hormone in the foetus life of cattle. *J. Exp. Zool.* **23,** 371–452.
Linares, T., King, W. A., Gustavsson, I., and Larsson K. (1981). Testicular feminization and XY gonadal dysgenesis in Suedish Red and White cattle. *Annu. Meet., 73rd, Am. Soc. Anim. Prod., Raleigh, N.C.* p. 160.
Logue, D. N. (1977). Meiosis in the domestic ruminants with particular reference to Robertsonian translocations. *Ann. Genet. Sel. Anim.* **9,** 493–507.
Logue, D. N., and Harvey, M. J. A. (1978). Meiosis and spermatogenesis in bulls heterozygous for a presumptive 1/29 Robertsonian translocation. *J. Reprod. Fertil.* **54,** 159–165.
Long, S. E. (1984). Autosomal trisomy. *Vet. Rec.* **115,** 16–17.
Long, S. E., and David, J. S. E. (1981). Testicular feminisation in an Ayrshire cow. *Vet. Rec.* **109,** 116–118.
Lyon, M. F. (1961). Gene action in the X chromosome of the mouse (*Mus musculus* L.). *Nature (London)* **190,** 372–373.
Marx, W. (1979). Des recherches cytogénétiques de la race Brune de l'Atlas au Maroc en considération spéciale de preuve des translocations 1 et 29. Inaugural Dissertation zur Erlangung des Doktorgrades, Leibig, Univ. zu Giessen.
Masuda, H., Okamoto, A., and Waide, Y. (1975). Autosomal abnormality in a swine. *Jpn. J. Zootech. Sci.* **46,** 671–676. (In Jpn.; Engl. Sum.)

Mayr, B., Krutzler, H., Auer, H., Schleger, W., Sasshofer, K., and Glawischnig, E. (1985). A viable calf with trisomy 22. *Cytogenet. Cell Genet.* **39**, 77–79.

Meyer, E. H. H., Harris, E. J., Maaczynski, I., and Weiermans, S. J. E. (1980). Preliminary results on Y chromosome dimorphism in South African cattle breeds. *Proc. Afr. Genet. Congr., 7th* pp. 2–8.

Miyake, Y. I., Kanagawa, H., and Ishikawa, T. (1984). Further chromosomal and clinical studies on the XY/XYY mosaic bull. *Jpn. J. Vet. Res.* **32**, 9–21.

Moraes, J. C. F., Erdtmann, B., Mattevi, M. S., and Salzano, F. M. (1979). Densitometric analysis of the C-band variability in chromosome 1 of cattle. *Vet. Rec.* **105**, 102–103.

Moraes, J. C. F., Mattevi, M. S., Salzano, F. M., Poli, J. L. E. H., and Erdtmann, B. (1980). A cytogenetic survey of five breeds of cattle from Brazil. *J. Hered.* **71**, 146–148.

Mori, M., Sasaki, M., Makino, S., Ishikawa, T., and Kawata, K. (1979). Autosomal trisomy in a malformed new born calf. *Proc. Jpn. Acad.* **45**, 955–959.

Nel, N. D., Harris, E. J., Weiermans, S. J. E., and Meyer, E. H. H. (1985). A 1/29 chromosome translocation in Southern African Nguni cattle. *Genet. Sel. Evol.* **17**, 293–302.

Nes, N. (1966). Testikulaer feminisering hos storfe. *Nord. Veterinaermed.* **18**, 19–29.

Niebuhr, E. (1972). Dicentric and monocentric Robertsonian translocations in man. *Humangenetik* **16**, 217–226.

Ohno, S., Truillo, J. M., Stenius, C., Christian, C. L., and Teplitz, R. L. (1962). Possible germ cell chimeras among newborn dizygotic twin calves *(Bos taurus)*. *Cytogenetics* **1**, 258–265.

Ohno, S., Christian, C. L., Wachtel, S. S., and Koo, G. C. (1976). Hormone like role of H-Y antigen in bovine freemartin gonad. *Nature (London)* **261**, 597–598.

Pinheiro, L. E. L., Ferrari, I., and Lobo, R. B. (1979). Robertsonian translocation in imported bulls utilized at artificial insemination centers in Brazil. *Rev. Bras. Genet.* **2**, 135–143.

Pinheiro, L. E. L., Moraes, J. C. F., Mattevi, M. S., Erdtmann, B., Salzano, F. M., and Mies Filho, A. (1980). Two types of Y chromosome in a Brazilian cattle breed. *Caryologia* **33**, 25–32.

Pinheiro, L. E. L., Ferrari, I., Ferraz, J. B. S., and Lobo, R. B. (1981). High frequency of Robertsonian translocation in a Brazilian cattle breed. *Rev. Bras. Genet.* **4**, 657–665.

Popescu, C. P. (1968). Observations cytogénétiques chez les bovins Charolais normaux et culards. *Ann. Genet.* **11**, 262–264.

Popescu, C. P. (1969). Idiograms of yak *(Bos, grunniens)*, cattle *(Bos taurus)* and their hybrid. *Ann. Genet. Sel. Anim.* **1**, 207–217.

Popescu, C. P. (1971). Deux cas nouveaux de fusion centrique chez les bovins. (Note). *Ann. Genet. Sel. Anim.* **3**, 521–526.

Popescu, C. P. (1973). L'hétérochromatine constitutive dans le caryotype bovin normal et anormal. *Ann. Genet.* **16**, 183–188.

Popescu, C. P. (1974a). Observations sur une fusion centrique chez les bovins *(Bos taurus* L.). *World Congr. Genet. Appl. Livestock Prod., 1st, Madrid* **3**, 165–168. Editorial Garsi, Madrid.

Popescu, C. P. (1974b). Etude du caryotype bovin par une nouvelle méthode cytogénétique: les bandes C. *World Congr. Genet. Appl. Livestock Prod., 1st, Madrid* **3**, 159–164. Editorial Garsi, Madrid.

Popescu, C. P. (1975a). L'étude du caryotype bovin *(Bos taurus* L.) par les méthodes des bandes. *Ann. Biol. Anim. Biochim. Biophys.* **15**, 751–756.

Popescu, C. P. (1975b). Essai d'identification des chromosomes bovins *(Bos taurus* L.) a l'aide du marquage au 5-bromodeoxiuridine (BUDR). *Eur. Kolloq. Zytogenet. (Chromosomenpathol. Veterinarmed. Tierzucht Saugetierkd., 2nd, Giessen* pp. 59–64.

Popescu, C. P. (1977). Les anomalies chromosomiques des bovins (*Bos taurus* L.): État actuel des connaissances. *Ann. Genet. Sel. Anim.* **9,** 463–470.

Popescu, C. P. (1978). A study of meiotic chromosomes in bulls carrying the 1/29 translocation. *Ann. Biol. Anim. Biochim. Biophys.* **18,** 383–389.

Popescu, C. P. (1980). Cytogenetics study on embryos sired by a bull carrier of 1/29 translocation. *Eur. Colloq. Cytogenet. Domest. Anim., 4th, Uppsala* pp. 182–186.

Popescu, C. P. (1989). "Cytogénétique des mammifères d'élevage." INRA, Paris.

Popescu, C. P., and Cribiu, E. P. (1982). L'étude cytogénétique de l'embryon bovin. *Congr. Int. Transfert Embryons Mammifères, Annecy, Fr.*

Popescu, C. P., Cribiu, E. P., Poivey, J. P., and Seitz, J. L. (1979). Etude cytogénétique d'une population bovine de Cote-d'Ivoire. *Rev. Elev. Med. Vet. Pays Trop.* **32,** 81–84.

Popescu, C. P., Gauthier, D., and Tambasco, A. J. (1987). Etude cytogénétique des bovins créoles élevés en Guadeloupe. *Rev. Elev. Med. Vet. Pays Trop.* **40,** 89–91.

Popescu, C. P., Cotinot, C., Boscher, J., and Kirszenbaum, M. (1988). Chromosomal localization of a bovine male specific probe. *Ann. Genet.* **31,** 39–42.

Queinnec, G., Darre, R., Berland, H. M., and Raynaud, J. C. (1974). Etude de la translocation 1/29 dans la population bovine du sud-ouest de la France: Conséquences zootechniques. *World Congr. Genet. Appl. Livestock Prod., 1st, Madrid* **3,** 131–151. Editorial Garsi, Madrid.

Rao, A. V. N. (1982). Causes and incidence of reproductive disorders among zebu × taurus crossbred cows in Andhra Pradesh. *Theriogenology* **17,** 189–191.

Refsdal, A. O. (1976). Low fertility in daughters of bulls with 1/29 translocation. *Acta Vet. Scand.* **17,** 190–195.

Rendel, J. M. (1980). Low calving rates in Brahman cross cattle. *Theor. Appl. Genet.* **58,** 207–210.

Rieck, G. W. (1971). Die testikulare Feminisierung beim Rind als Sterilitatsursache von Farsen. *Zuchthygiene* **6,** 145–154.

Rieck, G. W. (1984). XXY syndrome in domestic animals: Homologues to Klinefelter's syndrome in man. *In* "Klinefelter's Syndrome" (Bandmann and Breit, eds.). Springer-Verlag, Berlin.

Rieck, G. W., Hohn, H., and Herzog, A. (1968). Familial occurrence of centromerre chromosome fusion in cattle. *Zuchthygiene* **3,** 117–182. (In Ger.; Engl. sum.)

Rugiati, S., and Fedrigo, M. (1967). Alteratione cromosomica riscontrata in un toro acondroplasico di razza Romagnola. *Ateneo Parmense, Acta Bio-Med.* **38,** 3–7.

Sharma, A. K., and Popescu, C. P. (1986). The meiotic chromosomes of Creole from Guadeloupe. *Rev. Elev. Med. Vet. Pays Trop.* **38,** 353–357.

Sharma, A. K., Vijaykvmar, N. K., Khar, S. K., Verma, S. K., and Nugam, J. M. (1980). XY gonadal dysgenesis in a heifer *Vet. Rec.* **107,** 328–330.

Stafford, M. J. (1972). The fertility of bulls born co-twin to heifers. *Vet. Rec.* **90,** 146–148.

Taylor, K. M., Hungerford, D. A., and Snyder, R. L. (1967). The chromosomes of four artiodactyl and one perissodactyl. *Mamm. Chromosome Newsl.* **8,** 233–235.

Tschudi, P. (1984). 12 Years of cytogenetic investigation in AI bulls in Switzerland. *Eur. Colloq. Cytogenet. Domest. Anim., 6th, Zurich* pp. 40–42.

Tschudi, P., Ueltschi, G., Martig, J., and Kupfer, U. (1975). Autosomal trisomy as the cause of a defect of the interventricular septum in a Simmental calf. *Schweiz. Arch. Tierheilkd.* **117,** 335–340.

Vigier, B., Locatelli, A., Prepin, J., du Mesnil du Buisson, F., and Jost, A. (1976). Les premières manifestations du "freemartinisme" chez le foetus de veau ne dépendant pas du chimérisme chromosomique XX/XY. *C. R. Hebd. Seances Acad. Sci., Ser. D* **282,** 1355–1358.

Wachtel, S. S., Koo, G. C., Breg, W. R., Ellias, S., Boyse, E. A., and Miller, O. J. (1975). Expression of the H-Y antigen in human males with two Y chromosomes. *N. Engl. J. Med.* **293,** 1070–1073.

Wachtel, S. S., Hall, J. L., Muller, V., and Chaganti, R. S. K. (1980). Serum borne H-Y antigen in the foetal bovine freemartin. *Cell* **21,** 917–929.

Wintenberger-Torres, S., and Popescu, C. P. (1980). Transfer of cow blastocysts after sexing. *Theriogenology* **14,** 309–318.

Zartman, D. L., and Fechheimer, N. S. (1967). Somatic aneuploidy and polyploidy in inbred and line cross cattle. *J. Anim. Sci.* **26,** 678–682.

Chromosomes of the Pig

INGEMAR GUSTAVSSON

Department of Animal Breeding and Genetics, Swedish University of Agricultural Sciences, Uppsala, Sweden

    I. Introduction
   II. Evolutionary Aspects on the Pig Karyotype
  III. The Normal Mitotic and Meiotic Chromosomes
      A. Mitosis
      B. Meiosis
  IV. Polymorphism
      A. Heterochromatin
      B. Nucleolar Organizer Regions (NORs)
   V. Spontaneous Chromosome Aberrations and Their Phenotypic Effects
      A. Numerical Aberrations
      B. Structural Aberrations
      C. Undefined Aberrations
  VI. Intersexuality and Chimerism
 VII. Chromosomes of the General Population
VIII. Use of the Pig and Pig Chromosomes for Experimental Purposes
      A. Induction *in Vivo* of Chromosome Aberrations
      B. Cell Lines Established and Their Use in Different Experiments
  IX. Future Cytogenetic Research Work in the Pig
      References

I. Introduction

The domestic pig (*Sus scrofa*) is one of the most well-studied domestic animals from the point of view of cytogenetics. In spite of this, there are, as in all other domestic animals, cytogenetic aspects that still are almost untouched. The relatively large interest in domestic pig chromosomes is not only due to the importance of the pig as a domestic animal, but also due to the fact that the pig chromosomes are very attractive for use in detailed studies, owing to their small number and large size, which make them individually easily identifiable.

The domestic pig was one of the first domestic animals to be studied cytogenetically, but there were many analyses before the correct chromosome number was definitely established. The first report on *S. scrofa* chromosomes described a diploid chromosome number of 20 in females and 18 in males, due to an XX/O sex determination mechanism (Wodsedalek, 1913). In 1931, however, Krallinger (1931) described the correct number as 38, but later there were numerous works reporting deviating chromosome numbers, such as 40 (e.g., Makino, 1944; Spalding and Berry, 1956). For many years, there were disagreements about the correct chromosome number and the question was not solved definitely until modern techniques, e.g., treatment of cells with colchicine and hypotonic solutions (Gimenez-Martin *et al.*, 1962), and the use of tissue culture (Stone, 1963; McConnell *et al.*, 1963) were introduced. Later, with the introduction of banding techniques (see Gustavsson, 1980) and the establishment of an international standard for the detailed description of chromosomes [Committee for the Standardized Karyotype of the Domestic Pig (Committee), 1988], a more sophisticated background for further development became available.

Most work in pig cytogenetics has, of course, been devoted to clinical cytogenetics. By the 1950s, the pig was used for studies concerning the role of spontaneous chromosome aberrations in early embryonic mortality. Hermaphroditism has also long been of scientific and lay interest, but previously the most remarkable findings were cases of the reciprocal chromosome translocations often found in association with the production of decreased litter size. Pig chromosomes have also been used for experimental purposes, and lately the pig has also become a popular animal in gene mapping studies (see Fries *et al.*, this volume).

Cytogenetics of the domestic pig has been summarized in textbooks (Hare and Singh, 1979; Rieck, 1984; Eldridge, 1985; Popescu, 1989) as well as in articles (e.g., Gustavsson, 1973; Fechheimer, 1981). This article is an attempt to give a comprehensive description using the latest information, at least from the author's laboratory, concerning pig chromosomes. Throughout this article, only the international standard (Committee, 1988) for chromosome designation and arrangement will be used. As far as possible, old chromosome designations have been adapted to the accepted system.

II. Evolutionary Aspects on the Pig Karyotype

The family Suidae includes five living genera: *Babyrousa, Sus, Phacochoerus, Potamochoerus,* and *Hylochoerus*. The domestic pig is considered to originate from the wild form of *S. scrofa*. However, although the chromosome number is 38 in all breeds of the domestic pig previously studied, there are two polymorphic systems of the centric fusion type in the wild pig. One of them, due to a centric fusion of chromosomes 16 and 17, occurs in Asian wild pigs (Tikhonov and Troshina, 1975). The other one, due to a centric fusion of chromosomes 15 and 17, has been described in several countries, for example, the United States, the Federal Republic of Germany, Austria, Sweden, the USSR, the Netherlands, and France (McFee *et al.*, 1966a; Gropp *et al.*, 1969; Rittmannsperger, 1971; Gustavsson *et al.*, 1973; Tikhonov and Troshina, 1975; Bosma, 1976; Popescu *et al.*, 1980; respectively).

The original findings of the 15/17 polymorphic system (McFee *et al.*, 1966a; Rary *et al.*, 1968; McFee and Banner, 1969) encouraged belief that there had been crossings between wild and domestic pigs. Following scrutiny of investigations of wild pigs carried out in different parts of the world, as well as of the evolutionary information available, Bosma (1983) drew the conclusion that there is a polymorphic system in the wild pig. An apparent shift was found in chromosome number from 38 in the east (Muramoto *et al.*, 1965; Okamoto *et al.*, 1980), particularly in Japanese wild pigs (*Sus vittatus leucomystax* Temminck, a subspecies of *S. scrofa*), to 36 in the countries mentioned above. Investigation of the pigmy hog *Sus (Porsula) salvanius,* another member of the same genus, also supported the view of polymorphism, because the latter species had a karyotype very similar to and with the same chromosome number as the domestic pig (Bosma, 1983).

Other Suidae of the genera *Babyrousa, Phacochoerus, Potamochoerus,* and *Hylochoerus* demonstrate karyotypes deviating markedly from the domestic pig karyotype. *Babyrousa babyrussa* has a chromosome number of 38 but nevertheless has the most deviant karyotype (Bosma and de Haan, 1981). Some chromosome pairs have no direct equivalents in domestic or wild pigs. The wart hog (*Phacochoerus aethiopus*) has a chromosome number of 34 (Bosma, 1978; Melander and Hansen-Melander, 1980), the giant forest hog (*Hylochoerus meinertzhageni*) has a chromosome number of 32, and the bush pig (*Potamochoerus porcus*) has a chromosome number of 34 (Melander and Hansen-Melander, 1980).

The occurrence of two polymorphic systems, both including chromosome 17, indicates that there has been a centric fusion and not a centric fission process in the evolution of the domestic pig. It is also possible to draw the conclusion that centric fusion translocations, in general, have played an important role in the karyotype evolution of the family Suidae.

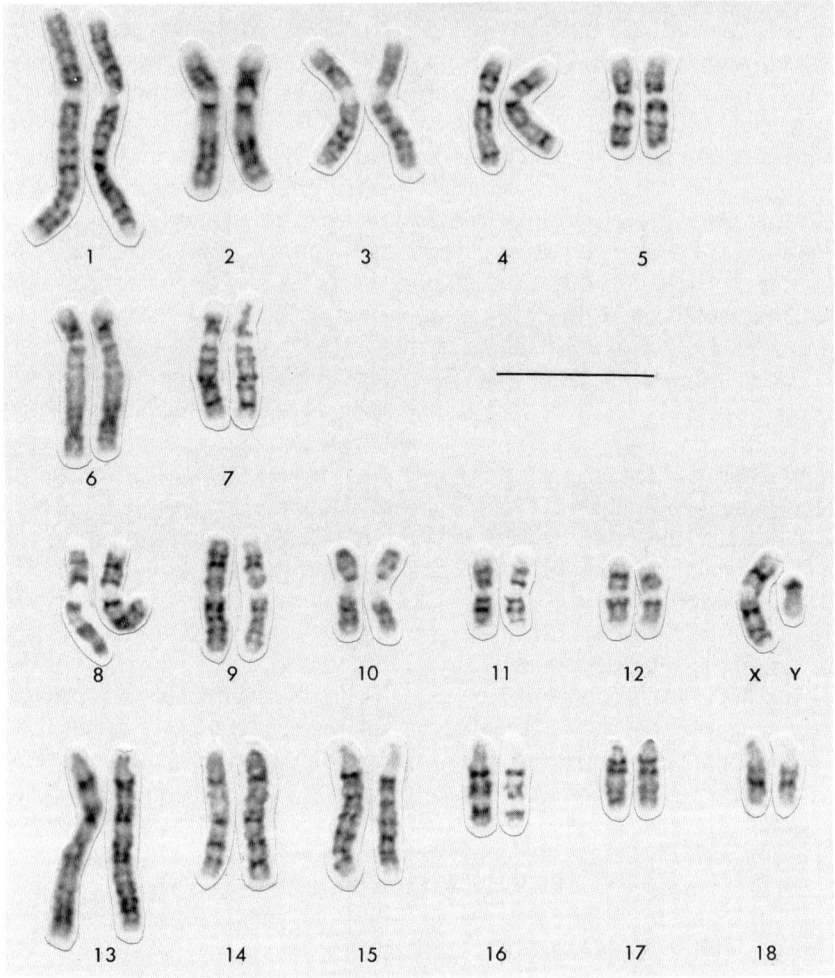

FIG. 1. GTG-banded karyotype of a normal boar. The chromosomes have been arranged according to the international standard. Bar indicates 10 μm. (Committee, 1988; courtesy of *Hereditas*.)

III. The Normal Mitotic and Meiotic Chromosomes

A. MITOSIS

The pig karyotype (Figs. 1 and 2) consists of 38 chromosomes—36 autosomes and 2 sex chromosomes. There are 13 biarmed and 6 uni-

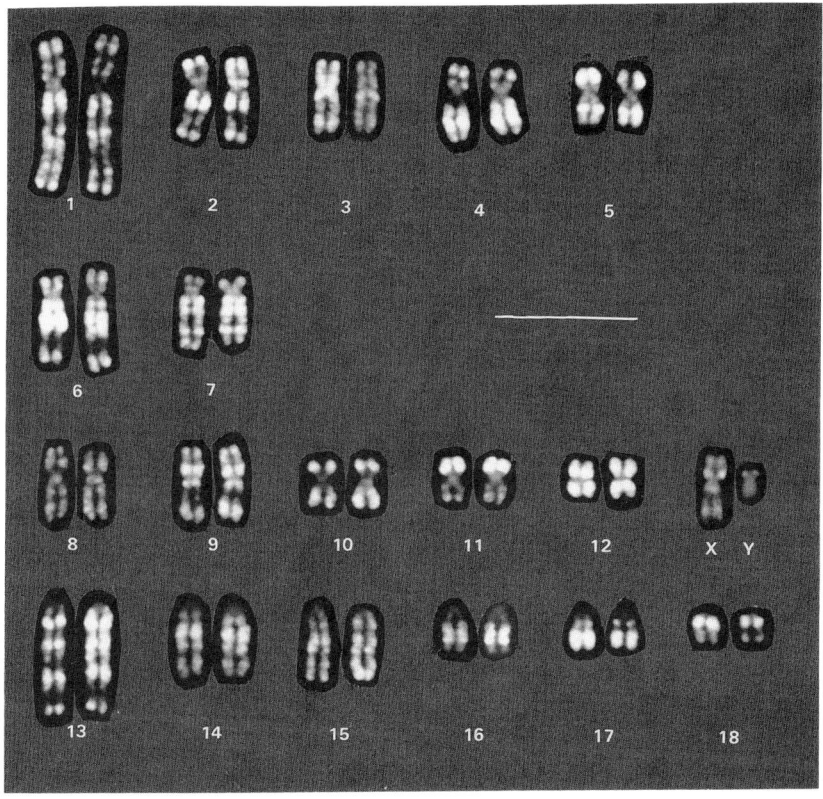

Fig. 2. RBA-banded boar karyotype. Bar indicates 10 μm.

armed pairs; of these, the X is a medium-sized biarmed chromosome and the Y is a very small biarmed chromosome. Specific banding patterns can be obtained by previously described techniques (Gustavsson, 1980), or by counterstaining techniques (Van de Sande et al., 1977; Sahar and Latt, 1978; Schweizer, 1981). By Q- (Caspersson et al., 1970), G- (Seabright, 1971), and R-banding (Dutrillaux et al., 1973) techniques, each individual chromosome pair can be identified. The pig chromosomes were first identified by Q-banding (Gustavsson et al., 1972; Hansen, 1972) and G-banding (Berger, 1972). These bandings (Fig. 1) give almost identical patterns and are almost the reverse of the banding patterns obtained by R-banding (Fig. 2) (Hansen, 1977).

In early studies, there were problems in distinguishing between chromosome 9 and the X chromosome (Hansen, 1972, 1977), but these problems now appear to be solved (Fries, 1980; Hansen 1980a,b). The most heat sensitive R-bands can be removed, and then so-called T-bands are obtained (Dutrillaux, 1973). In the pig, these occur specifically in the centromere regions of biarmed chromosomes and in some interstitial positions (Gustavsson, 1984a). International standards (Ford et al., 1980; Committee, 1988) are currently available for the description of normal pig chromosomes (Fig. 3), as well as for chromosome aberrations. Measurements of pig chromosomes have been carried out (Lin et al., 1980; Hansen, 1980b) and high-resolution studies of banded chromosomes are also available (Rönne et al., 1987).

The centromeric heterochromatin of the chromosomes, often demonstrating extensive polymorphism (see below), are Q-, G-, and R-band negative but stain positively (Hansen, 1982) with the C-banding technique (Sumner, 1972). The centromeric heterochromatin appears to be of different types. The guanine- and cytosine-rich heterochromatin, which is positively stained with chromomycin A_3, is located in the centromere regions of the biarmed chromosomes. However, heterochromatin that is less enriched with guanine and cytosine, and which is positively stained with distamycin A plus 4′,6-diamidino-2-phenylindole (DA–DAPI), is located in the centromere regions of the uniarmed chromosomes (Jorgensen et al., 1978; Schnedl et al., 1981; Mayr et al., 1984). It has been argued that the less guanine- and cytosine-rich or moderately adenine- and thymidine-rich centromere regions of the uniarmed chromosomes represent the original centromere regions of a primitive acrocentric karyotype (Mayr et al., 1984). Utilization of the guanine- and cytosine-specific fluorochrome, chromomycin A_3, and the adenine- and thymidine-specific fluorochrome, DAPI, in combination with C-banding, could reveal four major groups of heterochromatin (Lin et al., 1982). Adenine- and thymidine-rich (C-positive) heterochromatin was located in the centromeric regions of the uniarmed chromosomes, guanine- and cytosine-rich (C-positive) heterochromatin was located in the centromeric region of the biarmed chromosomes (although C-positive, this heterochromatin did not bind the base-pair-specific fluorochromes used), and a C-positive and a C-negative heterochromatin were found in the long arm and in the centromeric region, respectively, of the Y chromosome. The heterochromatin of the Y chromosome lacked available binding sites for either adenine-thymidine- or guanine-cytosine-specific fluorochromes.

There are nucleolar organizer regions identifiable by silver staining techniques (e.g., Bloom and Goodpasture, 1976) in chromosomes 8 and 10 (Lin et al., 1980), which often show polymorphism (see below).

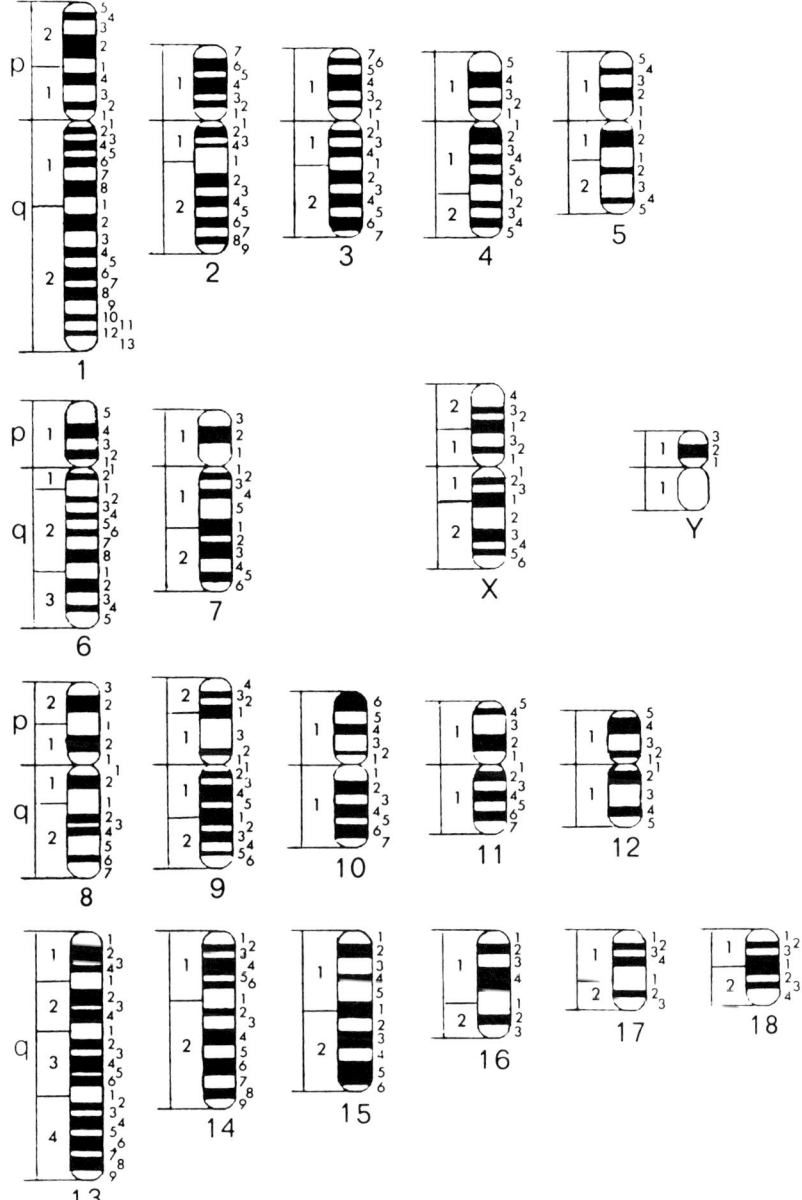

FIG. 3. Diagrammatic representation of the GTG-banded karyotype. The landmark system and the band designations follow the international agreements. (Committee, 1988; courtesy of *Hereditas*.)

B. Meiosis

In laboratory studies, many problems had long been encountered in obtaining good, conventional meiotic spreads from the domestic pig (I. Gustavsson, unpublished observations). The introduction of a technique by King (1981), adapted from Pathak (see Pathak et al., 1976), however, solved these problems. As was expected, there are 19 ring- and chain-shaped bivalents in normal male and female pigs, and in the male the XY bivalent constitutes a characteristic rod. By application of banding techniques it is possible to identify single bivalents as well as to study chiasma localization in different rearrangement configurations (I. Gustavsson, unpublished observations).

Synaptonemal complex analysis (Counce and Meyer, 1973) has also been applied to male pig chromosomes (e.g., Schwarzacher et al., 1984). During zygotene of the prophase I stage of meiosis, homologous chromosomes start pairing. The pairing is complete in the pachytene stage. The paired chromosomes form two strongly stained axes with a more weakly stained central element. The chromosome ends have strongly stained attachment plaques and the kinetochores form densely stained structures after phosphotungstic acid staining. The uniarmed bivalents form one or two chromocenters at their kinetochore ends. Chromosomes 8 and 10 form two pairs of nucleoli. With knowledge of size, arm index, and nucleolar organizing regions, it is possible to identify each individual chromosome pair. Recombination nodules, which represent the recombination sites, also can to some extent be identified (D. F. Villagomez, personal communication).

IV. Polymorphism

Chromosomal polymorphisms involving the amount of heterochromatin, particularly in the centromeric regions, and variability in the activity of the nucleolar organizer regions have been observed.

A. Heterochromatin

Hansen-Melander and Melander (1974) described polymorphism for the centromeric heterochromatin of chromosome pairs 1 and 14. By application of dual techniques, C-band polymorphism could be observed in chromosome pairs 2, 11, 14, and 17 (Hansen, 1982). Pairs 15 and 16 also have shown polymorphism (Christensen and Smedegård, 1978, 1979; Glahn-Luft et al., 1982). Sysa (1980) identified polymorphism in chromosome pairs 1, 8, 12, 13, 15, 16, and 18. In particular, uniarmed chromosomes showed polymorphism (Świtoński et al., 1983), with pairs 16, 17, and 18 showing most clearly. There appears to be a distinct Mendelian inheritance of the latter pairs. Thus, most pairs have demonstrated C-band polymorphism in their centromeric regions. Further, interstitial C-bands, which appear to be polymorphic, have also been observed in chromosome 16 (Glahn-Luft et al., 1982).

B. Nucleolar Organizer Regions (NORs)

There is a polymorphism for the NORs (ribosomal RNA genes) of the domestic pig (Czaker and Mayr, 1980; Lin et al., 1980; Mayr and Schleger, 1981). Both homologues of chromosome 10 are most often stained in conjunction with one chromosome 8. There are, however, cases in which only one chromosome 10 is stained and, even more rare, in which both chromosome 8 homologues are stained.

V. Spontaneous Chromosome Aberrations and Their Phenotypic Effects

A. Numerical Aberrations

1. Euploid Heteroploidy (Polyploidy)

Early studies on pig chromosomes revealed that triploidy in particular may be due to polyspermy or polygyny, both depending on mating time after ovulation. Delayed mating was shown to increase the frequency of polyandric fertilization and recovery of pronucleate ova from sows killed at 0, 24, 30, and 48 hours after mating (Hancock, 1959). Of the eggs recovered, 20 demonstrated more than 2 pronuclei; 19 of these originated from sows mated 30 to 48 hours after the onset of heat. It was proposed that polyspermy was largely responsible for these abnormalities. Another investigation (Bomsel-Helmreich, 1961) showed that at day 17 of gestation, 26% of the sows, which had been impregnated more than 44 hours after the onset of heat, had heteroploid, triploid, or mosaic embryos, with a frequency of 4.1%. It was concluded that fertilization must take place within 60 hours after the onset of heat, to avoid cytogenetically abnormal embryos. When fertilization was delayed (coitus more than 36 hours after the beginning of estrus), polygyny increased to 22% and polyspermy to 11% (Thibault, 1959). Hunter (1967) demonstrated an increase of 14.1% of the mean percentage of polyspermic eggs as the ova increased in age from 4 to 16 hours at the time of sperm penetration.

McFeely (1966, 1967) demonstrated the chromosomes XXXX and XXXY in three tetraploid zygotes (3.4% of all blastocysts) recovered from normal, healthy pigs. These zygotes probably arose because of suppression of the first cleavage division. In 88 10-day-old blastocysts that were recovered from seven gilts, 10% demonstrated chromosome defects. Additionally, 2.3% of the blastocysts were degenerated. All abnormal karyotypes were tetraploid, triploid, or mixed diploid/triploid, with the exception of a uniarmed deletion (see below). The triploids had sex chromosomes XXX, XXY, and XYY, respectively. The former two chromosomal types might have occurred from polyspermy or polygyny, but XYY can only have occurred through polyspermic fertilization. Moon et al. (1975) also found a high incidence of polyploids, particularly mixoploids. However, in another study of 169 10-day-old blastocysts (Dolch and Chrisman, 1981), only diploid cells were observed.

Cytogenetic investigations in early embryos of pigs have pointed to the fact that chromosome abnormalities might account for as much as one-third of the early embryonic mortality in normal pigs. Total embryonic mortality has been estimated to be about 33% of all embryos (Hanly, 1961). However, these early figures of chromosome abnormalities now have to be carefully reconsidered regarding more current information that the trophoblast cells of the normal embryo are polyploid (Long and Williams, 1982). All polyploid cells can not be attributed to trophoblast cells, but in the latter investigation, the incidence of triploidy was only 2.9%.

2. Aneuploid Heteroploidy

a. Sex Chromosomes. There are rare cases in which numerical variations in the sex chromosomes have been described. In 1968, Nes (1968) described the presumptive occurrence of 37,XO in four pigs. Three piglets, which were comparatively small at birth, developed into small, anestrous female pigs with infantile genitalia and small inactive gonads. The remaining piglet had ovaries, a uterus, and a rudimentary penis, and demonstrated atresia ani. Histologically, the ovary of the half-day-old piglet corresponded to the ovaries seen in females at day 90 of gestation. Clinically, the pigs described by Nes could be confused with pigs having rachitis. A similar case was later described by Lojda (1975).

Apparently coincidental cases (see below) of 39,XXY and 39,XXY/ 40,XXXY were found in studies of intersexuality (Breeuwsma, 1970)

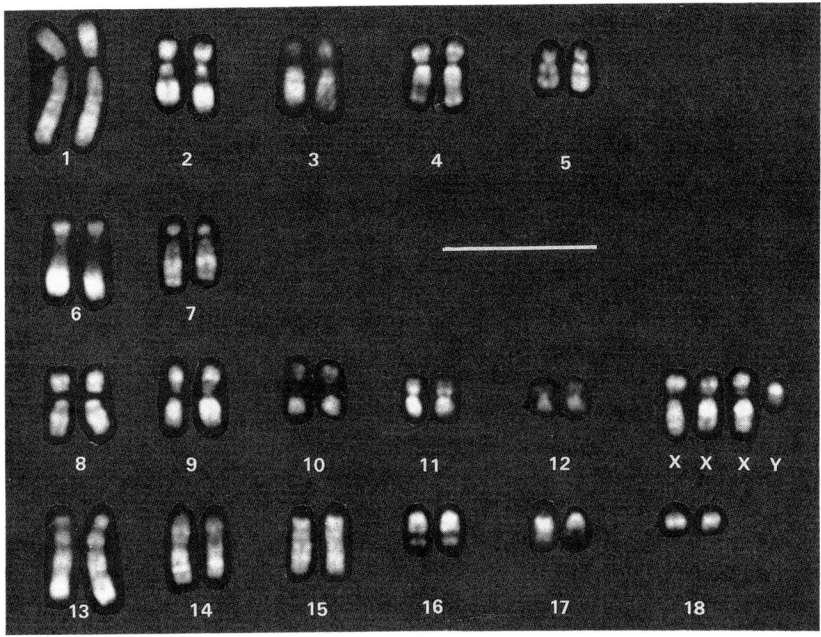

FIG. 4. Sex chromosome tetrasomy (40,XXXY) in a boar. The chromosomes have been stained with the QFQ-banding technique. Bar indicates 10 μm.

and lymphosarcoma (Harvey, 1968), respectively. In another case of XXY (Hancock and Daker, 1981), testicular hypoplasia was found. There was a total absence of spermatogenic tissue and the tubules were lined by Sertoli cells. Fortuitously, a case of 40,XXXY (Fig. 4) was found in an offspring group of a translocation carrier (Gustavsson, 1984b).

b. Autosomes. No pure cases of numerical variations of the normal autosomes have been found in liveborn pigs. The fact that they occur has, however, been proved in studies of early embryos (Smith and Marlowe, 1971). In 1 out of 76 embryos recovered from nine normal gilts, on day 25 following coitus, monosomy for pair 11 was observed. In another case, a presumptive double trisomy involving chromosomes 17 and 18 was found in one of the four embryos recovered (Ruzicska, 1968). Liveborn cases with mixoploid conditions for extra chromosomes and chromosome fragments have also been described. Thus, Vogt *et al.* (1974) described two full sibs, with 50% reduced litter size, to have the presumptive constitutions 37,XY, − 18/38,XY/39,XY + 18 and 37,XY, − 18/38,XY, respectively. These sibs also produced daughters with abnormal karyotypes (see below). Coincidentally, a pregnant true hermaphrodite was found to be a 38,XX/39,XX, + 14 mosaic, with an abnormal cell line occurring in 29% of the cells investigated (Bösch et al., 1985). Rare cases of tertiary monosomy and trisomy have also been observed (see below). The available evidence, however, points to the fact that cases with pure autosomal trisomies and monosomies do not survive beyond embryo stage.

B. Structural Aberrations

1. Translocations

a. Reciprocal Translocations. Reciprocal translocations (Fig. 5) seem to be common in the domestic pig. Approximately 45 different translocations have been described in the literature, and of these, 24 have been found by the present author in a recent survey of boars with reproductive problems (Gustavsson, 1990). The Swedish survey has demonstrated that at least 50% of all boars in Sweden, which were removed from the breeding population because they were producing decreased litter size, are carrying reciprocal translocations. In other European countries there also appear to be high incidences of reciprocal translocations in boars producing decreased litter size. Several translocations have been found in France (Popescu and Legault, 1979; Popescu et al., 1983, 1984, 1988; Popescu and Boscher, 1986) and Finland (Mäkinen and Remes, 1986; Kuokkanen and Mäkinen, 1987, 1988; Mäkinen et al., 1987), and a single case each was reported in Belgium (Bouters et al., 1974), Yugoslavia (Ločniškar et al., 1976), Britain (Madan et al., 1978), the Federal Republic of Germany (Förster et al., 1981), the Germany Democratic Republic (Golisch et al., 1982a), and Italy (Tarocco et al., 1987).

The overwhelming majority of translocations described have been new mutations—only a few were inherited. They have most often been easy to detect due to unequal exchange of chromosome material. There appears to be a nonrandom distribution of participating chromosomes; chromosomes 1 and 14 are often involved and most breaks have occurred in segments close to the centromere and/or the telomere. A nonrandom distribution according to type of band is evident; most breaks have occurred in R-positive bands. There appear to be "hot spots" in the pig karyotype, with some chromosome segments more prone to breakage than others. In fact, breaks in the same chromosome band have been observed in several different translocations.

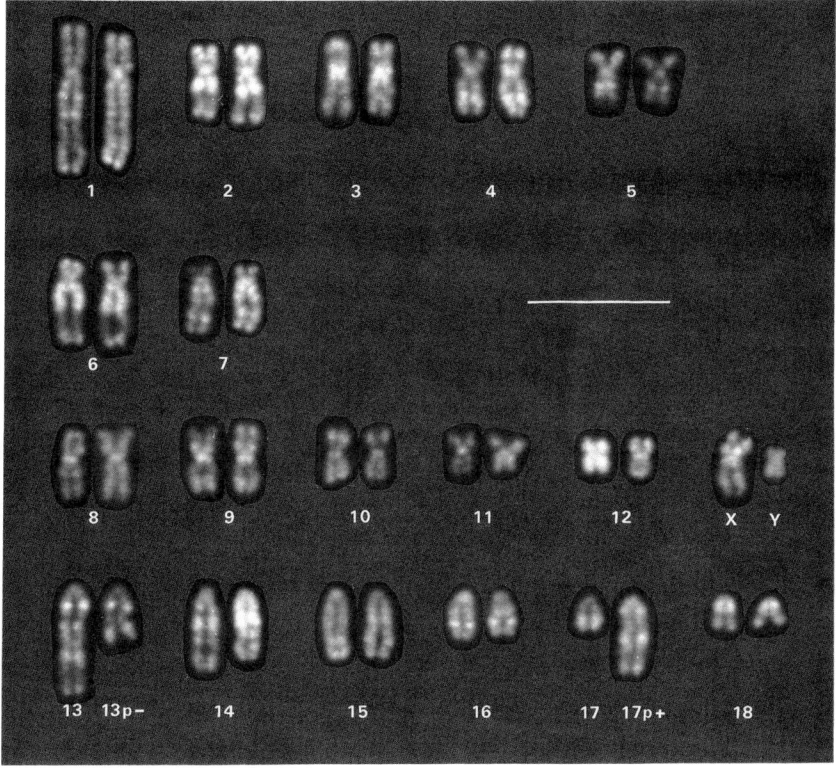

FIG. 5. An rcp(13q−;17q+) of a boar producing decreased litter size. In six litters the boar produced 4.4 piglets on an average. Bar indicates 10 μm.

The mechanisms causing reduced litter size in translocation carriers are similar for all reciprocal translocations and in both sexes, although the meiotic behavior of the chromosomes (Fig. 6) and their ultimate effects may vary. At the pachytene stage of the first meiotic prophase, there is pairing of homologous chromosome segments and a crosslike configuration (quadrivalent) is formed (Gustavsson et al., 1988; Gabriel-Robez et al., 1988). The prophase stages can be studied in great detail with electron microscopy (Fig. 7). At metaphase I, the quadrivalent can be of different morphology, depending on the size of translocated segments, size and centromere position of the chromosomes involved, and the chiasmata formed. For each translocation, a variety of balanced and unbalanced types of segregational products is formed

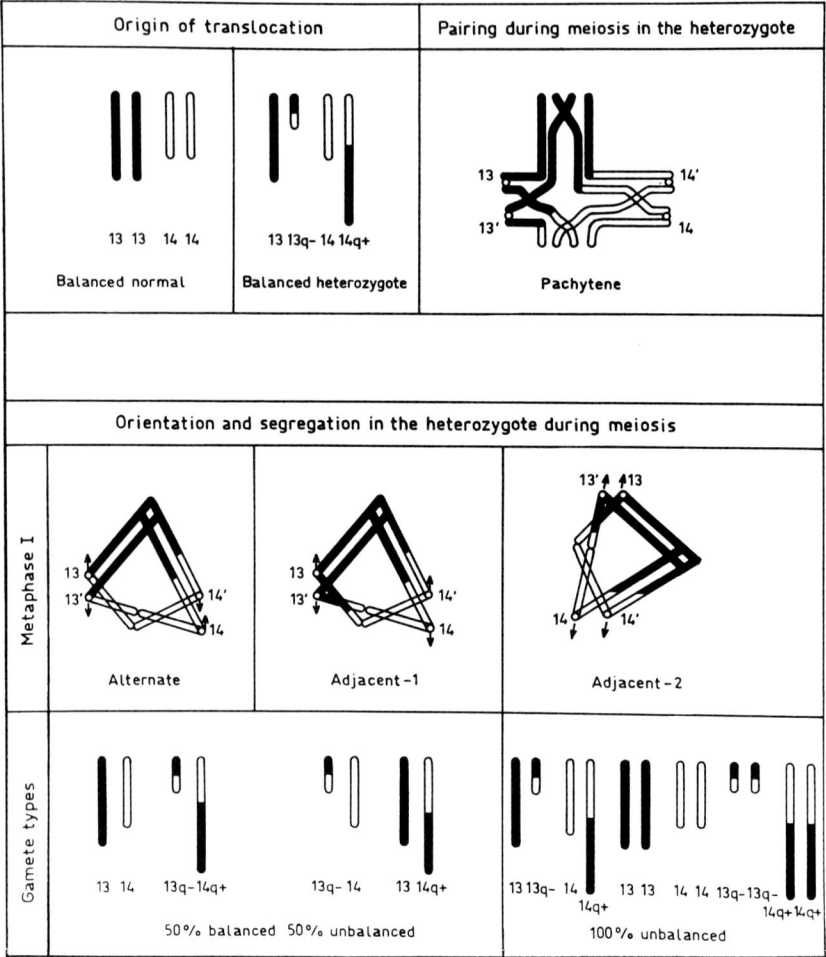

FIG. 6. Schematic drawing of an rcp(13q−;14q+) and its behavior in meiosis. For details, see text. (Courtesy of Dr. W. A. King; King, 1980.) The translocation has earlier been described in detail in somatic cells (Hageltorn et al., 1976), in meiosis (King, 1981), and in zygotes (King et al., 1981).

(Ford and Clegg, 1969). There are three types (Fig. 6) of 2:2 disjunctions: alternative, adjacent-1, and adjacent-2 (McClintock, 1945). The alternative type produces balanced products—normal and balanced heterozygous haploid karyotypes. In the adjacent-1 and adjacent-2 types, nonhomologous and homologous centromeres disjoin to the op-

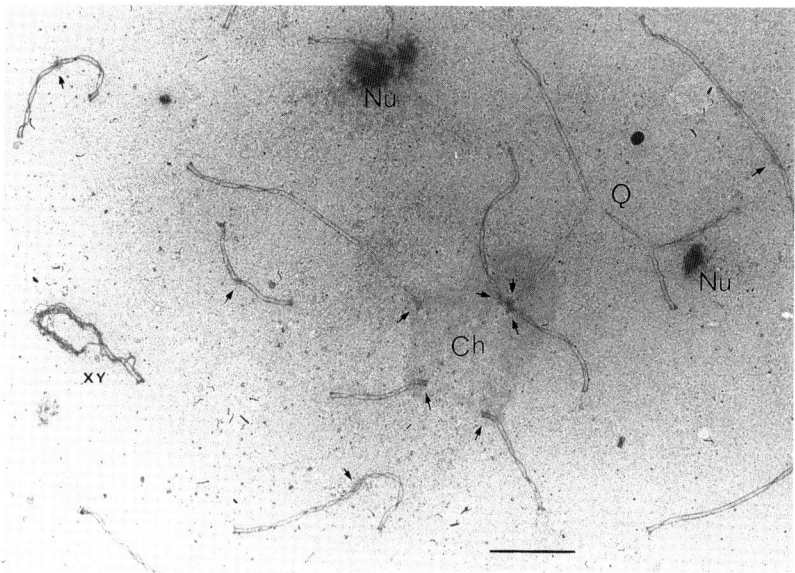

FIG. 7. Partial synaptonemal complex analysis of the pachytene stage in a spermatocyte of a boar with an rcp(8q+;14q−) The chromosomes are completely paired, including heterologous pairing in the quadrivalent (Q). The sex bivalent (XY) is easy to identify and the telocentric bivalents and chromosomes 14 and 14q− of the quadrivalent are associated by their kinetochore ends to a chromocenter (Ch). The nucleoli (Nu) organized by the chromosome bivalent 10 and chromosomes 8 and 8q+ of the quadrivalent are strongly stained. The kinetochores form densely stained structures (arrows). Bar indicates 4 μm.

posite and the same poles, respectively, and give chromosomally unbalanced products. Chiasma formation in the interstitial segments (segments between the centromere and breakage/rejoining points) gives exclusively alternative and adjacent-1 disjunction (50% of each type). If there is regular chiasma formation between the translocated at their homologous nontranslocated (terminal) segments, a ring-shaped quadrivalent forms, which will result in an orientation giving preferential alternative and adjacent-1 disjunction. With a 2:2 disjunction (see Fig. 4), the number of segregation products will consequently be 10, of which 8 are chromosomally unbalanced. The relative frequency of the different products will vary according to the nature of the translocation. Other disjunctions (3:1 and 4:0) can also occur, especially when the translocation concerns segments highly asymmetrical in size, sometimes with an absence of chiasmata, resulting in the formation of a chain quadrivalent or a trivalent and a univalent. With 3 : 1 or 4 : 0 segregations, the number of segregation products will increase to 36 or even 64, respectively. Adjacent-2 disjunctions, which produce exclusively unbalanced gametes, together with numerical nondisjunctions, account for the more than 50% increase in unbalanced gametes. As mentioned above, chromosomally balanced gametes are also formed, which means that a translocation is inherited from a carrier in approximately 50% of its offspring.

Although serious malformations were described in a stillborn piglet that was mosaic for a presumptive balanced rcp(1q − ;11q +) translocation (Hansen-Melander and Melander, 1970), it is considered that autosomal translocation carriers have a normal body conformation. Most often, the semen is also normal but the litter size is still reduced from 25 (Ločniškar et al., 1976) to 100% (Bouters et al., 1974). As a general rule, there appears to be an early, most often before embryo implantation, elimination of chromosomally unbalanced translocation zygotes. In 1972, reduced litter size of an rcp(11q + ;15q −) [later described as a rcp(-11p + ;15q −) by Hageltorn et al., (1976)] was demonstrated to be due to elimination of chromosomally unbalanced zygotes (Åkesson and Henricson, 1972). The litter size reduction was about 30% and five different types of unbalanced karyotypes could be found as late as 80 days after breeding (normal time of pregnancy is 114 days). There also appeared to be a differential mortality, depending on the unbalanced karyotype. The most comprehensive investigation in early embryonic mortality of translocation carriers (King et al., 1981) demonstrated that chromosomally unbalanced zygotes carrying an rcp(13q − ;14q +) were eliminated before or at implantation. Of the expected gamete types at a 2 : 2 segregation, 9 out of 10 could be identified. Similarly, 11 embryos (41% of all recovered) at the 9- to 10-day stage of crossings, in which one of the parents was a carrier of an rcp(4q + ;14q −), demonstrated an unbalanced karyotype (Popescu and Boscher, 1982). Six different unbalanced karyotypes could be distinguished. The early elimination of unbalanced karyotypes could also be seen (Gustavsson et al., 1983) in a t(9p- +;11q −). At implantation, a few apparently degenerating zygotes could be observed to be monosomic for the larger part of chromosome arm 11q.

It is also expected that reciprocal translocations in males sometimes cause degenerative changes in the testicles, thereby reducing gametic production (Chandley et al., 1972). Degenerations were seen in some testicular tubules of a carrier with an rcp (2p + ;4q −). Of the cells investigated with electron microscopy, 50% demonstrated associations between the translocation quadrivalent and the sex bivalent (Gustavsson et al., 1990). Nevertheless, the semen picture was normal. An abnormal semen picture was, however, seen in a boar with an rcp(2p+;14q−). There were degenerations in the testicles and electron microscopy demonstrated extensively unpaired and heterologously paired chromosome segments (Villagomez et al., in preparation). These deviations appeared to be induced by some inflammatory processes. Degenerative changes and complete meiotic arrest were observed (Gustavsson et al., 1989b) in a family with an rcp(Xq+;13q−). The translocation, which was inherited from a female carrier, caused complete sterility with testicular hypoplasia in the male carrier offsprings.

b. *Centric Fusion Translocations.* Centric fusion translocations between chromosomes 13 and 17 have been described in pigs with normal phenotypes (Alonso and Cantu, 1982). The same translocation was also found in an intersex piglet (Masuda et al., 1975) and in a malformed female piglet and three phenotypically normal littermates (Miyake et al., 1977). It was concluded, however, that an association between the malformations and the balanced centric fusion translocation was unlikely. The fact that the 13/17 translocations give up to 10% reduced litter size was, however, proved by Golisch et al. (1986) for a similar translocation described in the German Democratic Republic (Schwerin et al., 1986). Also, a recently found 13/17 translocation female carrier demonstrated reduced litter size (McFeeley et al., 1988).

2. *Duplications and Deletions*

No clear-cut examples of duplications and deletions in normal chromosomes have been described in liveborn animals. However, in 10-day-old embryos of normal parents, a whole-arm deletion of a medium-sized biarmed chromosome was observed (McFeely, 1966). Translocations or inversions may result in formation of gametes with duplications and deletions. After fertilization, however, most of these zygotes die at an early stage (see above). Recently, however, one boar with an rcp(7q+;17q−) translocation was found to produce gametes that, after fertilization, yielded offspring with tertiary trisomy and monosomy (Fig. 8). According to the farmer, the monosomic piglets have specific malformations and die early. The trisomic piglets appear to have a fairly normal appearance and can survive. Careful investigations of these cases are under way (Gustavsson et al., in preparation).

C. UNDEFINED ABERRATIONS

Unspecific numerical and structural aberrations appear to arise spontaneously, with a rate that is variable, depending on the popula-

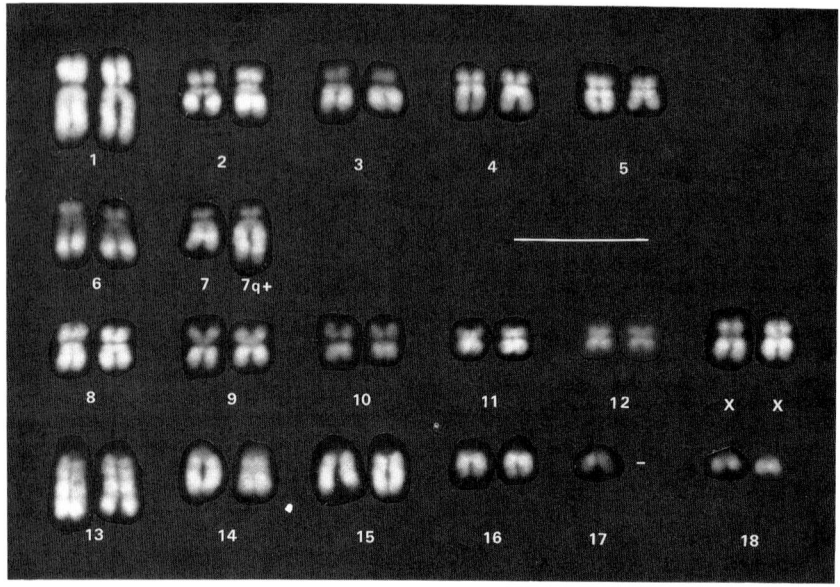

FIG. 8. Tertiary monosomy in an offspring of an rcp(7q+;17q−) boar. The liveborn female piglet lacking the derivative 17 was malformed and died soon after birth. Bar indicates 10 μm.

tion, the phenotypic performance, etc. (Michelmann et al., 1977; Hanada et al., 1979; Golisch et al., 1982a). Two female offspring of the mixoploid full male siblings described above (Vogt et al., 1974) also produced decreased litter size and showed an extra undefined centric fragment having the chromosome constitutions 39,XX, + cen and 38,XX/39,XX, + cen, respectively. Also, a boar with a normal body conformation produced litters with a high mortality rate, including stillborn and congenitally abnormal offspring, and was reported to have 24% cells containing undefined structural chromosomal abnormalities (Oprescu et al., 1976). One offspring of the latter boar, with severe phenotypical disturbances, demonstrated cells with an extra chromosome fragment.

VI. Intersexuality and Chimerism

The pig hermaphrodite shows a variable phenotype ranging from almost female to almost male, but the most typical hermaphrodite phenotypic pattern is characterized by organ structures derived both from Wolffian and Müllerian ducts (Maik and Jáskowski, 1968). Often, epididymis, ductus deferens, seminal vesicles, penis, vagina, and uterus are found. Presence of a well-developed uterus has been considered the ultimate characteristic of the "classical" pig hermaphrodite, distinguishing them from cattle freemartins (see below).

Often a separate ovary and testis or the two combined into an ovotestis are also found and the individual is then classified as a true hermaphrodite (e.g., Basrur and Kanagawa, 1971). In the unilateral type of true hermaphroditism, the left gonad is constantly an ovary. Rarely, however, true intersexual pigs become pregnant (Bösch et al., 1985). In the testis or the testicular part of the ovotestis, there is a hypoplasia of the seminiferous tubules with no spermatogonia and thus no spermatogenesis. Sertoli as well as Leydig cells are present. The ovotestis usually has ovarian tissue in the cortex and testicular tissue in the medulla (Maik and Jáskowski, 1968). Folliculogenesis suggests apparently normal ovarian activity (Basrur and Kanagawa, 1971), but usually no ovulation is observed in the ovaries or in the ovarian portion of the gonads. Instead, the follicles become atretic or cystic.

Male pseudohermaphroditism is the next common type of pig hermaphroditism, characterized by testes but with reproductive organs having some of the characteristics of the opposite sex (e.g., Makino et al., 1962). Some extreme cases of male pseudohermaphrodites have been described with an overall male picture but having a well-formed uterus with body and horns (e.g., Gerneke, 1964). In such cases it was found that the testes were easily palpable and sometimes of nearly normal size, the vas deferens opened into the cornu of the uterus, and the penis was rudimentary, with the urethral orifice located dorsally. The seminiferous tubules were atrophic, with very few germ cells and no evidence of spermatogenesis. There was a hyperplasia of the interstitial cells. Histology of the epididymis showed a rather normal structure of the epididymal tubules. Such a case, but with the pig lacking internal female sex organs, was proposed to be a sterile male with XX sex chromosomes (Hard and Eisen, 1965). Single cases of female pseudohermaphrodites have also been described (e.g., Maik and Jáskowski, 1968).

A great majority of hermaphrodite pigs have been determined to be chromosomally female (e.g., Makino et al., 1962; Gerneke, 1967; Melander et al., 1971; Miyake, 1973), and only in a few cases has the male karyotype been observed. No apparent correlation has been observed between the phenotypic appearance and the chromosomal sex. There are indications that swine hermaphroditism has a genetic background

(Hulot, 1970; Lojda, 1975), but in the work by Breeuwsma (1970) the adrenal glands and crowding of the embryos were suggested to have important effects on the diffusion of hormones, thus resulting in masculinization of gonads. Some research workers have also indicated that deletions in the X or Y chromosome, or translocation of the Y chromosome to an autosome (e.g., Hard and Eisen, 1965), may cause hermaphroditism.

Some hereditary cases of testicular hermaphroditism are reminiscent of testicular feminization in humans (Lojda, 1968). Testicular feminization was definitely established in a pig with a female phenotype and a male karyotype (Wensing et al., 1975).

Cases of XX/XY chimerism (McFee et al., 1966b; Bruère et al., 1968; Vogt, 1968; Breeuwsma, 1970; Somlev, et al., 1970; Toyama, 1974) apparently are most often due to intrauterine placental fusion; vascular anastomoses between female and male pigs, have been described. It is interesting to note that females selected according to inguinal hernia invariably demonstrate XX/XY chimerism in blood, but XX sex chromosome constitution in other cells (Bosma et al., 1975). Phenotypically, these animals have a normal female appearance, e.g., clitoris and vulva are of normal size and conformation (Colenbrander and Wensing, 1975). Preputial development is the only sign of masculinization. However, the genital apparatus is abnormal and similar to that seen in cattle freemartins. There is a malelike vaginal process and a well-developed cremaster muscle, an absence of ovarian tissue and sometimes the presence of hypoplastic testes without germ cells, severe hypoplasia or total aplasia of the Müllerian and Wolffian ducts, and an absence of male accessory glands other than the underdeveloped vesicular glands. A similar case, but also showing chimerism for a balanced reciprocal translocation, was described by King et al. (1980).

Cases of whole-body XX/XY (Basrur and Kanagawa, 1971) and XX/XXY (Toyama, 1974) chimerism have been seen. Intersexuality in a case with an XXY chromosome constitution (see below) has also been described (Breeuwsma, 1968). The fact that XX/XY chimerism in the female does not necessarily give intersexuality was shown by Christensen and Bräuner Nielsen (1980).

VII. Chromosomes of the General Population

Almost nothing is known about the distribution of chromosomal polymorphisms in different breeds and populations. At present, there is also little information on chromosome aberrations in the general pig population. Michelmann et al. (1977), in the Federal Republic of Germany, investigated 156 breeding and slaughter pigs by using banding techniques, but found no constant aberrations. In a similar study in the German Democratic Republic, Golish et al. (1982b) found one translocation carrier among 273 boars investigated. This gives an overall incidence of 0.23% translocations in the general pig populations studied. The mouse is the only polytoccous animal in which there is some information available about the incidence of spontaneously occurring aberrations. In 3,531 mice tested, 3 (0.09%) were semisterile, presumably due to reciprocal translocations (Ford, 1970). In humans, there is an incidence of 0.10% balanced reciprocal translocations found in newborns (van Dyke et al., 1983). These initial comparative figures indicate a relatively high incidence of translocations in the general pig population.

There are, however, indications from coincidental findings that aberrations may be fairly common in the pig population. Such cases include a 37,XX,cf(13;17) (Masuda et al., 1975), an rcp(6p+;14q−)(Madan et al., 1978), a 38,XX/39,XX,+14 mosaic (Bösch et al., 1985), and two cases of a 39,XXY (Breeuwsma, 1970) found when studying the chromosomes in relation to hermaphroditism. The incidence of XXY chromosomes in newborn human males is approximately 1 in 1,000 (Hook and Hamerton, 1977) and 1 in 5,000 in mice (Ford, 1970). Another case involved a male pig with an XXY/XXXY sex chromosome constitution; the pig was investigated because of a suspected lymphosarcoma (Harvey, 1968). To this group of unexpected findings should be added the cases of an rcp(1p−;8q+) and 40,XXXY found in two offspring groups of the boars included in the Swedish survey conducted by Gustavsson (1990). The rcp(1p−;8q+) occurred in the same family that had the rcp(9p+;11q−). In humans, the occurrence of two translocations in the same family is not common and has only occasionally been described (e.g., Bijlsma et al., 1978). There are no reliable figures for the incidence of XXXY in other species, but there are subjective estimations of 1 in 25,000–30,000 human newborns (Taylor and Moores, 1976).

VIII. Use of the Pig and Pig Chromosomes for Experimental Purposes

A. INDUCTION *in vivo* OF CHROMOSOME ABERRATIONS

The incidence of chromosome aberrations in tissue-cultured blood cells can be increased by treating pigs with various agents, for example, live vaccine against swine fever (Lojda and Rubes, 1977) and aflatoxin B_1 (Petříčková et al., 1976; Lojda and Petříčková, 1977). Halothane, commonly used for investigating stress susceptibility in the pig, is another potent mutagen. There is a common belief, however, that the doses applied do not induce mutations (Förster and von Butler, 1983). The pig does not appear to have an increased sensitivity to mutations of the chromosomes in peripheral blood lymphocytes when compared with several other mammals studied by the sister chromatid exchange (SCE) test (A. F. McFee personal communication). There also appears to be a fairly low sensitivity to γ irradiation of the testes (Erickson and Martin, 1984). However, chromosome abberrations can be induced fairly easily by treating semen with X irradiation, before insemination; this sensitivity has been proposed to be ascribable to an aerobic metabolism of the boar spermatozoa (Nevo et al., 1970). This approach has been utilized in two experiments to induce chromosome aberrations in the pig.

Zartman et al. (1969) exposed fresh semen to 600 R of X irradiation before inseminating sows. Of the 31 offspring studied, 4 (12.8%) had consistent aberrations; three were translocations and one was a pericentric inversion. The mosaic condition of breakage–deletion of the same chromosome was seen in three of the pigs studied. Two of these deletions were inherited. There were also delayed effects of the X irradiation, such as aneuploidy, fragments, chromatid breaks, and chromosome gaps. It was found that the X irradiation had a threshold effect, which probably was due to the fact that with too much accumulated chromosome damage, the cells could not retain their viability. The delayed effects, in the form of aneuploidy and breaks, could be studied in cells of stillborn piglets (Zartman et al., 1971). There was no consistent aberration and the aneuploidy appeared to be randomly distributed in the karyotype. In contrast, the breaks were nonrandomly distributed and occurred particularly often in chromosomes 1 and 16.

In a similar experiment, Fries and Stranzinger (1982) found eight translocations, two pericentric inversions, and one paracentric inversion in 8 (26.7%) of the 30 phenotypically normal pigs derived from semen irradiated at 800 R. In this experiment, no chromosomal mutations were observed at an irradiation dose of 600 R. By application of different banding techniques, it was possible to study the details of the chromosome aberrations. It was observed that five of the translocations had no visible reciprocal exchange, which in fact might indicate breaks and unions at the telomeric regions. Minor deletions could, however, not be ruled out. Carriers of the aberrations demonstrated reduced fertility in mating experiments. In summary, it was concluded that chromosomes 1 and 15 appear to be frequently involved in rearrangements.

B. Cell Lines Established and Their Use in Different Experiments

Several cell lines derived from pigs have been used in different experiments and have been described in the literature. The most famous is the pig kidney cell line, PK-2a, established in 1955 by Dr. E. Stice of Cutter Laboratories, Berkeley, California; PK-2a has given rise to three clone lines, PK(13), PK(14), and PK(15) (Ruddle, 1961). PK-2a, growing in an epitheloid fashion, had a diploid chromosome number of 38 with a karyotype similar to that of the normal pig, although a large component of the cell population has a hypotetraploid number (Ruddle, 1961). The PK(13) (PK 1-1) clone was heteroploid, and probably originated from the heteroploid component of the PK-2a line. A diploid component also occurred, however. Whether this was due to chromosome loss from the heteroploid type or due to contamination from an outside source could not be determined (Ruddle, 1961). The PK(14) (PK 1-2) clone initially demonstrated a modal chromosome number of 38. Later, the modal value increased to 78 due to an increase in cells of high ploidy. When compared with the normal pig karyotype, distinct morphological deviations were observed. A third clone, PK(15) (PK 1-3), demonstrated a karyotype similar to that of PK-2a but with a modal number of 39 (Ruddle, 1961). A cell line of PK(15) is currently commercially available [American Type Culture Collection (ATCC) cell repository number CCL 33].

From the PK(15) cell line, two lines, R344 and R338, resistant to 2,6-diaminopurine and 8-azaguanine, respectively, were established (Harris and Ruddle, 1960). The chromosome range for R388 was 36–38, with a mode at 38. The nine clones established showed the following patterns: six were of low ploidy (mode 35–38) and three were of high ploidy. Three of the clones demonstrated uniform deviations from the parental line, with characteristic marker chromosomes. Although fairly unstable, the R344 line appeared hypodiploid, with modal values of 32 and 35. The low numbers were apparently due to loss of chromosomes. The clones derived from R 344 were unstable at the low ploidy level and shifted upward into the heteroploid region. The experiment could not provide evidence that chromosomal changes are necessary for the development of drug resistance.

With the use of X irradiation, several clones, having well-defined marker chromosomes present in all cells, were established from the PK(14) (PK 1-2) clone line (Ruddle, 1961). The marker chromosomes were large, telocentric, subtelocentric, and metacentric chromosomes, probably originating from reciprocal translocations and tandem and centric fusions. In at least one clone, a minute chromosome was found. The chromosomes behaved very stably for more than a year, even as isolated drug-resistant variants (see below). This probably reflected the importance of certain gene blocks for the clones. The clones were typically epithelioid in appearance, but in one case round cell variants appeared and became the dominant cell type. Several isolated subclones of epithelioid and round cell type showed a very long, peculiar telocentric chromosome, which excluded the possibility of cellular contamination by human cell lines as an explanation for the chromosomal pattern. Similar to the PK(15) clone, the PK(14) clone was used to establish drug-resistant lines (Harris and Ruddle, 1961). From X-irradiated PK(14), two drug-resistant variants, C23 and C26, were isolated as clonal derivatives. Two clonal sublines, R206 and R208, were isolated with aminopterin and 2,6-diaminopurine from variants C23 and C26, respectively. By comparison with the PK(15) cells, they showed higher resistance to the drug concerned. The isolated R206 contained a long acrocentric marker. The modal number of R206 was, however, 34, due to the loss of small chromosomes. Subline R208 exhibited a modal chromosome number of 33, evidently also due to the loss of small chromosomes. One long acrocentric and one very minute chromosome were found in the R208 subline. It was concluded that the loss of chromosomes might be related to the acquisition of resistance by deletion of gene material that is responsible for incorporation of the metabolic antagonists into sensitive cells.

The commercial ATCC PK(15) cell line mentioned herein was compared with another cell line, the NADL, also originating from the PK(15) clone (Pirtle, 1966). Both lines were mixoploid, showing subdiploid to tetraploid chromosome counts with the modal chromosome numbers 37 and 38 in the ATCC and the NADL lines, respectively. Most cells were clustered in the range 36–38. One outstanding large metacentric marker chromosome was common for both lines. By banding techniques (Echard, 1974), it was demonstrated that the large metacentric chromosome in the NADL cell line is due to a fusion of chromosomes 14 and 15. Another biarmed chromosome is due to a fusion of chromosomes 16 and 18. There is also some marker chromosomes of unknown origin. Although having almost the same modal chromosome number, the NADL and ATCC cell lines can be distinguished from each other by different marker chromosomes and different nutritional requirements (Pirtle and Woods, 1967). Some experiments with the NADL and ATCC PK(15) cell lines that were infected with the Ames strain of virulent hog cholera (HC) virus gave results difficult to interpret cytogenetically. The NADL cell line was studied before and after infection with the HC virus (Pirtle, 1966). The noninfected cell line showed, before infection, a modal chromosome number of 38, with an extra large metacentric marker chromosome. There were also some additional chromosomes and some chromosomes missing, when compared to the normal pig karyotype. After infection, the culture demonstrated a lower number (37) than did the noninfected cells. As no chromatid breaks, telomeric associations, and quadriradial arrangements were observed, the decreased modal number indicated the occurrence of centric fusion translocation and might reflect an adaptation by the cells to establish a host–virus relationship, resulting in the preservation of essential chromatin material. In another experiment, anti-HC viral serum was added to the culture medium of the chromosomes of the ATCC cell line, which was persistently infected with the HC virus (Pirtle and Woods, 1968). Shortly after the initial infection, the line underwent a burst of endoreduplication. Other cell populations remained fairly stable when compared to normal cell propagated in parallel, but a relatively high incidence of chromosomal pulverization was evident. At the end of the 16 passages propagated in the medium containing the anti-HC viral serum, the infected line as well as the noninfected line demonstrated approximately 98% of the cells at a near-tetraploid level. Endoreduplication occurred rarely and the incidence of chromosomal pulverization decreased. The final eight passages were cultured without the addition of anti-HC viral serum. Then, the high incidence of endoreduplication remained, but the endoreduplication phenomenon disappeared. There was also a marked increase in the incidence of chromosomal pulverization. The selective advantage of higher ploidy values was considered to be definitely substantiated in this experiment.

There are also other established cell lines, such as PTF (Genest and Bouillant, 1985) and ENS 122 (de Noronha, 1963), but these have been used to a lesser extent in different experiments.

IX. Future Cytogenetic Research Work in the Pig

Techniques are available today that can increase our knowledge of the domestic pig and its chromosomes. High-resolution banding techniques make possible detailed studies of chromosome polymorphisms and aberrations. Molecular cytogenetics is another technique to be utilized for further detailed studies. We still know very little about the chromosomes in the general population. Polymorphisms can provide information on genetic relationships and can be used to trace lineages, estimate the degree of inbreeding, and verify parentage of individual animals. There is an increasing body of information about pigs with reproductive disturbances, for example, decreased litter size, and about their possible association with chromosomal aberrations. However, for other disturbances, such as repeat breeding, we still know almost nothing about the chromosomal relationship and the impact of events occurring at the meiotic level. Increased knowledge of these things will be important for veterinary diagnostics in the future and thus are of economic importance in pig breeding. It is suspected that there is an increased chromosomal mutation rate in the pig population. If this is correct—and proof will require population studies—it is urgent that we identify possible mutagens and their effects, in the pig environment, and rule them out.

Although normal karyotypes have been demonstrated in malformations such as atresia ani (Vogt, 1967; Bosma and Neetson, 1977), cyclops (Arakaki and Vogt, 1976), aplasia of the vulva (Hansen-Melander and Melander, 1972), polymelia meningocele, double muscle and cryptorchidism (Oprescu *et al.*, 1972), it would be worthwhile to investigate malformed and stillborn animals with new banding techniques, including high-resolution techniques.

There is an increasing interest in mapping the genes of the domestic pig (see Fries *et al.*, this volume). The somatic cell hybridization technique has been used and until now some genes have also been mapped with *in situ* hybridization techniques. Spontaneous as well as induced aberrations provide excellent material for detailed mapping. The use of flow cytometry for sorting out interesting normal or rearranged chromosomes can speed up the analysis. Thus, the derivative $14q^+$ of the $rcp(13q^-;14q^+)$ mentioned previously could be sorted as easily as the normal chromosome 13 (Matsson *et al.*, 1986). It is now possibile to compare the physical maps with available genetic maps based on gene recombination rates. In this regard it would be interesting and important to know more about chiasma frequencies and locations. This can be done using conventional studies of diplotene chromosomes as well as electron microscope studies of recombination nodules in pachytene chromosomes.

As probably has become clear in the present article, the domestic pig has a karyotype that is easy to work with from the analytical point of view and thus represents a very attractive animal for research work, serving also as a good model for other species. It is hoped that new young scientists, particularly cytogeneticists working with molecular geneticists, can further reveal this interesting karyotype.

ACKNOWLEDGMENTS

The author wants to express gratitude to Dr. B. P. Chowdhary for correcting the English; Dr. W. A. King, Department of Biomedical Science, Ontario Veterinary College of Guelph, Guelph, Ontario, Canada for supplying Fig. 6; and Ms. Gudrun Mellberg-Wieslander for excellent typing. The work was financed by the Swedish Council of Agricultural Research.

REFERENCES

Åkesson, A., and Henricson, B. (1972). Embryonic death in pigs caused by unbalanced karyotype. *Acta Vet. Scand.* **13,** 151–160.

Alonso, R. A., and Cantu, J. M. (1982). A Robertsonian translocation in the domestic pig *(Sus scrofa).* 37, XX—13–17, t.rob. (13;17). *Ann. Genet.* **25,** 50–52.

Arakaki, D. J., and Vogt, D. W. (1976). A porcine cyclops with normal female karyotype. *Am. J. Vet. Res.* **37,** 95–96.

Basrur, P. K., and Kanagawa, H. (1971). Sex anomalies in pigs. *J. Reprod. Fertil.* **26,** 369–372.

Berger, R. (1972). Étude du caryotype du porc avec une nouvelle technique. *Exp. Cell Res.* **75,** 298–300.

Bijlsma, J. B., de France, H. F., Bleeker-Wagemakers, L. M., and Dijkstra, P. F. (1978). Double translocation t(7;12), t(2;6) heterozygosity in one family. A contribution to the trisomy 12p syndrome. *Hum. Genet.* **40,** 135–147.

Bloom, S. E., and Goodpasture, C. (1976). An improved technique for selective silver staining of nucleolar organizer regions in human chromosomes. *Hum. Genet.* **34,** 199–206.

Bösch, B., Höhn, H., and Rieck, G. W. (1985). Hermaphroditismus verus bei einem gravidem Mutterschwein mit einem 39,XX,14+ − Mosaik. *Zuchthygiene* **20,** 161–168.

Bomsel-Helmreich, O. (1961). Hétéroploidie expérimentale chez la truie. *Proc. Int. Congr. Anim. Reprod., 4th, The Hague* **3,** 578–581.

Bosma, A. A. (1976). Chromosomal polymorphism and G-banding patterns in the wild boar *(Sus scrofa* L.) from the Netherlands. *Genetica* **46,** 391–399.

Bosma, A. A. (1978). The chromosomal G-banding pattern in the wart hog, *Phacochoerus aethiopicus* (Suidae, Mammalia) and its implications for the systematic position of the species. *Genetics* **49,** 15–19.

Bosma, A. A. (1983). The karyotype, including G- and C-banding patterns, of the pigmy hog *Sus (Porcula) salvanius* (Suidae, Mammalia). *Genetica* **61,** 99–106.

Bosma, A. A., and de Haan, N. A. (1981). The karyotype of *Babyrousa babyrussa* (Suidae, Mammalia). *Acta Zool. Pathol. Antverp.* No. 76, 17–27.

Bosma, A. A., and Neetson, F. A. (1977). G-banding patterns in chromosomes of pigs with atresia ani. *Genen Phaenen* **19,** 41–44.

Bosma, A. A., Colenbrander, B., and Wensing, C. J. G. (1975). Studies of phenotypically female pigs with hernia inguinalis and ovarian aplasia. II. Cytogenetical aspects. *Proc. K. Ned. Akad. Wet., Ser. C* **78,** 43–46.

Bouters, R., Bonte, P., Spincemaille, J., and Vandeplassche, M. (1974). Het chromosomenonderzoek bij de huisdieren II. De afwijkingen in de geslachtschromosomen alsoorzakelijke of begeleidnede factor van onvruchtbaarheid. *Vlaams Diergeneeskd. Tijdschr.* **43**, 85–91.

Breeuwsma, A. J. (1968). A case of XXY chromosome constitution in an intersex pig. *J. Reprod. Fertil.* **16**, 119–120.

Breeuwsma, A. J. (1970). Studies on intersexuality in pigs. Ph.D. Thesis, Res. Inst. Anim. Husb. "Schoonord," Ziest, Netherlands.

Bruère, A. N., Fielden, E. D., and Hutchings, H. (1968). XX/XY mosaicism in lymphocyte cultures from a pig with freemartin characteristics. *N.Z. Vet. J.* **16**, 31–38.

Caspersson, T., Zech, L., Johansson, C., and Modest, E. J. (1970). Identification of human chromosomes by DNA-binding fluorescent agents. *Chromosoma* **30**, 215–227.

Chandley, A., Christie, S., Fletcher, J., Frackiewicz, A., and Jacobs, P. A. (1972). Translocation heterozygosity and associated subfertility in man. *Cytogenetics* **11**, 516–533.

Christensen, K., and Bräuner Nielsen, P. B. (1980). A case of blood chimerism (XX, XY) in pigs. *Anim. Blood Groups Biochem. Genet.* **11**, 55–57.

Christensen, K., and Smedegård, K. (1978). Chromosome marker in domestic pigs. C-band polymorphism. *Hereditas* **88**, 269–272.

Christensen, K., and Smedegård, K. (1979). Chromosome markers in domestic pigs. A new C-band polymorphism. *Hereditas* **90**, 303–304.

Colenbrander, B., and Wensing, C. J. G. (1975). Studies on phenotypically female pigs with hernia inguinalis and ovarian aplasia. I. Morphological aspects. *Proc. K. Ned. Akad. Wet., Ser. C* **78**, 33–42.

Committee for the Standardized Karyotype of the Domestic Pig. (1988). Standard karyotype of the domestic pig. *Hereditas* **109**, 151–157.

Counce, S. J., and Meyer, G. F. (1973). Differentiation of the synaptonemal complex and the kinetochore in *Locusta* spermatocytes studies by whole mount electron microscopy. *Chromosoma* **44**, 231–253.

Czaker, R., and Mayr, B. (1980). Detection of nucleolar organizer regions in the chromosomes of the domestic pig (*Sus scrofa domestica* L.). *Experientia* **36**, 1356–1357.

de Noronha, F. (1963). Chromosomenuntersuchungen an einem latent mit Teschen-Virus infizierten Zellstamm aus Schweinenieren. *Zentralbl. Bakteriol., Abt. 1, Orig.* **190**, 7–25.

Dolch, K. M., and Chrisman, C. L. (1981). Cytogenetic analysis of preimplantation blastocysts from prepuberal gilts treated with gonadotropins. *Am. J. Vet. Res.* **42**, 344–346.

Dutrillaux, B. (1973). Nouveau système de marquage chromosomique: Les bandes T. *Chromosoma* **41**, 395–402.

Dutrillaux, B., Laurent, C., Couturier, J., and Lejeune, J. (1973). Coloration des chromosomes humains par l'acridine orange après traitement par le 5-bromodeoxyuridine. *C. R. Hebd. Seances Acad. Sci., Ser. D* **276**, 3179–3181.

Dyke, D. L. van, Weiss, L., Robertson, J. R., and Babu, V. R. (1983). The frequency and mutation rate of balanced autosomal rearrangements in man estimated from prenatal genetic studies for advanced maternal age. *Am. J. Hum. Genet.* **35**, 301–308.

Echard, G. (1974). Chromosomal banding patterns and karyotype evolution in three pig kidney cell strains (PK 15, F and RP). *Chromosoma* **45**, 133–149.

Eldridge, F. E. (1985). "Cytogenetics of Livestock." AVI, Westport, Connecticut.

Erickson, B. H., and Martin, P. G. (1984). Stem-spermatogonial at survival and incidence of reciprocal translocations in the γ-irradiated boar. *Environ. Mutagen.* **6**, 219–227.

Fechheimer, N. S. (1981). Cytogenetics in pig production. *Commonw. Agric. Bur.* **2,** 387–391.
Förster, M., and von Butler, I. (1983). Lymphozytenteilungsaktivität in Abhängigkeit von der *in vivo* Halothanreakiton. *Zuechtungskunde* **55,** 100–105.
Förster, M., Willeke, H., and Richter, L. (1981). Eine autosomale, reziproke 1/16 Translokation bei Deutschen Landrasse Schweinen. *Zuchthygiene* **16,** 54–57.
Ford, C. E. (1970). The population cytogenetics of other mammalian species. *In* "Human Population Cytogenetics," Vol. 5, pp. 222–239. Pfizer Med. Monogr., Edinburgh.
Ford, C. E., and Clegg, H. M. (1969). Reciprocal translocation. *Br. Med. Bull.* **25,** 110–114.
Ford, C. E., Pollock, D. L., and Gustavsson, I. (eds.). (1980) Proceedings of the First International Conference for the Standardization of Banded Karyotype of Domestic Animals, University of Reading, Reading, England, 2–6 August, 1976. *Hereditas* **92,** 145–162.
Fries, R. (1980). A contribution to the identification of the X-chromosome in swine. *Proc. Eur. Colloq. Cytogenet. Domest. Anim., 4th* pp. 354–358.
Fries, R., and Stranzinger, G. (1982). Chromosomal mutations in pigs derived from X-irradiated semen. *Cytogenet. Cell Genet.* **34,** 55–56.
Gabriel-Robez, O., Jaafar, H., Ratomponirina, C., Boscher, J., Bonneau, J., Popescu, C. P., and Rumpler, Y. (1988). Heterosynapsis in a heterozygous fertile boar carrier of a 3;7 translocation. *Chromosoma* **97,** 26–32.
Genest, P., and Bouillant, A. M. P. (1985). Chromosomes et cancérogenèse. Étude de l'évolution d'une lignée cellulaire épithéliale d'origine porcine (PFT). *Ann. Genet.* **28,** 25–31.
Gerneke, W. H. (1964). The karyotype of a gonadal male pig intersex. *S. Afr. J. Sci.* **60,** 347–352.
Gerneke, W. H. (1967). Cytogenetic investigations on normal and malformed animals, with special reference to intersexes. *Onderstep. J. Vet. Res.* **34,** 219–300.
Gimenez-Martin, G., Lopez-Saez, J. F., and Monge, F. G. (1962). Somatic chromosomes of the pig. *J. Hered.* **53,** 281, 290.
Glahn-Luft, B., Dzapo, V., and Wassmuth, R. (1982). Polymorphism of C-banding in swine. *Proc. Eur. Colloq. Cytogenet. Domest. Anim., 5th* pp. 312–313.
Golisch, D., Ritter, E., and Schwerin, M. (1982a). Zytogenetische Untersuchungen von Spontanaberrationen bei Ebern. *Arch. Tierz.* **25,** 537–547.
Golisch, D., Ritter, E., and Schwerin, M. (1982b). Zytogenetische Untersuchungen von Ebern unterschiedlicher genetischer Konstruktionen. *Arch. Tierz.* **25,** 337–344.
Golisch, D., Ritter, E., and Schwerin, M. (1986). Die 13/17-Fusionstranslokation beim Schwein und ihre phänotypischen Auswirkungen. *Arch. Tierz.*
Gropp, A., Giers, D., and Tettenborn, O. (1969). Das Chromosomenkomplement des Wildschweins *(Sus scrofa). Experientia* **25,** 778.
Gustavsson, I. (1973). Chromosomal errors in the reproduction of the domestic pig. *In* "Les accidents chromosomiques de la reproduction." INSERM, Paris.
Gustavsson, I. (1980). Banding techniques in chromosome analysis of domestic animals. *Adv. Vet. Sci. Comp. Med.* **24,** 245–289.
Gustavsson, I. (1984a). The THA technique as applied to porcine chromosomes. *Hereditas* **99,** 311–313.
Gustavsson, I. (1984b). Reciprocal translocations in the domestic pig (an interim report of a Swedish survey). *Proc. Eur. Colloq. Cytogenet. Domest. Anim., 6th* pp. 80–86.
Gustavsson, I. (1990). Reciprocal translocations in the pig: Common occurrence in boars producing decreased litter size. *Vet. Rec.,* in press.

Gustavsson, I., Hageltorn, M., Johansson, C., and Zech, L. (1972). Identification of the pig chromosomes by quinacrine mustard fluorescence technique. *Exp. Cell Res.* **70,** 471–474.

Gustavsson, I., Hageltorn, M., Zech, L., and Reiland, S. (1973). Identification of the chromosomes in centric fusion/fission polymorphic system of the pig (*Sus scrofa* L.). *Hereditas* **75,** 153–155.

Gustavsson, I., Settergren, I., and King, W. A. (1983). Occurrence of two different reciprocal translocations in the same litter of domestic pigs. *Hereditas* **99,** 257–267.

Gustavsson, I., Świtoński, M., Larsson, K., Plöen, L., and Höjer, K. (1988). Chromosome banding studies and synaptonemal complex analyses of four reciprocal translocations in the domestic pig. *Hereditas* **109,** 169–184.

Gustavsson, I., Larsson, K., Świtoński, M., and Plöen, L. (1990). Spontaneous chromosome translocation, rcp(2;4)(p17;q11), in a boar demonstrating impaired gametogenesis and decreased litter size. *Hereditas,* in press.

Gustavsson, I., Świtoński, M., Iannuzzi, L., Plöen, L., and Larsson, K. (1989b). Banding studies and synaptonemal complex analyses of an X-autosome translocation in the domestic pig. *Cytogenet. Cell Genet.,* **50,** 188–194.

Hageltorn, M., Gustavsson, I., and Zech, L. (1976). Detailed analysis of a reciprocal translocation (13q−;14q+) in the domestic pig by G- and Q-staining techniques. *Hereditas* **83,** 268–272.

Hanada, H., Muramatsu, S., and Himeno, K. (1979). Frequency of spontaneous chromosome aberrations in peripheral lymphocytes of swine. *Bull. Natl. Inst. Anim. Ind. (Jpn).* **35,** 27.

Hancock, J. L. (1959). Polyspermy of pig ova. *Anim. Prod.* **1,** 103–106.

Hancock, J. L., and Daker, M. G. (1981). Testicular hypoplasia in a boar with abnormal sex chromosome constitution (39 XXY). *J. Reprod. Fertil.* **61,** 395–397.

Hanly, S. (1961). Prenatal mortality in farm animals. *J. Reprod. Fertil.* **2,** 182–194.

Hansen, K. M. (1972). The karyotype of the pig *(Sus scrofa domestica),* identified by quinacrine mustard staining and fluorescence microscopy. *Cytogenetics* **11,** 286–294.

Hansen, K. M. (1977). Identification of the chromosomes of the domestic pig *(Sus scrofa domestica).* An identification key and a landmark system. *Ann. Genet. Sel. Anim.* **9,** 517–526.

Hansen, K. M. (1980a). Identification of the X chromosome of the domestic pig *(Sus scrofa domestica).* *Ann. Genet. Sel. Anim.* **12,** 225–232.

Hansen, K. M. (1980b). The relative length of pig chromosomes and a suggestion for a karyotype system. *Ann. Genet. Sel. Anim.* **12,** 313–320.

Hansen, K. M. (1982). Sequential Q- and C-band staining of pig chromosomes, and some comments on C-band polymorphism and C-band technique. *Hereditas* **96,** 183–189.

Hansen-Melander, E., and Melander, Y. (1970). Mosaicism for translocation heterozygosity in a malformed pig. *Hereditas* **64,** 199–202.

Hansen-Melander, E., and Melander, Y. (1972). A malformed pig with a normal female karyotype. *Hereditas* **70,** 154.

Hansen-Melander, F., and Melander, Y. (1974). The karyotype of the pig. *Hereditas* **77,** 149–158.

Hard, W. L., and Eisen, J. D. (1965). A phenotypic male swine with a female karyotype. *J. Hered.* **56,** 254–258.

Hare, W. C. D., and Singh, E. L. (1979). "Cytogenetics in Animal Reproduction." Commonw. Agric. Bur., Farnham Royal, England.

Harris, M., and Ruddle, F. H. (1960). Growth and chromosome studies on drug resistant lines of cells in tissue culture. *In* "Cell Physiology of Neoplasia," pp. 521–526. Univ. of Texas Press, Austin.

Harris, M., and Ruddle, F. H. (1961). Clone strains of pig kidney cells with drug resistance and chromosomal markers. *J. Natl. Cancer Inst.* **26**, 1405–1411.

Harvey, M. J. A. (1968). A male pig with an XXY/XXXY sex chromosome complement. *J. Reprod. Fertil.* **17**, 319–324.

Hook, E. B., and Hamerton, J. L. (1977). The frequency of chromosome abnormalities detected in consecutive newborn studies—differences between studies—results by sex and by severity of phenotypic involvement. *In* "Population Cytogenetics: Studies in Humans" (E. B. Hook and I. H. Porter, eds), pp. 63–79. Academic Press, New York.

Hulot, F. (1970). Analyse chromosomique de deux porcs intersexués *(Sus scrofa domesticus)*. *Ann. Genet. Sel. Anim.* **2**, 355–361.

Hunter, R. H. F. (1967). The effects of delayed insemination on fertilization and early cleavage in the pig. *J. Reprod. Fertil.* **13**, 133–147.

Jorgenson, K. F., Van de Sande, J. H., and Lin, C. C. (1978). The use of base specific DNA binding agents as affinity labels for the study of mammalian chromosomes. *Chromosoma* **68**, 287–302.

King, W. A. (1980). Spontaneous chromosome translocations in cattle and pigs: A study of the causes of their fertility reducing effects. Ph.D. Thesis, Swedish Univ. Agric. Sci., Uppsala.

King, W. A. (1981). Meiotic behaviour of a rcp(13q − ;14q +) translocation in heterozygous pigs. *Hereditas* **94**, 235–240.

King, W. A., Linares, T., and Hageltorn, M. (1980). A case of chi 38,XX,rcp(13q − ;14q +)/ 38,XY in pigs *Proc. Eur. Colloq. Cytogenet. Domest. Anim., 4th* pp. 124–128.

King, W. A., Gustavsson, I., Popescu, C. P., and Linares, T. (1981). Gametic products transmitted by rcp(13q − ;14q +) translocation heterozygous pigs, and resulting embryonic loss. *Hereditas* **95**, 239–246.

Krallinger, H. F. (1931). Cytologische Studien in einigen Haussäugetieren. Habilitationsschrift. *Arch. Tierernaehr. Tierz., Abt. B* **5**.

Kuokkanen, M.-T., and Mäkinen, A. (1987). A reciprocal translocation (7q − ;12q +) in the domestic pig. *Hereditas* **106**, 147–149.

Kuokkanen, M.-T., and Mäkinen, A. (1988). Reciprocal translocations, (1p − ;11q +) and (1p + ;15q −), in domestic pigs with reduced litter size. *Hereditas* **109**, 69–73.

Lin, C. C., Biederman, B. M., Jamro, H. K., Hawthorne, A. B., and Church, R. B. (1980). Porcine *(Sus scrofa domestica)* chromosome identification and suggested nomenclature. *Can. J. Genet. Cytol.* **22**, 103–116.

Lin, C. C., Joyce, E., Biederman, B. M., and Gerhart, S. (1982). The constitutive heterochromatin of porcine chromosomes. *J. Hered.* **73**, 231–233.

Ločniškar, F., Gustavsson, I., Hageltorn, M., and Zech, L. (1976). Cytological origin and points of exchange of reciprocal chromosome translocation (1p − ;6q +) in the domestic pig. *Hereditas* **83**, 272–275.

Lojda, L. (1968). Das chromosomale Bild des Testikulären Hermaphroditismus bei Schweinen und die Vererbung dieser Störung. *Congr. Int. Reprod. Anim. Insemin. Artif., 6th, Paris* pp. 897–899.

Lojda, L. (1975). The cytogenetic pattern in pigs with hereditary intersexuality similar to the syndrome of testicular feminization in man. *Doc. Vet. (Brno)* **8**, 71–82.

Lojda, L., and Petříčková, V. (1977). The effect of feeding various levels of aflatoxin B_1 on the chromosome pattern of rats and pigs. *Ann. Genet. Sel. Anim.* **9**, 539.

Lojda, L., and Rubes, J. (1977). Chromosome aberrations in pigs after vaccination with living vaccin against swine fever. *Ann. Genet. Sel. Anim.* **9**, 540.

Long, S. E., and Williams, C. V. (1982). A comparison of the chromosome complement of inner cell mass and trophoblast cells in day 10 pig embryos. *J. Reprod. Fertil.* **66**, 645–648.

McClintock, B. (1945). *Neurospora*. I. Preliminary observations of the chromosomes of *Neurospora crassa*. *Am. J. Bot.* **32**, 671–678.

McConnell, J., Fechheimer, N. S., and Gilmore, L. O. (1963). Somatic chromosomes of the domestic pig. *J. Anim. Sci.* **22**, 374–379.

McFee, A. F., and Banner, M. W. (1969). Inheritance of chromosome number in pigs. *J. Reprod. Fertil.* **18**, 9–14.

McFee, A. F., Banner, M. W., and Rary, J. M. (1966a). Variation in chromosome number among European wild pigs. *Cytogenetics* **5**, 75–81.

McFee, A. F., Banner, N. W., and Rary, J. H. (1966b). An intersex pig with XX/XY leucocytes mosaicism. *Can. J. Genet. Cytol.* **8**, 502–505.

McFeely, R. A. (1966). A direct method for the display of chromosomes from early pig embryos. *J. Reprod. Fertil.* **11**, 161–163.

McFeely, R. A. (1967). Chromosome abnormalities in early embryos of the pig. *J. Reprod. Fertil.* **13**, 579–581.

McFeely, R. A., Klunder, L. R., and Goldman, J. B. (1988). A Robertsonian translocation in a sow with reduced litter size. *Proc. Eur. Colloq. Cytogenet. Domest. Anim., 8th* pp. 35–37.

Madan, K., Ford, C. E., and Polge, C. (1978). A reciprocal translocation, t(6p+;14q−) in the pig. *J. Reprod. Fertil.* **53**, 395–398.

Mäkinen, A., and Remes, E. (1986). Low fertility in pigs with rcp(4q+;13q−) translocation, *Hereditas* **104**, 223–229.

Mäkinen, A., Kuokkanen, M.-T. Niini, T., and Perttola, L. (1987). A complex three breakpoint translocation in the domestic pig. *Acta Vet. Scand.* **28**, 189–196.

Maik, H., and Jáskowski, L. (1968). Chromosome sex determination of intersexual pigs. *Congr. Int. Reprod. Anim. Insemin. Artif., 6th, Paris* **2**, 909–911.

Makino, S. (1944). The chromosome complex of the pig *(Sus scrofa)*. (Chromosome studies in domestic mammals, III.) *Cytologia* **13**, 170–178.

Makino, S., Sasaki, M. S., Sofumi, T., and Ishikawa, T. (1962). Chromosome condition of an intersex swine. *Proc. Jpn. Acad.* **38**, 686–689.

Masuda, H., Okamoto, A., and Waide, Y. (1975). Autosomal abnormality in a swine. *Jpn. J. Zootech. Sci.* **46**, 671–676.

Matsson, P., Annerén, G., and Gustavsson, I. (1986). Flow cytometric karyotyping of mammals, using blood lymphocytes: Detection and analysis of chromosomal abnormalities. *Hereditas* **104**, 49–54.

Mayr, B., and Schleger, W. (1981). Cytogenetic investigations in Austrian bulls and boars. *Zentralbl. Veterinaermed., Reihe A* **23**, 70–75.

Mayr, B., Schweizer, D., and Geber, G. (1984). NOR activity, heterochromatin differentiation, and the Robertsonian polymorphism in *Sus scrofa* L. *J. Hered.* **75**, 79–80.

Melander, Y., and Hansen-Melander, E. (1980). Chromosome studies in African wild pigs (Suidae, Mammalia). *Hereditas* **92**, 283–289.

Melander, Y., Hansen-Melander, E., Holm, L., and Somlev, B. (1971). Seven swine intersexes with XX chromosome constitution. *Hereditas* **69**, 51–58.

Michelmann, H. W., El-Nahass, E. M., and Paufler, S. (1977). Vergleichende Chromosomenuntersuchung bei Zucht- und Mastschweinen mit Hilfe der Giemsa-Färbung und der Bänderungstechnik. *Zuechtungskunde* **49**, 294–300.

Miyake, Y.-I. (1973). Cytogenetical studies on swine intersexes. *Jpn. J. Vet. Res.* **21**, 41–49.

Miyake, Y.-I., Kawata, K., Ishikawa, T., and Umezu, M. (1977). Translocation heterozygosity in a malformed piglet and its normal littermates. *Teratology* **16**, 163–168.

Moon, R. G., Rashad, M. N., and Mi, M. P. (1975). An example of polyploidy in pig blastocysts. *J. Reprod. Fertil.* **45**, 147–149.

Muramoto, J., Makino, S., Ishikawa, T., and Kanagawa, H. (1965). On the chromosomes of the wild boar and the boar–pig hybrids. *Proc. Jpn. Acad.* **41,** 236–239.
Nes, N. (1968). Betydningen av kromosomaberrasjoner hos dyr. *Forsk. Fors. Landbruket* **19,** 393–410.
Nevo, A. C., Polge, C., and Frederick, G. (1970). Aerobic and anaerobic metabolism of boar spermatozoa in relation to their motility. *J. Reprod. Fertil.* **22,** 109–118.
Okamoto, A., Shiobara, H., Tomita, T., and Ohmi, H. (1980). Chromosome studies of the wild boar and Ohmini pigs. *Bull. Coll. Agric. Utsunomiya Univ.* **11,** 1–8.
Oprescu, S., Baicoianu, C., Dinu, M., Câmpean, C., Oprescu, S., and Câmpean, N. (1972). Comparative cytogenetic investigations into some somatic anomalies and reproductive disorders in swine. *Proc. Int. Congr. Anim. Reprod. Artif. Insemin., 7th, Munich* **2,** 1118–1122.
Oprescu, S., Voiculescu, I., Oprescu, S., and Gessner, E. (1976). Cytogenetic investigations on a phenotypically normal boar responsible for repeated abortions and on his progeny. *Proc. Int. Congr. Anim. Reprod. Artif. Insemin., 8th, Cracow* **4,** 738–741.
Pathak, S., Hsu, T. C., and Markvong, A. (1976). Pachytene mapping of the male Chinese hamster. *Cytogenet. Cell Genet.* **17,** 1–8.
Petříčková, V., Lojda, L., Rubeš, J., and Štavíková, M. (1976). Effect of aflatoxin B on the chromosomal pattern and reproduction of rats and pigs. *Proc. Int. Congr. Anim. Reprod. Artif. Insemin., 8th, Cracow* **4,** 617–619.
Pirtle, E. C. (1966). Chromosomal variations in a pig kidney cell line persistently infected with hog cholera virus. *Am. J. Vet. Res.* **27,** 737–745.
Pirtle, E. C., and Woods, L. K. (1967). Dissimilarities in two PK-15 swine kidney cell lines. *Mamm. Chromosome Newsl.* **8,** 93–94.
Pirtle, E. C., and Woods, L. K. (1968). Cytogenetic alterations in swine kidney cells persistently infected with hog cholera virus and propagated with and without anitserum in the medium. *Am. J. Vet. Res.* **29,** 153–164.
Popescu, C. P. (1989). "Cytogénétique des mammifères d'élevage." INRA, Paris.
Popescu, C. P., and Boscher, J. (1982). Cytogenetics of preimplantation embryos produced by pigs heterozygous for the reciprocal translocation (4q+;14q-). *Cytogenet. Cell Genet.* **34,** 119–123.
Popescu, C. P., and Boscher, J. (1986). A new reciprocal translocation in a hypoprolific boar. *Genet. Sel. Evol.* **18,** 123–130.
Popescu, C. P., and Legault, C. (1979). Une nouvelle translocation réciproque t(4q-+;14q-) chez le porc domestique *(Sus scrofa domestica)*. *Ann. Genet. Sel. Anim.* **11,** 361–369.
Popescu, C. P., Quéré, J. P., and Franceschi, P. (1980). Observations chromosomiques chez le sanglier français *(Sus scrofa scrofa)*. *Ann. Genet. Sel. Anim.* **12,** 395–400.
Popescu, C. P., Boscher, J., and Tixier, M. (1983). Une nouvelle translocation réciproque t, rcp(7q-;15q+) chez un verrat "hypoprolifique." *Genet. Sel. Evol.* **15,** 179–488.
Popescu, C. P., Bonneau, M., Tixier, M., Bahri, I., and Boscher, J. (1984). Reciprocal translocation in pigs. Their detection and consequences on animal performance and economic losses. *J. Hered.* **75,** 448–452.
Popescu, C. P., Boscher, J., and Zhang, S. (1988). Cytogenetic evaluation of boars with low prolificacy: Two new types of chromosome translocation. *Ann. Genet.* **31,** 75–80.
Rary, J. M., Henry, V. G., Matschke, G. H., and Murphree, R. L. (1968). The cytogenetics of swine in the Tellico Wildlife Management Area, Tennessee. *J. Hered.* **59,** 201–204.
Rieck, G. W. (1984). "Allgemeine veterinärmedizinische und allgemeine Teratologie." Enke, Stuttgart.
Rittmannsperger, C. (1971). Chromosomenuntersuchungen bei Wild- und Hausschweinen. *Ann. Genet. Sel. Anim.* **3,** 105–107.

Rönne, M., Stefanova, V., Di Berardino, D., and Strandby Poulsen, B. (1987). The R-banded karyotype of the domestic pig *(Sus scrofa domestica* L.). *Hereditas* **106**, 219–231.

Ruddle, F. H. (1961). Chromosome variation in cell populations derived from pig kidney. *Cancer Res.* **21**, 885–894.

Ruzicska, P. (1968). Double trisomy in a pig embryo. *Mamm. Chromosome Newsl.* **9**, 240–241.

Sahar, E., and Latt, S. A. (1978). Enhancement of banding patterns in human chromosomes by energy transfer. *Proc. Natl. Acad. Sci. U.S.A.* **75**, 5650–5654.

Schnedl, W., Abraham, R., Förster, M., and Schweizer, D. (1981). Differential fluorescent staining of porcine heterochromatin by chromomycin A3/distamycin A/DAPI and D287/170. *Cytogenet. Cell Genet.* **31**, 249–253.

Schwarzacher, T., Mayr, B., and Schweizer, D. (1984). Heterochromatin and nucleolus-organizer-region behaviour at male pachytene of *Sus scrofa domestica*. *Chromosoma* **91**, 12–19.

Schweizer, D. (1981). Counterstain-enhanced chromosome banding. *Hum. Genet.* **57**, 1–14.

Schwerin, M., Golisch, D., and Ritter, E. (1986). A Robertsonian translocation in swine. *Genet. Sel. Evol.* **18**, 367–374.

Seabright, M. (1971). A rapid banding technique for human chromosomes. *Lancet* **ii**, 971–972.

Smith, J. H., and Marlowe, T. J. (1971). A chromosomal analysis of 25-day-old pig embryos. *Cytogenetics* **10**, 385–391.

Somlev, B., Hansen-Melander, E., Melander, Y., and Holm, L. (1970). XX/XY chimerism in leucocytes of two intersexual pigs. *Hereditas* **64**, 203–210.

Spalding, J. F., and Berry, R. O. (1956). A chromosome study of the wild pig *(Pecari angulatus)* and the domestic pig *(Sus scrofa)*. *Cytologia* **21**, 81–84.

Stone, L. (1963). A chromosome analysis of the domestic pig *(Sus scrofa)* utilizing a peripheral blood culture technique. *Can. J. Genet. Cytol.* **5**, 38–42.

Sumner, A. T. (1972). A simple technique for demonstrating centromeric heterochromatin. *Exp. Cell Res.* **75**, 304–306.

Świtoński, M., Fries, R., and Stranzinger, G. (1983). C-band variants of telocentric chromosomes in swine: Evidence and inheritance studies *Genet. Sel. Evol.* **15**, 469–478.

Sysa, P. S. (1980). Polymorphism of metaphase chromosomes in swine (*Sus scrofa* L.). *Genetica* **52/53**, 312–315.

Tarocco, C., Franchi, F., and Croci, G. (1987). A new reciprocal translocation involving chromosomes 1/14 in a boar. *Genet. Sel. Evol.* **19**, 381–386.

Taylor, A. I., and Moores, E. C. (1967). A sex chromatin survey of newborn children in two London hospitals. *J. Med. Genet.* **4**, 258–259.

Thibault, C. (1959). Analyse de la fécondation de l'oeuf de la truie après accouplement ou insémination artificielle. *Colloq. Reprod. Artif. Insemin. Pig, Inst. Natl. Rech. Agron., Paris* pp. 165–188.

Tikhonov, V. N., and Troshina, A. I. (1975). Chromosome translocations in the karyotype of wild boars *Sus scrofa* L. of the European and the Asian areas of USSR. *Theor. Appl. Genet.* **45**, 304–308.

Toyama, Y. (1974). Sex chromosome mosaicisms in five swine intersexes. *Jpn. J. Zootech. Sci.* **45**, 551–557.

Van de Sande, J. H., Lin, C. C., and Jorgensen, K. F. (1977). Reverse banding on chromosomes produced by a guanosine–cytosine specific DNA binding antibiotic: olivomycin. *Science* **195**, 400–402.

Vogt, D. W. (1967). Chromosome condition of two atresia ani pigs. *J. Anim. Sci.* **26,** 1002–1004.

Vogt, D. W. (1968). Sex chromosome mosaicism in a swine intersex. *J. Hered.* **59,** 166–167.

Vogt, D. W., Arakaki, D. T., and Brooks, C. C. (1974). Reduced litter size associated with aneuploid cell lines in a pair of full-brother Duroc boars. *Am. J. Vet. Res.* **35,** 1127–1130.

Wensing, C. J. G., Colenbrander, B., and Bosma, A. A. (1975). Testicular feminisation syndrome and gubernacular development in a pig. *Proc. K. Ned. Akad. Wet., Ser. C* **78,** 402–405.

Wodsedalek, J. E. (1913). Spermatogenesis of the pig with special reference to the accessory chromosomes. *Biol. Bull.* **25,** 8–32.

Zartman, D. L., Fechheimer, N. S., and Baker, L. N. (1969). Chromosomal aberrations in cultured leukocytes from pigs derived form X-irradiated semen. *Cytogenetics* **8,** 355–368.

Zartman, D. L., Fechheimer, N. S., and Baker, L. N. (1971). Chromosomal aberrations in cultured porcine fibroblasts after X-irradiation of male progenitors. *J. Anim. Sci.* **32,** 1–9.

Chromosomes of Sheep and Goats

SUSAN E. LONG

Department of Animal Husbandry, School of Veterinary Science, University of Bristol, Bristol, England

I. Normal Chromosome Complement
   A. Goat
   B. Sheep
II. Chromosome Abnormalities in Sheep
   A. Centric Fusion (Robertsonian) Translocations
   B. Reciprocal Translocations
   C. Deletions
   D. Miscellaneous Structural Abnormalities
   E. XO (Turner) Syndrome
   F. XXY (Klinefelter) Syndrome
   G. XYY
   H. Intersexes
III. Chromosome Abnormalities in Goats
   A. Centric Fusion Translocations
   B. Sex Chromosome Anomalies
   C. Intersexes
IV. Goat–Sheep Hybrids
   References

I. Normal Chromosome Complement

A. Goat

The goat *(Capra hircus)* has the basic Bovidae chromosome complement with a diploid number of 60. All the autosomes and the X chromosome are acrocentric, whereas the Y chromosome is an extremely small metacentric chromosome (Fig. 1). The X chromosome was identified as the third longest acrocentric chromosome by means of autoradiographic studies (Evans, 1965) and as the second longest when identified by G-banding (Bunch *et al.*, 1976a). This confusion merely illustrates how difficult it is to make accurate measurements of chromosomes.

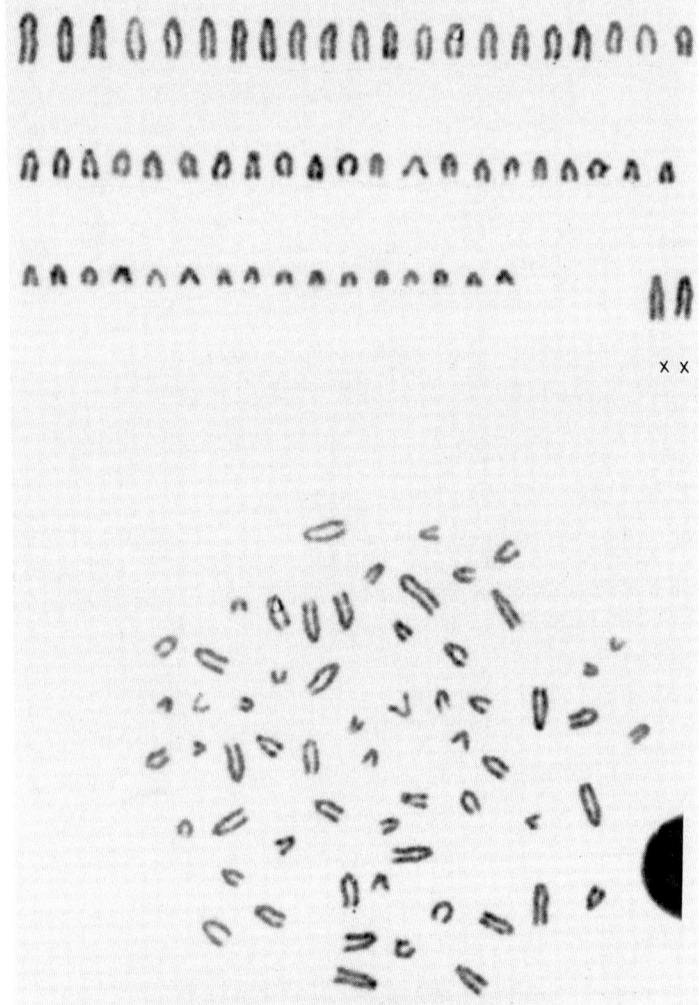

FIG. 1. The karyotype and spread from a female goat, *Capra hircus;* 2n = 60,XX. Conventional Giemsa staining.

The karyotype was first examined with differential staining using Q-bands (Hansen, 1973a). There is very close correlation between the Q-band pattern of goats, cattle, and sheep, indicating that speciation in the Bovidae has taken place by means of gene mutations and centric fusion translocations. The major differences between cattle and goats are in chromosome number 9 and the X and Y chromosomes (Second International Conference for the Standardization of Domestic Animal Karyotypes, 1989). G-banding has been done using the acid/saline/ Giemsa (ASG) method (Evans *et al.*, 1973; Schnedl and Czaker, 1974) and the trypsin method (Schnedl and Czaker, 1974; Arruga and Lopez, 1988). The nomenclature for a standard G-band karyotype was developed at the First International Conference for the Standardization of Banded Karyotypes of Domestic Animals (Ford *et al.*, 1980). R-banding, by both the 5-bromodeoxyuridine/acridine orange (RBA) and fluorescent-plus-Giemsa (FPG) methods, has been examined by Di Berardino *et al.* (1987).

All of the autosomes have blocks of heterochromatin at the centromere, which give positive C-bands, whereas the X and Y chromosomes are negative for C-banding (Evans *et al.*, 1973; Schnedl and Czaker, 1974). There is some evidence of a natural polymorphism in the size of the centromeric heterochromatin in some autosomes (Arruga and Lopez, 1988). The nucleolar organizer regions are located on the telomeres of chromosomes 2, 3, 4, 5, and 28 (Henderson and Bruere, 1979; Mayr and Czaker, 1981).

B. Sheep

The chromosome complement of the domestic sheep *(Ovis aries)* differs from that of cattle and goats in that the diploid number is 54 and there are three pairs of metacentric chromosomes. The other autosomes are all acrocentric. The X chromosome is the largest acrocentric chromosome (McFee *et al.*, 1965) and has marked, short arms. The Y chromosome is similar to that of the goat and is a small metacentric chromosome (Fig. 2). Comparison of the banding patterns of sheep chromosomes with those of cattle and goats shows that the largest metacentric chromosome in sheep is formed by the centric fusion of cattle chromosomes 3 and 1, the second sheep metacentric chromosome is formed by centric fusion of cattle chromosomes 8 and 2, and the third sheep metacentric chromosome is formed by centric fusion of cattle chromosomes 11 and 5 (Second International Conference, 1989). The Q-band karyotype has been reported by Hansen (1973b) and the G-band karyotype was studied by Zartman and Bruere (1974), Schnedl and Czaker (1974), and Matejka and Cribiu (1987). The nomenclature

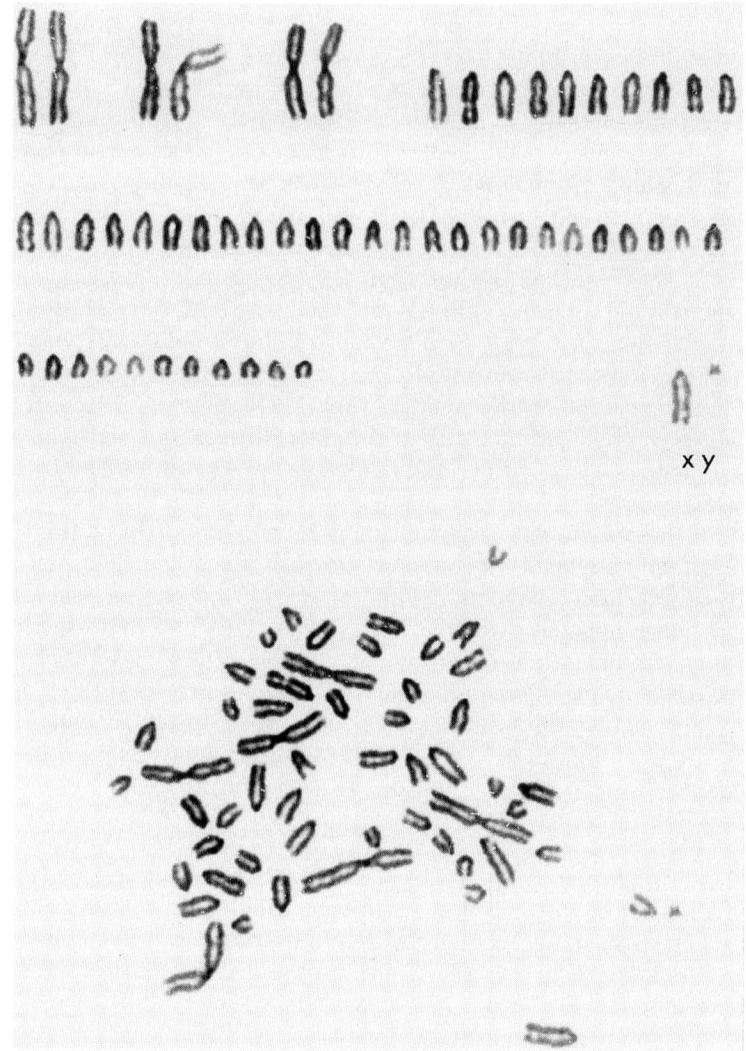

FIG. 2. The karyotype and spread from a ram, *Ovis aries;* $2n = 54$,XY. Conventional Giemsa staining.

for the G-band karyotype was developed at the First International Conference for the Standardization of Banded Karyotypes of Domestic Animals (Ford et al., 1980) and was updated by the Committee for Standardized Karyotype of *Ovis aries* (1985). R-banding, using the RBA method (Matejka et al., 1988; Hayes et al., 1988; Di Berardino et al., 1989) and 5-bromodeoxyuridine/Giemsa (RBG) method (Hayes et al., 1988), has been reported.

As in the goat, all autosomes of sheep have blocks of centromeric heterochromatin, but those in the three pairs of metacentric chromosomes are very small (Evans et al., 1973; Schnedl and Czaker, 1974), particularly in chromosome 3 (Long, 1975). The nucleolar organizer regions are located on the telomeres of the short arm of chromosome 1, the long arms of chromosomes 2 and 3, and telomeres of chromosomes 4 and 25 (Henderson and Bruere, 1977, 1979; Mayr and Czaker, 1981).

Although the diploid number of all breeds of domestic sheep *(O. aries)* has been found to be 54, there is a range of chromosome number in the different species of wild sheep. Urial sheep *(Ovis vignei)* have a diploid number of 58, with one pair of metacentric chromosomes corresponding to chromosome 1 in domestic sheep; arkhar/argali sheep *(Ovis ammon)* have 56 chromosomes, with two pairs of metacentric chromosomes corresponding to pairs 1 and 2 in domestic sheep, and snow sheep *(Ovis nivicola)* have four pairs of metacentric chromosomes (Bunch, 1978). It is difficult to tell from the published work which chromosomes have fused to form the fourth metacentric chromosome in *O. nivicola*. However, there is some suggestion that the long arm may be either chromosome 6 or 7 (note: numbering conforms to the sheep standardization; see Committee for Standardized Karyotype, 1985). Other wild sheep, such as the mouflon (*Ovis musimon* and *Ovis orientalis*) and North American wild sheep (*Ovis canadensis* and *Ovis dalli*), have 54 chromosomes and the karyotype appears identical to that of domestic sheep (Bunch, 1978). Within some populations of wild sheep there are hybrid populations with chromosome numbers of 55 and 57 (Nadler et al., 1971).

II. Chromosome Abnormalities in Sheep

A. Centric Fusion (Robertsonian) Translocations

Three different centric fusion translocations have been identified in sheep. These are the Massey I (t_1) (Bruere, 1969), Massey II (t_2) (Bruere and Mills, 1971), and Massey III (t_3) (Bruere et al., 1972) (Fig.

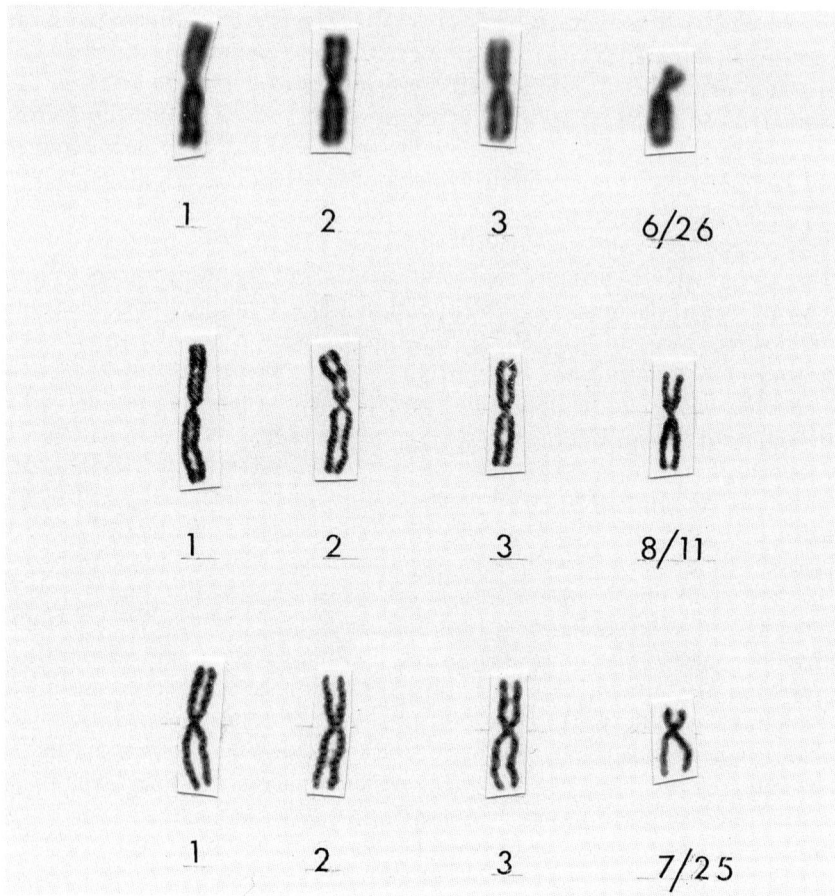

FIG. 3. Centric fusion translocations in the sheep. Partial karyotypes showing the size of the translocation chromosomes relative to the first three pairs of metacentric chromosomes in the normal chromosome complement. Conventional Giemsa staining.

3). The name derives from Massey University in New Zealand, where the translocations were first discovered. Differential staining has identified them as 6/26 (originally designated 5/26, but the new nomenclature makes the designation 6/26), 8/11, and 7/25 translocations, respectively (Bruere et al., 1974). All three translocations have two blocks of centromeric heterochromatin, one on either side of the centromere. This and their general morphology make them easily distinguishable from the normal metacentric chromosomes of the sheep karyotype.

The 6/26 translocation was first identified in the New Zealand Romney breed. This breed was developed in New Zealand from the imported British Romney Marsh sheep in the middle and late nineteenth century (Bruere et al., 1976). Subsequent investigation of Romney Marsh sheep in Britain showed that the translocation was indeed present in this breed (Bruere et al., 1978).

The 8/11 translocation was also found in the New Zealand Romney breed (Bruere et al., 1972), but has not been found in British Romney Marsh sheep. The 7/25 translocation has been found in three New Zealand breeds (New Zealand Romney, Drysdale, and Perendale) (Bruere et al., 1972), but has never been found in sheep of any other country.

The effect of these translocations on fertility has been widely investigated. Specific breeding trials were designed to check conception rates and lambing percentages (Bruere and Chapman, 1974; Bruere, 1974, 1975; Long, 1978a). These involved single and multiple heterozygous and homozygous male and female animals. No deleterious effects of the translocations could be determined.

Analyses of meiosis in heterozygous rams showed that nondisjunction (ND) was taking place and that unbalanced secondary spermatocytes were being formed (Chapman and Bruere, 1975; Long, 1978b). However, examination of a limited number of preimplantation embryos from normal ewes mated to rams heterozygous for the 6/26 translocation failed to find any with an unbalanced karyotype (Long, 1977). The conclusion was that either the unbalanced spermatozoa were not taking part in fertilization (i.e., the secondary spermatocytes failed to mature or, having matured, were incapable of fertilization) or aneuploid embryos were dying before the late preimplantation stage. The latter possibility was thought to be unlikely, because this would have been revealed in the mating programs as a reduction in the lambing percentage. It was therefore concluded that prezygotic selection was occurring and that this was why no effect of the translocations on fertility could be detected.

B. Reciprocal Translocations

Two different reciprocal translocations have been identified in sheep. The first was a $1p-;20q+$ (Fig. 4) found in a ram in Germany. Breeding studies indicated that there was a reduction in the number of twins and triplets in offspring from affected animals, which was attributed to early embryonic death of embryos with unbalanced chromosome complements (Glahn-Luft and Wassmuth, 1980).

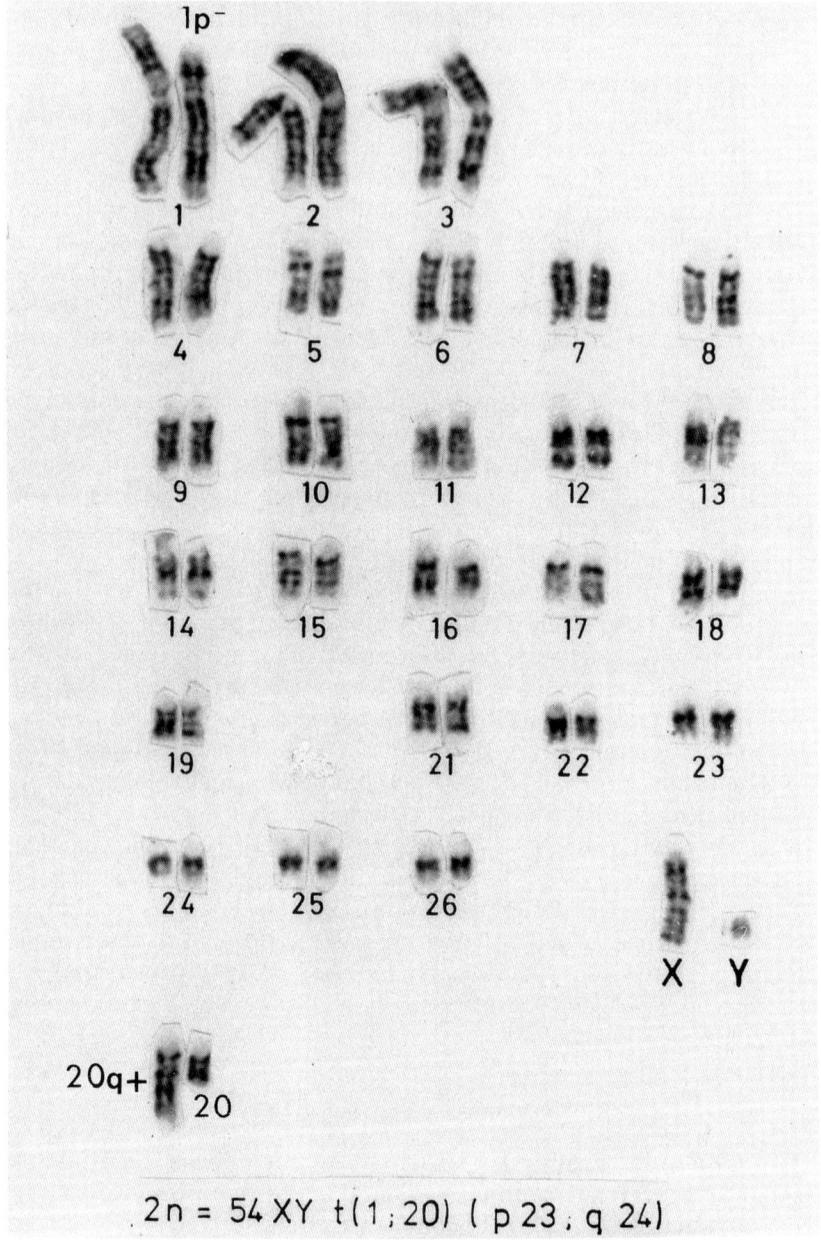

FIG. 4. Karyotype of a ram heterozygous for the 1p−;20q+ reciprocal translocation; $2n = 54,XY$. Giemsa/trypsin G-band (GTG) staining. (Karyotype supplied by courtesy of Dr. Glahn-Luft and Prof. Wassmuth, University of Giessen.)

The second translocation was in Icelandic sheep. It had been noted that a particular line of Icelandic sheep, which were large for the breed, had a low lambing percentage (Adalsteinsson and Hallgrimsson, 1977). Subsequent meiotic studies on a ram that consistently produced high return rates demonstrated the presence of a reciprocal translocation (K. A. Jonsson, S. Long, P.-K. Basrur, and S. Adalsteinsson, unpublished observations). Banding studies on mitotic chromosomes suggested that the translocation was a 13q−;20q+.

C. Deletions

There have been a number of reports of animals with apparent deletions in one of the chromatids. In some cases the deleted fragment has been visible in certain cells (Luft, 1973). Sometimes the chromosome anomaly has been associated with morphological abnormalities such as brachygnathia superior or agnathia (Henry et al., 1966; Luft, 1972; Glahn-Luft et al., 1978), whereas in other cases no phenotypic abnormalities were detected (Luft, 1973; Moraes et al., 1980). Confident diagnosis of a deletion requires the application of differential staining techniques. Deletions and secondary constrictions are known to arise in some instances as cultural artifacts (Palmer and Funderburk, 1965; Sasaki and Makino, 1963; Bruere and McLaren, 1967) so that association of these chromosomal anomalies with phenotypic abnormalities has to be made with caution.

D. Miscellaneous Structural Abnormalities

Chromosome 20 has also been implicated in another structural variation (Matejka and Cribiu, 1989). This was in a population of Ile-de-France sheep and consisted of an extra, heterochromatic block on the short arm of the chromosome. No information was given as to the possible effects of this variant.

E. XO (Turner) Syndrome

This condition is presumed to be rare in sheep, but because few barren ewes are examined cytogenetically it may be more common than is realized. One of three barren ewes in a flock of 200 was found to be a 53,XO ewe (Zartman et al., 1981). The external phenotype was female but unfortunately the internal genitalia were not examined. In another case a barren ewe was found to be a 53,XO/54,XX mosaic (Baylis et al., 1984). It had a normal vagina, uterus, fallopian tubes, and right ovary, but the left ovary was undeveloped and was only 2 mm in diameter.

F. XXY (Klinefelter) Syndrome

This chromosome complement has been found in five New Zealand Romney rams and one Cheviot ram from New Zealand (Bruere et al., 1969a; Bruere and Kilgour, 1974). The affected animals all showed bilateral testicular hypoplasia. Histologically the seminiferous tubules were small and were lined only by Sertoli cells. No spermatogenesis was present. The libido was normal despite the fact that plasma testosterone levels were low. Behavioral tests could detect no difference between the Klinefelter and normal rams (Kilgour and Bruere, 1970; Bruere and Kilgour, 1974). To what extent this chromosome anomaly is responsible for primary testicular hypoplasia in rams is not known.

G. XYY

There has been one report of a Polwarth ram in Brazil with a 54,XY/55,XYY chromosome complement (Moreas et al., 1980). The extra Y chromosome was found in 20 of 130 cells examined. No information was given on the fertility of the ram but scrotal palpation revealed no abnormalities.

H. Intersexes

1. Freemartins

Freemartins do occur in sheep but with much less frequency than in cattle because fusion of major placental blood vessels seems to be relatively uncommon in multiple pregnancies in sheep. Freemartinism has been variously estimated to occur in 5% (Stormont et al., 1953) and 1.2% (Dain, 1971) of twin conceptuses. Long (1980) found three freemartins in 261 ewes (1.1%) bought at market.

Anatomically, ovine freemartins demonstrate the same variation in development of the Wolffian duct system and inhibition of the Müllerian duct system as is seen in cattle (Fig. 5). Cytogenetically they show sex chromosome chimerism on peripheral blood cultures but are, of course, 54,XX in all nonhemopoetic tissue. Although freemartins are infertile, the incidence in sheep is so low that the condition is not of great commercial importance.

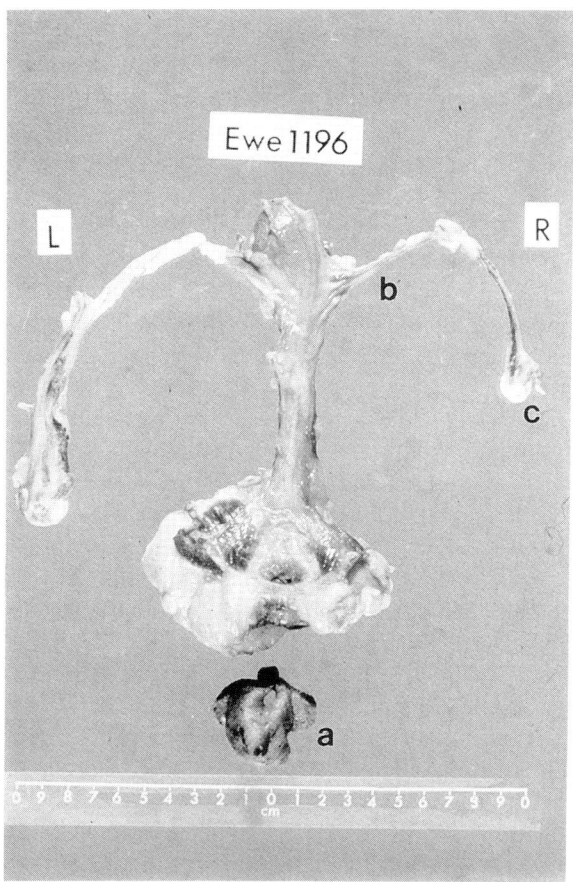

FIG. 5. Reproductive tract of a freemartin sheep showing (a) normal vulva, (b) tubular genitalia resembling a vas deferens, and (c) a small, testislike gonad.

2. Testicular Feminization

This is a very rare condition caused by an X-linked gene, the testicular feminizing gene (Tfm) (Lyon and Hawkes, 1970), which results in an inability of the target organs to respond to the secretion of testosterone. The animal is a genetic male but has a female external phenotype and abdominal testes. One such case has been reported by Bruere et al. (1969b). The animal appeared to be an overfat, barren ewe. There was a vagina but no clitoris. The vagina was shorter than normal and blind ending. Internally there were two large testes in an ovarian position. The head of the epididymis was present in each case but other parts of the efferent duct system were absent. There were no Müllerian duct derivatives nor internal accessory glands. Because the condition is X linked, it is inherited through the dam and the breeder should be advised to cull accordingly.

3. *Miscellaneous*

There have been a couple of reports of intersex animals that do not fit into the above classifications. Dain (1972) mentions in passing that she examined an intersex sheep. The animal was a genetic female but had well-developed testes and masculine genitalia. This would appear to be a case of male pseudohermaphroditism similar to that seen in polled goats. Gerneke (1967) described a single-born Karakul sheep that had anatomical features of a freemartin, but no Y chromosome was found in bone marrow cultures. However, this could have been an incidence of a freemartin with a low level of XY cells.

III. Chromosome Abnormalities in Goats

A. Centric Fusion Translocations

The first centric fusion translocation was identified in a Saanen goat that was also, coincidentally, a freemartin (Padeh *et al.*, 1965). Subsequently, translocations were reported in normal animals (Soller *et al.*, 1966; Hulot, 1969; Sohrab *et al.*, 1973; Elmiger and Stranzinger, 1982; Dolf and Hediger, 1984). There has also been a centric fusion translocation reported in a Toggenburg goat. It is not clear from the reports whether all these cases involve the same translocation, because not all of the preparations were banded.

In the Saanen goat, the translocation has been identified as 2q;13q (Popescu, 1972) and 1q;17q (S. E. Long, unpublished observations) on the basis of length alone and as 6q;17q (Elmiger and Stranzinger, 1982) and 6q;15q (Burguete *et al.*, 1987) on the basis of G-banding and RBA banding, respectively. Comparison of the banding patterns of the chromosomes in the latter two reports shows that the same chromosomes are involved but they have been numbered differently. Only a limited amount of data are available on the reproductive performance of translocation-bearing Saanen goats. Furthermore, some of the data are confounded by the presence of the polling (P) gene in some of the animals. In homozygous females this leads to intersexuality and in homozygous males it may lead to sterility (see later). Nevertheless, heterozygosity for a centric fusion translocation in Saanen goats does appear to be associated with a reduction in litter size, particularly when normal females are mated to heterozygous males (Padeh et al., 1971). Similarly, Ricordeau (1972) reported a reduction in litter size in heterozygous females with one of eight heterozygous females being barren. Offspring with unbalanced karyotypes were not found in either study. Although trivalent configurations have been seen at meiotic diakinesis (Pedeh et al., 1971; Popescu, 1972) metaphase II figures were not reported, thus no information is available on nondisjunction rates. No comparable data are available for Toggenburg goats.

B. Sex Chromosome Anomalies

1. X Chromosome Polyploidy

Three polled goats with a phenotype similar to that seen in cases of Klinefelter syndrome were reported by Gluhovschi et al. (1975). These animals had hypoplastic testes and gynecomastia with lactation. However, they showed normal male libido. They produced normal volumes of ejaculates that were completely azoospermic. The chromosome complement was said to be 2A+XXXY/XXXXY, but it was not clear whether this was in one or all three animals.

2. Y Chromosome Anomaly

Rieck et al. (1975) reported another fertile male goat that had gynecomastia and was lactating. This animal was mosaic for a deleted Y and was described as 60,XY/60,X,delY/59,XO.

C. Intersexes

1. Intersexuality in Polled Goats

Reports of intersexuality in goats have appeared in the literature since 1888 (Morot, 1888), but it was not until 1944 that the connection with the absence of horns was appreciated (Asdell, 1944). Affected animals show a wide range of external phenotype but the gonads are usually testes, although in rare instances they may be ovotestes. The gonads are most commonly abdominal, but may come to lie in a normal scrotal position. In general, the larger the ano-genital distance the more likely it is that the testes will be in a scrotal position (Fig. 6). Some animals have quite a female phenotype with only an enlarged

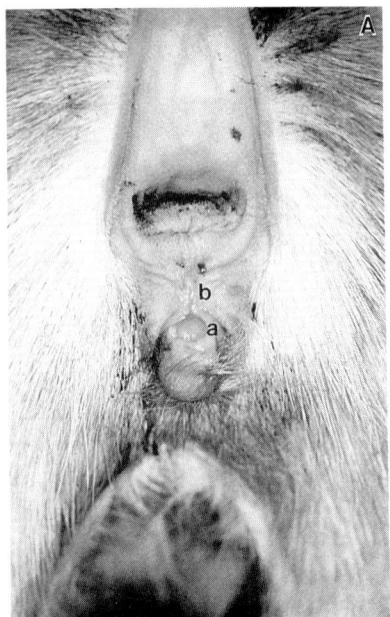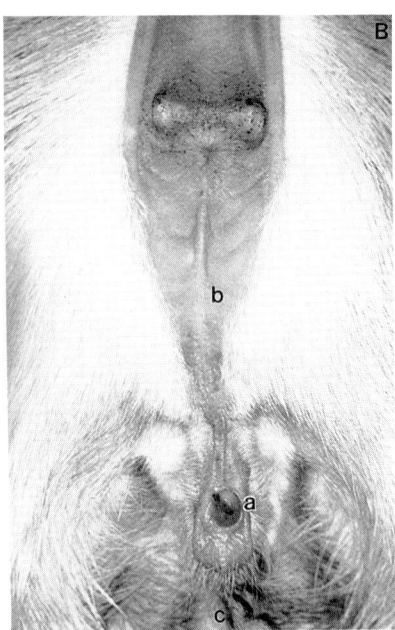

FIG. 6. (A) Rear end of an intersex polled goat showing (a) enlarged clitoris in prepucelike vulva, (b) short ano-genital distance, and no evidence of scrotal testes. (B) Rear end of an intersex polled goat showing (a) enlarged clitoris in prepucelike vulva, (b) long ano-genital distance, and (c) testes in a scrotal position.

clitoris, whereas others may be so masculine that they are mistaken for normal males.

The gene for hornlessness (polling gene) is an autosomal dominant and breeding studies suggest that intersex goats are probably homozygous for the polling gene. Cytogenetic examination of intersex polled goats show that they are genetic females (for a review of the early literature, see Hamerton et al., 1969). Females heterozygous for the polling gene are normal and fertile. Males heterozygous for the polling gene are normal. Males homozygous for the polling gene are usually normal but between 10 and 30% may be sterile due to tubular blockage in the head of the epididymis (Widmaier, 1957).

Interest in intersex goats has been rekindled in recent years following the identification in mice of a sex reversal *(Sxr)* gene (Cattanach et al., 1971). This gene is the testis-determining *(Tdy)* gene from a Y chromosome that has been translocated to an X chromosome to produce an X_{Sxr} (Evans et al., 1982; Singh and Jones, 1982). It causes genetic females to develope as phenotypic but sterile males, a situation very similar to that in the goat. It is now thought that in the goat a gene very closely linked to the polling gene acts in a manner similar to the *Sxr* gene action in mice, i.e., it causes testicular development in genetic females. In goats, the condition is inherited as an autosomal, sex-limited recessive and the masculinization is incomplete, resulting in intersexuality.

A male-specific antigen, designated H-Y antigen, is found on the cell surface of male mammalian species (Wachtel *et al.*, 1974). This is a different gene from the testis-detemining gene, but is usually found in animals with testicular development because it is closely linked to the *Tdy* gene. The 60,XX intersex goats are usually H-Y positive (Wachtel *et al.*, 1978; Shalev *et al.*, 1980). This is further indication that the intersex gene in goats is similar to the *Tdy* gene in mice.

2. Freemartins

Freemartins do occur in goats but appear to be even rarer than in sheep. There are three reports of animals with a 60,XX/60,XY lymphocyte chromosome chimerism and 60,XX in nonhemopoetic tissue (Ilbery and Williams, 1967; Soller *et al.*, 1969; Smith and Dunn, 1981). Two animals were known to have been born with male sibs and both had testicular-like gonads at the external inguinal ring and a vulva with an enlarged clitoris. Only one animal, a Saanen, was examined internally and this had a pseudovagina, vas deferens, and seminal vesicles. No Müllerian duct derivatives were present.

There are a number of reports of XX/XY chimerism, but without confirmation of an XX complement in nonhemopoetic tissue (Lojda, 1968; Basrur and Kanagawa, 1969; Hamerton *et al.*, 1969; Bondurant *et al.*, 1980).

3. True Hermaphrodites

Bongso *et al.* (1982) reported a true hermaphrodite animal that had a 60,XX/60,XY complement in blood, bone marrow, and skin tissue. It was born with three normal sibs (two males and one female). The hermaphrodite had a female external phenotype but with an enlarged clitoris. She would come into heat at approximately 20-day intervals but in between these cycles would mount other estrous females. Internally, the right gonad was found to be an ovotestis with two mature Graafian follicles. The left gonad was a testis. The testicular areas of the gonads were hypoplastic with Sertoli cells and spermatogonia but no spermatogenesis. Active Leydig cells were present between the tubules.

A second animal with bilateral ovotestes was reported by Lojda (1968). The animal had a hypoplastic vulva and vagina and a small uterus. The chromosome complement was XX/XY/XO.

IV. Goat–Sheep Hybrids

Popular belief in goat–sheep hybrids has existed for many centuries and in countries all over the world. Males of one species would be seen to mount females of the other species and when a slightly different or abnormal offspring was produced it would have been logical to conclude that this was a hybrid. However, proof of hybridization was difficult before chromosome analyses could be made and it is likely that most of these designations were incorrect. For example, some "hybrids" born to sheep are believed to have been sheep with a gene mutation resulting in a new, silky fleece (for review of the early literature, see McGovern, 1969).

Because the chromosome complements of goats and sheep are so similar, it might be thought that they would easily interbreed and produce hybrids comparable to mules and hinnies. However, this is not so. Attempts to deliberately create hybrids have usually not met with success.

If a billy goat is mated to an ewe, the goat semen usually fails to fertilize the sheep ovum (Warwick and Berry, 1948; Lopyrin and Loginova, 1953). In contrast, when a ram is mated to a nanny goat, fertilization and early embryonic development frequently do take place. This was established by Warwick in the 1930s by a series of experiments (for review, see McGovern, 1969). However, the pregnancy rarely goes to term and the embryo is aborted after about 2 months. Numerous investigations have been made as to why this should occur. Such things as maternal antigens (McGovern, 1973a), sensitivity to heterologous sperm (McGovern, 1973b), and volume of fetal fluids (McGovern, 1977) have all been studied. However, to date no satisfactory explanation has been found as to why the embryos are lost. There have been reports from Bulgaria (Bratanov *et al.*, 1980) of artificial manipulations of semen that have resulted in hybrid production, but the rationale for the treatments is not entirely clear. The work in Bulgaria indicated that hybrids could be made both by crossing rams with nanny goats and by crossing ewes with billy goats.

Despite the apparent problems, there are a few well-documented cases of goat–sheep hybrids having been produced by natural matings and confirmed by cytogenetic analysis (Roca and Rodero, 1971; Bunch *et al.*, 1976b; Eldridge *et al.*, 1983). The hybrid chromosome complement consists of 57 chromosomes with three unpaired matecentrics. One such hybrid, a female produced from a mating of a nanny goat with a ram, was fertile. When the hybrid was mated back to a ram it produced one stillborn offspring and one ram lamb whose karyotype was 54,XY (Cribiu *et al.*, 1988). Why these animals should have survived to term when others abort is not known.

References

Adalsteinsson, S., and Hallgrimsson, S. (1977). Inherited fertility depression in Icelandic sheep. *J. Agric. Res. Icel.* **9**, 77–82.
Arruga, M. V., and Lopez, N. L. (1988). Cytogenetic studies in two samples of Spanish goat breeds. *Proc. Colloq. Cytogenet. Domest. Anim., 8th Bristol, Eng.* pp. 39–52.
Asdell, S. A. (1944). The genetic sex of intersexual goats and a probable linkage with the gene for hornlessness. *Science* **99**, 124.
Basrur, P.-K., and Kanagawa, H. (1969). Anatomic and cytogenetic studies on 19 hornless goats with sexual disorders. *Ann. Genet. Sel. Anim.* **1**, 349–378.
Baylis, M. S., Wayte, D. M., and Owen, J. B. (1984). An XO/XX mosaic sheep with associated gonadal dysgenesis. *Res. Vet. Sci.* **36**, 125–126.
Bondurant, R. H., McDonald, M. C., and Trommershausen-Bowling, A. (1980). Probable freemartin in a goat. *J. Am. Vet. Med. Assoc.* **177**, 1024–1125.
Bongso, T. A., Thavalingam, M., and Mukherjee, T. K. (1982). Intersexuality associated with XX/XY mosaicism in a horned goat. *Cytogenet. Cell Genet.* **34**, 315–319.
Bratanov, K., Dikov, V., Somlev, B., and Efremova, V. (1980). Chromosome complement and fertility of sheep–goat hybrids. *Eur. Colloq. Cytogenet. Domest. Anim., 4th, Uppsala* pp. 262–266.
Bruere, A. N. (1969). Male sterility and an autosomal translocation in Romney sheep. *Cytogenetics* **8**, 209–218.
Bruere, A. N. (1974). The segregation patterns and fertility of sheep heterozygous and homozygous for three different Robertsonian translocations. *J. Reprod. Fertil.* **41**, 453–464.
Bruere, A. N. (1975). Further evidence of normal fertility and the formation of balanced gametes in sheep with one or more different Robertsonian translocations. *J. Reprod. Fertil.* **45**, 323–331.
Bruere, A. N., and Chapman, H. M. (1974). Double translocation heterozygosity and normal fertility in domestic sheep. *Cytogenet. Cell Genet.* **13**, 342–351.
Bruere, A. N., and Kilgour, R. (1974). Normal behaviour patterns and libido in chromatin-positive Klinefelter sheep. *Vet. Rec.* **95**, 436–439.
Bruere, A. N., and McLaren, R. D. (1967). The idiogram of the sheep with particular reference to secondary constrictions. *Can. J. Genet. Cytol.* **9**, 543–553.
Bruere, A. N., and Mills, R. A. (1971). Observations on the incidence of Robertsonian translocations and associated testicular changes in a flock of New Zealand Romney sheep. *Cytogenetics* **10**, 260–272.
Bruere, A. N., Marshall, R. B., and Ward, D. P. J. (1969a). Testicular hypoplasia and XXY sex chromosome complement in two rams: The ovine counterpart of Klinefelter's syndrome in man. *J. Reprod. Fertil.* **19**, 103–108.
Bruere, A. N., McDonald, M. F., and Marshall, R. B. (1969b). Cytogenetic analysis of

an ovine male pseudohermaphrodite and the possible role of the Y chromosome in cryptorchidism of sheep. *Cytogenetics* **8**, 148–157.

Bruere, A. N., Chapman, H. M., and Wyllie, D. R. (1972). Chromosome polymorphism and its possible implications in the select Drysdale breed of sheep. *Cytogenetics* **11**, 233–246.

Bruere, A. N., Zartman, D. L., and Chapman, H. M. (1974). The significance of the G-bands and C-bands of three different Robertsonian translocations of domestic sheep *(Ovis aries)*. *Cytogenet. Cell Genet.* **13**, 479–488.

Bruere, A. N., Chapman, H. M., Jaine, P. M., and Morris, R. M. (1976). Origin and significance of centric fusions in domestic sheep. *J. Hered.* **67**, 149–154.

Bruere, A. N., Evans, E. P., Burtenshaw, M. D., and Brown, B. B. (1978). Centric fusion polymorphism in Romney Marsh sheep of England. *J. Hered.* **69**, 8–10.

Bunch, T. D. (1978). Fundamental karyotype in domestic and wild species of sheep. *J. Hered.* **69**, 77–80.

Bunch, T. D., Foote, W. C., and Spillett, J. J. (1976a). Translocations of acrocentric chromosomes and their implications in the evolution of sheep *(Ovis)*. *Cytogenet. Cell Genet.* **17**, 122–136.

Bunch, T. D., Foote, W. P., and Spillet, J. J. (1976b). Sheep–goat hybrid karyotypes. *Theriogenology* **6**, 379–385.

Burguete, I., Di Beradino, D., Lioi, M. B., Taibi, L., and Matassino, D. (1987). Cytogenetic observations on a Robertsonian translocation in Saanen goats. *Genet. Sel. Evol.* **19**, 391–398.

Cattanach, B. M., Pollard, C. E., and Hawkes, S. G. (1971). Sex reversed mice: XX and XO males. *Cytogenetics* **10**, 318–337.

Chapman, H. M., and Bruere, A. N. (1975). The frequency of aneuploidy in the secondary spermatocytes of normal and Robertsonian translocation-carrying rams. *J. Reprod. Fertil.* **45**, 333–342.

Committee for Standardized Karyotype of *Ovis aries* (1985). Standard nomenclature for the G-band karyotype of the domestic sheep *(Ovis aries)*. *Hereditas* **103**, 165–170.

Cribiu, E. P., Matejka, M., Denis, B., and Malher, X. (1988). Etude chromosomique d'un hybride chèvre-mouton fertile. *Genet. Sel. Evol.* **20**, 379–386.

Dain, A. R. (1971). The incidence of freemartinism in sheep. *J. Reprod. Fertil.* **24**, 91–97.

Dain, A. R. (1972). Differences in chromosome lengths between male and female sheep. *Nature (London)* **237**, 455–457.

Di Berardino, D., Rønne, M., Burgete, I., Lioi, M. B., Taibi, L., and Matassino, M. (1987). The R-banding pattern of the prometaphase chromosomes of the goat *(Capra hircus* L). *J. Hered.* **78**, 225–230.

Di Berardino, D., Lioi, M. B., Miranda, C., Di Milia, A., D'Agostino, M. G., and Matassino, D. (1989). R-banding pattern of the prometaphase chromosomes of the domestic sheep *Ovis aries* L. *Genet. Sel. Evol.* **21**, 1–10.

Dolf, J., and Hediger, R. (1984). Comparison of centric fusions in Toggenburg and Saanen goats. *Proc. Eur. Colloq. Cytogenet. Domest. Anim., 6th, Zurich* pp. 311–312.

Eldridge, F., Leipold, W., and Harris, N. (1983). Sheep–goat hybrid: an additional case. *J. Dairy Sci.* **66**, 253.

Elmiger, B., and Stranzinger, G. (1982). Identification of a centric fusion in the G-banding karyotype of a Saanen goat. *Proc. Eur. Colloq. Cytogenet. Domest. Anim., 5th, Milan* pp. 407–409.

Evans, E. P., Burtenshaw, M. D., and Cattanach, B. M. (1982). Meiotic crossing-over between the X and Y chromosomes of male mice carrying the sex-reversing (S_{xr}) factor. *Nature (London)* **300**, 443–445.

Evans, H. J. (1965). A simple micro-technique for staining human chromosome preparations with some comments on DNA replication in sex chromosomes of the goat, cow and pig. *Exp. Cell Res.* **38,** 511–516.

Evans, H. J., Buckland, R. A., and Sumner, A. T. (1973). Chromosome homology and heterochromatin in goat, sheep and ox studied by banding techniques. *Chromosoma* **42,** 383–402.

Ford, C. E., Pollock, D. L., and Gustavsson, I. (1980). Proceedings of the First International Conference for the Standardization of Banded Karyotypes of Domestic Animals. *Hereditas* **92,** 145–162.

Gerneke, W. H. (1967). Cytogenetic investigations on normal and malformed animals with special reference to intersexes. *Onderstepoort J. Vet. Res.* **34,** 219–300.

Glahn-Luft, B., and Wassmuth, R. (1980). The influence of the 1/20 translocation in sheep on the efficiency of reproduction. *Proc. Annu. Meet. Eur. Assoc. Anim. Prod., 31st.*

Glahn-Luft, B., Schneider, H., Schneider, J., and Wassmuth, R. (1978). Chromosomal aberrations and Hb-deficiency in agnathic sheep. *Dtsch. Tieraerzti. Wochenschr.* **85,** 457–496.

Gluhovschi, M., Bistriceanu, M., and Palicia, R. (1975). Les troubles de la reproduction chez les animaux domestiques dus a des modifications du genome. *Cah. Med. Vet.* **44,** 155–163.

Hamerton, J. L., Dickson, J. M., Pollard, C. E., Grieves, S. A., and Short, R. V. (1969). Genetic intersexuality in goats. *J. Reprod. Fertil., Suppl.* No. 7, 25–51.

Hansen, K. M. (1973a). Q-band karyotype of the goat *(Capra hircus)* and the relation between goat and bovine Q-bands. *Hereditas* **75,** 119–130.

Hansen, K. M. (1973b). The karyotype of the domestic sheep *(Ovis aries)* identified by quinacrine mustard staining and fluorescence microscopy. *Hereditas* **75,** 233–240.

Hayes, H., Matejka, M., and Cribiu, E. P. (1988). Comparison of diagrammatic representations of the GTG, RBA and RHG band patterns in sheep chromosomes. *Proc. Eur. Colloq. Cytogenet. Domest. Anim., 8th, Bristol, Eng.* pp. 15–22.

Henderson, L. M., and Bruere, A. N. (1977). Association of nucleolus organiser chromosomes in domestic sheep *(Ovis aries)* shown by silver staining. *Cytogenet. Cell Genet.* **19,** 326–334.

Henderson, L. M., and Bruere, A. N. (1979). Conservation of nucleolus organizer regions during evolution in sheep, goat, cattle and aoudad. *Can. J. Genet. Cytol.* **21,** 1–8.

Henry, T. A., Ingalls, T. M., and Binns, W. (1966). Teratogenesis of craniofacial malformations in animals. IV. Chromosomal anomalies associated with congenital malformations of the central nervous system in sheep. *Arch. Environ. Health* **13,** 715–718.

Hulot, F. (1969). Nouveau cas de fusion centrique chez la chèvre domestique *(Capra hircus* L.). *Ann. Genet. Sel. Anim.* **1,** 175 176.

Ilbery, P. L. T., and Williams, D. (1967). Evidence of the freemartin condition in the goat. *Cytogenetics* **6,** 276–285.

Kilgour, R., and Bruere, A. N. (1970). Behaviour patterns in chromatin-positive Klinefelter's syndrome in sheep. *Nature (London)* **225,** 71–72.

Lojda, A. (1968). Der chromosomale, klinische und sektionsbefund bei einigen fallen der intersexualitat gvon ziegen und mud. *Proc. Int. Congr. Anim. Reprod. Artif. Insemin., 6th, Paris* **2,** 901–903.

Long, S. E. (1975). An investigation of a centric fusion (Robertsonian) translocation of sheep. Ph.D Thesis, Univ. of Glasgow.

Long, S. E. (1977). Cytogenetic examination of pre-implantaion blastocysts of ewes mated to rams heterozygous for the Massey I (t_1) translocation. *Cytogenet. Cell Genet.* **18,** 82–89.

Long, S. E. (1978a). Reproductive performance of ewes mated to rams heterozygous for the Massey I (t_1) centric fusion (Robertsonian) translocation. *Vet. Rec.* **102**, 399–401.
Long, S. E. (1978b). Chiasma counts and non-disjunction frequencies in a normal ram and in rams carrying the Massey I (t_1) Robertsonian translocation. *J. Reprod. Fertil.* **53**, 353–356.
Long, S. E. (1980). Some pathological conditions of the reproductive tract of the ewe. *Vet. Rec.* **106**, 175–176.
Lopyrin, A. I., and Loginova, N. V. (1953). Remote hybridization of animals. *Anim. Breed. Abstr.* **22**, No. 1019.
Luft, B. (1972). Autosomal deletion of two ewes and two rams with brachygnathia superior. *Dtsch. Tieraerztl. Wochenschr.* **79**, 327–330.
Luft, B. (1973). An autosomal deletion with the appearance of fragments in a ram. *Zuchthygiene* **8**, 125–129.
Lyon, M. F., and Hawkes, S. G. (1970). X-linked gene for testicular feminization in the mouse. *Nature (London)* **227**, 1217–1219.
McFee, A. F., Banner, M. W., and Murphree, R. L. (1965). Chromosome analysis of peripheral leucocytes of the sheep. *J. Anim. Sci.* **24**, 551–555.
McGovern, P. T. (1969). Goat and sheep hybrids. *Anim. Breed. Abstr.* **37**, 1–11.
McGovern, P. T. (1973a). The effect of maternal immunity on the survival of goat–sheep hybrid embryos. *J. Reprod. Fertil.* **34**, 215–220.
McGovern, P. T. (1973b). The fate of goat–sheep hybrid embryos in goats treated parenterally with sheep semen. *J. Reprod. Fertil.* **34**, 221–225.
McGovern, P. T. (1977). The volume and composition of amniotic and allantoic fluid in goat–sheep hybrid conceptuses. *Br. Vet. J.* **133**, 33–36.
Matejka, M., and Cribiu, E. P. (1987). Idiogramme et représentation schématique des bandes G des chromosomes du mouton domestique (*Ovis aris* L.). *Genet. Sel. Evol.* **19**, 113–126.
Matejka, M., and Cribiu, E. P. (1989). Observation d'un nouveau variant chromosomique chez le mouton domestique (*Ovis aries* L). *Genet. Sel. Evol.* **21**, 11–15.
Matejka, M., Cribiu, E. P., and Popescu, C. P. (1988). Diagrammatic representation of RBA-banded karyotype of domestic sheep *(Ovis aries)*. *J. Hered.* **79**, 71–74.
Mayr, B., and Czaker, R. (1981). Variable positions of nucleolus organizer regions in *Bovidae*. *Experientia* **37**, 564–565.
Moraes, J. C. F., Mattevi, M. S., and Ferreira, J. M. M. (1980). Chromosome studies in Brazilian rams. *Vet. Rec.* **107**, 489–490.
Morot, C. (1883). Quoted in Boyajean, D. Intersexualité associée a l'absence de cornes chez la chèvre d'origine alpine. *Ann. Genet. Sel. Anim.* **1**, 447–463 (1969).
Nadler, C. F., Lay, D. M., and Hassinger, J. S. (1971). Cytogenetic analyses of wild sheep populations in northern Iran. *Cytogenetics* **10**, 137–152.
Padeh, B., Wysoki, I., Ayalon, N., and Soller, M. (1965). An XX/XY hermaphrodite in the goat. *Isr. J. Med. Sci.* **1**, 1008–1012; *Anim. Breed. Abstr.* **34**, 3091.
Padeh, B., Wysoki, M., and Soller, M. (1971). Further studies on a Robertsonian translocation in the Saanen dairy goat. *Cytogenetics* **10**, 61–69.
Palmer, C. G., and Funderburk, S. (1965). Secondary constrictions in human chromosomes. *Cytogenetics* **4**, 261–276.
Popescu, C. P. (1972). Mode de transmission d'une fusion centrique dans la descendance d'un bouc (*Capra hircus* L.) hétérozygote. *Ann. Genet. Sel. Anim.* **4**, 355–361.
Ricordeau, G. (1972). Observations sur les caracteres de reproduction des produits male et femelles issus d'un bouc porteur d'une fusion centrique. *Ann. Genet. Sel. Anim.* **4**, 593–598.

Rieck, von G. W., Hohn, H., Loeffler, K., Marx, D., and Bohm, S. (1975). Gynakomastic bie einem Ziegenbock. II. Zytogenetische Befunds: XO/XY-Mosaik mit variablen Deletionen des Y-chromosoms. *Zuchthygiene* 10, 159–168.

Roca, R., and Rodero, A. (1971). The chromosomes of a sheep–goat hybrid. *Arch. Zootec.* 20, 235–247.

Sasaki, M. S., and Makino, S. (1963). The demonstration of secondary constrictions in human chromosomes by means of a new technique. *Am. J. Hum. Genet.* 15, 24–33.

Schnedl, W., and Czaker, R. (1974). Centromeric heterochromatin and comparison of G-banding in cattle, goat and sheep chromosomes *(Bovidae)*. *Cytogenet. Cell Genet.* 13, 246–255.

Second International Conference for the Standardization of Domestic Animal Karyotypes, Paris (1990). *Cytogenet. Cell Genet.* in press.

Shalev, A., Short, R. V., and Hamerton, J. L. (1980). Immunogenetics of sex determination in the polled goat. *Cytogenet. Cell. Genet.* 28, 195–202.

Singh, L., and Jones, K. W. (1982). Sex reversal in the mouse *(Mus musculus)* is caused by a recurrent nonreciprocal crossover involving the X and an aberrant Y chromosome. *Cell* 28, 205–216.

Smith, M. C., and Dunn, H. O. (1981). Freemartin condition in a goat. *J. Am. Vet. Med. Assoc.* 178, 735–737.

Sohrab, M., McGovern, P. T., and Hancock, J. L. (1973). Two anomalies of the goat karyotype. *Res. Vet. Sci.* 15, 77–81.

Soller, M., Wysoki, M., and Padeh, B. (1966). A chromosomal abnormality in phenotypically normal Saanen goats. *Cytogenetics* 5, 88–93.

Soller, M., Padeh, B., Wysoki, M., and Ayalon, N. (1969). Cytogenetics of Saanen goats showing abnormal development of the reproductive tract associated with the dominant gene for polledness. *Cytogenetics* 8, 51–67.

Stormont, C., Wier, W. C., and Lane, I. L. (1953). Erythrocyte mosaicism in a pair of sheep twins. *Science* 118, 695–696.

Wachtel, S. S., Koo, G. C., Zucherman, E. E., Hammerling, U., Scheid, M. P., and Boyse, E. A. (1974). Serological cross reactivity between H-Y (male) antigens of mouse and man. *Proc. Natl. Acad. Sci. U.S.A.* 71, 1215–1218.

Wachtel, S. S., Basrur, P., and Koo, G. C. (1978). Recessive male determining genes. *Cell* 15, 279–281.

Warwick, B. L., and Berry, R. O. (1948). Genetic relationship of domestic and wild species of sheep and goats based on hybridization and on comparative susceptibility to drugs. *Anim. Breed. Abstr.* 19, No. 715.

Widmaier, R. (1957). Untersuchungen an intersexuellen Ziegenlammern im Hinblick auf die Unfruchtbarkeit der Bucke. *Wiss. Z. Martin-Luther-Univ. Halle–Wittenberg* 6, 67–96.

Zartman, D., and Bruere, A. N. (1974). Giemsa banding of the chromosomes of the domestic sheep *(Ovis aries)*. *Can. J. Genet. Cytol.* 16, 555–564.

Zartman, D. L., Hinesley, L. L., and Gnatkowski, M. W. (1981). A 53,X female sheep *(Ovis aries)*. *Cytogenet. Cell Genet.* 30, 54–58.

Chromosomes of the Horse

MONICA M. POWER

Irish Equine Centre, Johnstown, Naas, County Kildare, Ireland

I. Historical Introduction
II. Techniques for the Study of Horse Chromosomes
    A. Mitotic Chromosomes
    B. Meiotic Chromosomes
    C. Banding Techniques Applied to Horse Chromosomes
III. The Normal Horse Karyotype
    A. Chromosome Morphology
    B. Reading Conference (1976)
    C. Measurement and Idiograms of Chromosomes
    D. Paris Conference (1989)
    E. Variants in the Karyotype
IV. Clinical Application of Cytogenetics in the Horse
    A. Introduction
    B. Chromosome Abnormalities Reported in the Horse
V. Horse Breeds and Interspecific Hybrids
    A. The Evolution of the Domestic Horse
    B. The Domestic Horse Breeds
    C. Comparative Equine Studies
    D. Hybridization in the Equidae
    References

I. Historical Introduction

Before the advent of modern techniques for chromosome preparation, a few attempts were made using testicular tissue to establish the chromosome number in the horse. Painter (1924) examined spermatogonial and primary spermatocyte divisions in the horse. Spermatogonial counts ranged from 57 to 60 and there were approximately 30 spermatocytes, suggesting a diploid number of 60. Painter quoted earlier studies by Kirillow (1912), who reported a haploid number of 10–16, Wodsedalek (1914), who reported a diploid number of 37 and a haploid number of 19, and Masui (1919), who also indicated a haploid number of 19 and a probable diploid number of 37. Makino (1942) reported a diploid number of 66 and a haploid number of 33. Despite this incorrect modal number he correctly identified the XY bivalent, confirming the horse XY sex chromosome status, which, up to then, had been in doubt.

Hsu (1952) fortuitously happened on one of the major breakthroughs in modern cytogenetics. This was the use of hypotonic treatment in the harvesting of cultured cells to improve the spreading of chromosomes. By this time somatic tissue was also being used for chromosome analysis. Rothfels et al. (1959), using kidney cell cultures from five horses, described, for the first time, the correct modal number of 64 for the horse. In 1960, Moorhead et al. published a simple routine technique for the culture of peripheral blood lymphocytes for chromosome analysis. Using this new technique, three further reports from Benirschke et al. (1962), Trujillo et al. (1962), and Makino et al. (1963) confirmed the chromosome modal number as 64 in the horse.

The first studies of Q- and G-banding in the horse was reported by Hageltorn and Gustavsson (1974). Up to 1975, only three papers had reported chromosome abnormalities, without banding, in three cases of very deviant sexual development in the horse (Payne et al., 1968; Basrur et al., 1970; Dunn et al., 1974). Using the new banding techniques, Chandley et al., (1975b) prompted an interest in the clinical application of equine cytogenetics by reporting the first chromosome abnormalities in seven mares out of nine who had been isolated because of poor reproductive performance. These included the genotypes 63,X, 65,XXX, 63,X/64,XX, and 64,XY sex reversal, which still represent the majority of types of chromosome abnormalities reported in the horse.

II. Techniques for the Study of Horse Chromosomes

A. Mitotic Chromosomes

1. Lymphocyte Cultures

Some modifications of the original method by Moorhead et al. (1960) are required for successful lymphocyte culture in the horse. The use of the mitogen phytohemagglutinin (PHA) in whole blood cultures causes a drastic agglutination of the red cells that is unresponsive to subsequent hypotonic treatment and impairs the eventual quality of the chromosomes (Power, 1987a). Equine red cells form rouleaux four times faster than those of man (Jeffcott, 1977). Alternatively, whole blood cultures using pokeweed mitogen (PWM), such as those of Ryder *et al.* (1978), seem to be the most successful and widely used methods. Other techniques using lymphocyte separation by Ficoll–diatrizoate gradient and subsequent culture with PHA (Hare and Singh, 1979) or the use of a lymphocyte-rich supernatant achieved by sedimentation and subsequent culture with PHA and PWM (Chaudhary and Kovacs, 1987) have also been reported to be successful in the horse.

2. Fibroblast Culture

Fibroblast cultures from skin, connective tissue, kidney, and testis have been reported to be successful for chromosome analysis in the horse. Individual authors seldom publish methodologies as they are not species specific and usually represent a routine method available in most cytogenetic laboratories based on the original methods of Paul (1975). Details of a method for growing skin and connective tissue in the horse are outlined by Power (1987a).

From the living animal, lymphocyte culture, because of its simplicity, will usually be the first method of choice for chromosome analysis. However, when clinically indicated, fibroblast culture may be established to provide chromosomes from an alternate cell line. When chromosome studies are to be performed using dead animals or abortion material tissue, culture may be established successfully from somatic tissues up to 72 hours post mortem (Hohn, 1967).

3. Amniotic Cell Culture

There has been only one report of amniocentesis in a horse, an onager, and a donkey. Successful culture of the amniocytes allowed the preparation of G- and C-banded karyotypes, providing the first prenatal chromosome analysis in the Equidae (Lear *et al.*, 1989).

4. Embryo Culture

Blue (1981b) reported no chromosome abnormality from cultures of 22 surgically removed equine embryos aged 28–64 days. Murer-Orlando *et al.* (1982b) used the whole blastocyst for cytogenetic sex determination of 21 9 to 15-day-old preattachment embryos collected transcervically. Romagnano *et al.* (1985) has described a technique for the preparation of chromosomes from early embryos. The R-banding technique described was further used by Romagnano *et al.* (1986) in the culture of 41 female embryos aged 6–28 days to determine the timing of X chromosome inactivation in preattachment equine embryos. The results indicated that X inactivation started around day 7.5 and was predominant by day 12.5 in both trophoblastic and embryonic disc cells.

5. Bone Marrow Culture

Bone marrow cells obtained by sternal puncture were the source of actively dividing cells in only one reported case in the horse. Gerneke and Coubrough (1970) reported a normal female chromosome pattern in this tissue in an Arabian intersex horse.

B. MEIOTIC CHROMOSOMES

1. Conventional Meiosis

Studies of meiotic chromosomes in the male equine were reported by Chandley et al. (1975a). These were done on testicular biopsies from an Arab stallion and a domestic mare/Prezwalski horse hybrid and from testicular material obtained after surgical castration of a mule and a hinny. The study included investigation of all stages of spermatogenesis, from spermatogonia to spermatozoa, to compare the behavior of meiotic chromosomes in the normal and hybrid animals (see Section V,D). To establish the normal pattern in the horse, Scott and Long (1980) reported results of conventional meiosis from eight stallions with normal spermatogenesis.

King et al. (1987) has reported on the meiotic stage of preovulatory oocytes from 16 mares in a study to determine the timing of ovulation of oocytes in domestic horses. It was concluded that horse oocytes, like those of most mammals studied, are ovulated after completion of the first meiotic division and formation of the first polar body.

2. Synaptonemal Complex Analysis

Conventional meiotic chromosome studies are mainly useful for visualizing postsynaptic stages, from which synaptic stages can only indirectly be inferred (Section II,B,1). In contrast, synaptonemal complex (SC) analysis, described by Moses et al. (1975) using a surface spreading technique for electron and light microscopy, allows detailed chromosome studies at high resolution of synaptic events, particularly at zygotene and pachytene. It can reveal meiotic behavior and the effect of chromosome abnormality and its possible effect on gametogenesis. One such study on the testes of a horse with trisomy 28 has been reported by Power et al. (1990). SC analysis was performed to examine the behavior of the extra chromosome at meiosis and to examine its possible contribution to the impaired fertility in this case (Fig. 1a and b) (see also Section IV,B,3,c).

C. BANDING TECHNIQUES APPLIED TO HORSE CHROMOSOMES

The codes used to describe banding techniques are according to Harnden and Klinger (1985). (For an overview of general banding techniques and their applications, see Long, "Chromosome Methodology," this volume.)

1. Q-Banding

Q-Banding with quinacrine fluorescence (QFQ) was reported by Hageltorn and Gustavsson (1974) and Buckland et al. (1976). This technique has not subsequently been used routinely for horse chromosomes, as the band definition achieved is not very good. However, it is still the method of choice for preidentification of chromosomes in the consecutive QFQ/Giemsa staining required for chromosome measurement (see Section III,c).

2. G-Banding

G-Banding studies of metaphase chromosomes using the trypsin/Glemsa (GTG) technique have been reported by Hageltorn and Gustavsson (1974), Buckland et al. (1976), Melchior and Hohn (1976), Ryder et al. (1978), and Power (1987a) and on prometaphase chromosomes by Maciulis et al. (1984) and Power (1987a). A study using the bromodeoxyuridine (BrdU)/Giemsa technique (GBG) was reported by Richer and Romagnano (1985). In the horse, as reported for other species, the G-bands are equivalent to the Q-bands and each chromosome pair has a distinctive banding pattern (Figs. 1a, 2, and 3).

3. R-Banding

An R-banding study of metaphase chromosomes using a heat denaturation technique (RHG) was reported by Murer-Orlando et al. (1982a) and using BrdU incorporation with Giemsa staining (RBG) by Molteni et al. (1982), Romagnano et al. (1987), and Power (1987a). The R-banding pattern of prometaphase chromosomes has been reported by Romagnano et al. (1987) and Power (1987a). An RBH technique using BrdU incorporation with Hoechst 33258 fluorescence was reported by Power (1987a). These are dynamic techniques that distinguish early and late replication of DNA both within and between chromosomes. They result in a distinctive banding pattern for each autosomal pair and clearly identify the early and late-replicating X

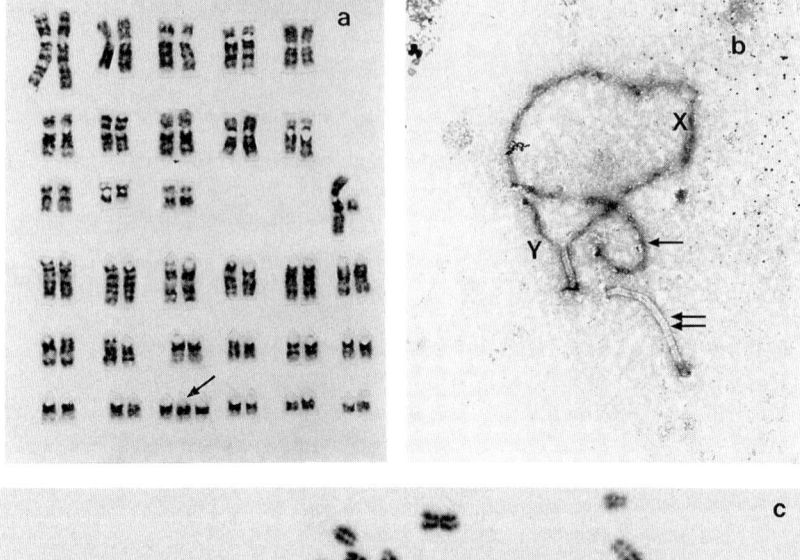
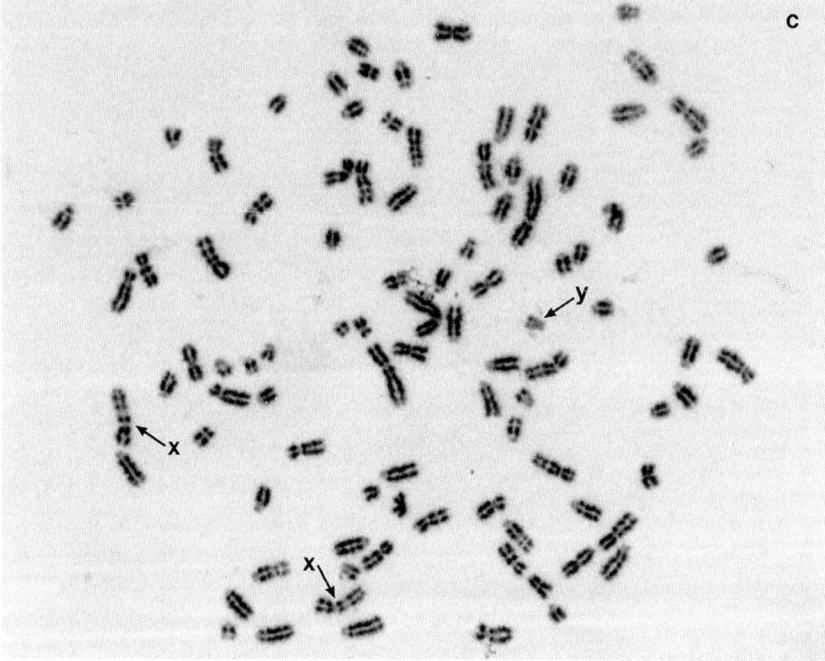

FIG. 1. (a) 65,XY, + 28 karyotype. (b) Detail of electron micrograph of synaptonemal complex from the trisomy 28 horse showing the XY sex bivalent and the trivalent with two paired (two arrows) and one unpaired (one arrow) number 28 chromosomes. (c) Triploid cell (96,XXY) from an intersex foal.

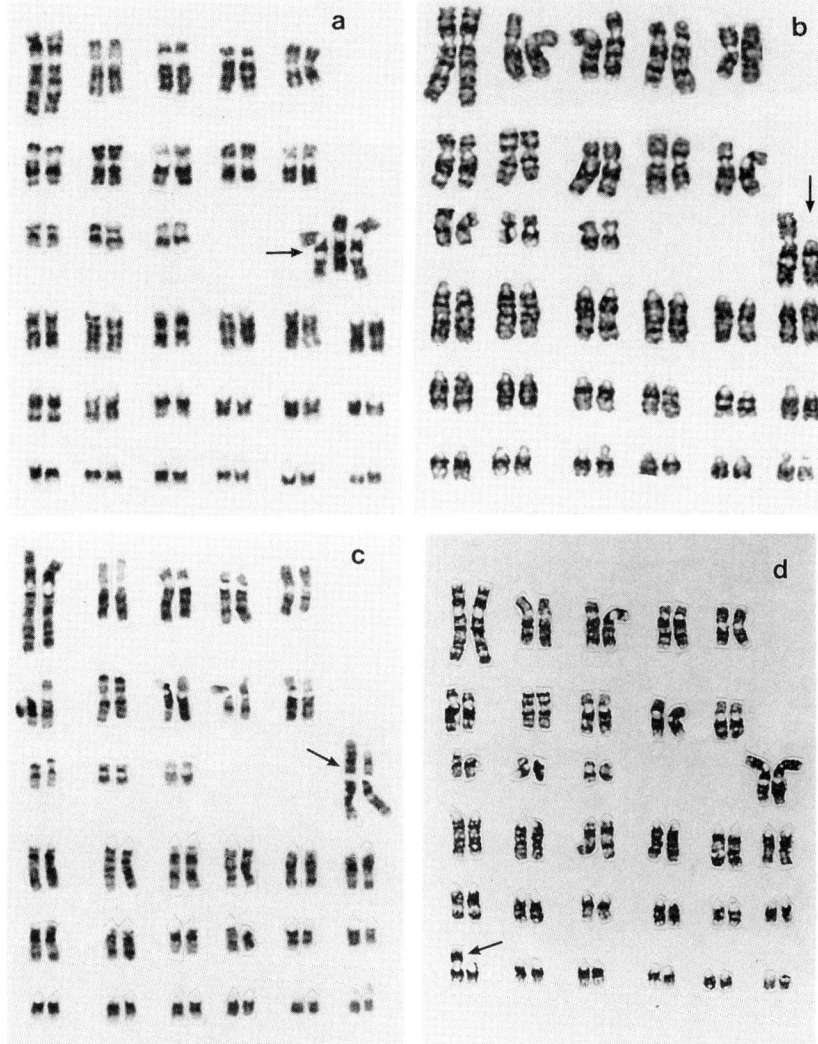

FIG. 2. (a) 65,XXX karyotype. (b) 64,X,del(Xp) karyotype. (c) 64,X, − X, + der(X), t(Xp;15q) karyotype. (d) 64,XX, − 26, + t(26q26q) karyotype (b and d karyotypes courtesy A. Bowling).

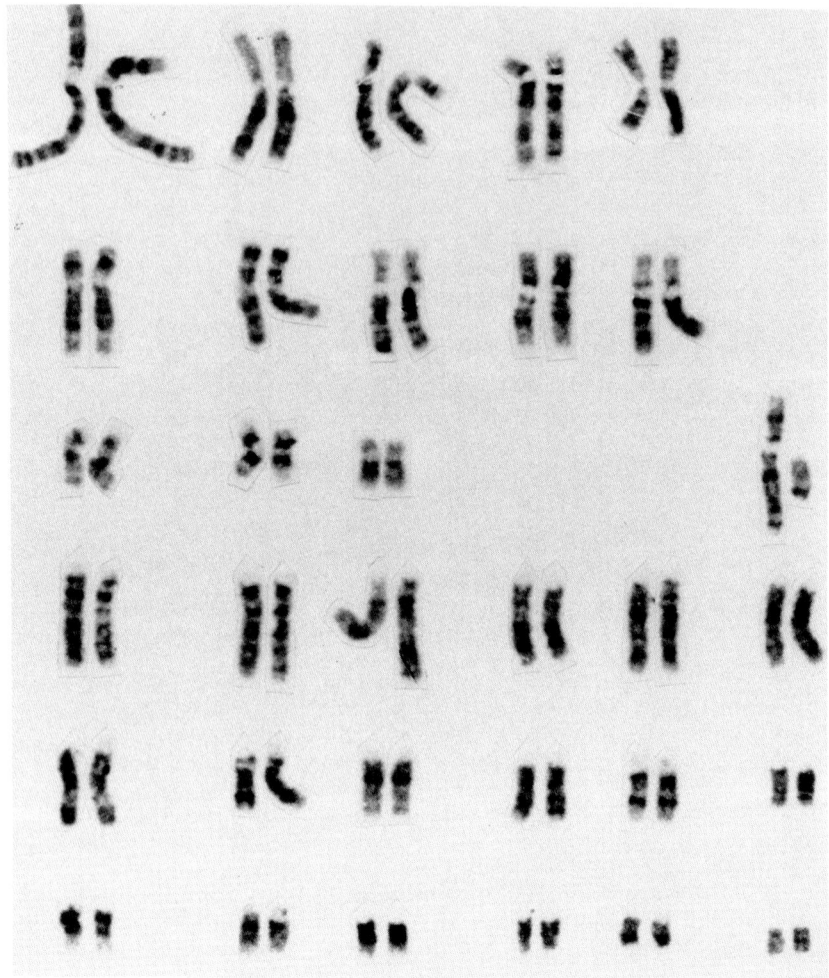

FIG. 3. A GTG-banded normal male karyotype.

chromosome in the female (Figs. 4 and 5b). Consecutive QFQ/RBG banding has been applied to identify homologous chromosomes with Q-, G-, and R-banding (see Section III,b).

4. C-Banding

Reports of C-banding of centromeric heterochromatin by techniques using barium hydroxide (CBG) were reported by Melchior and Hohn

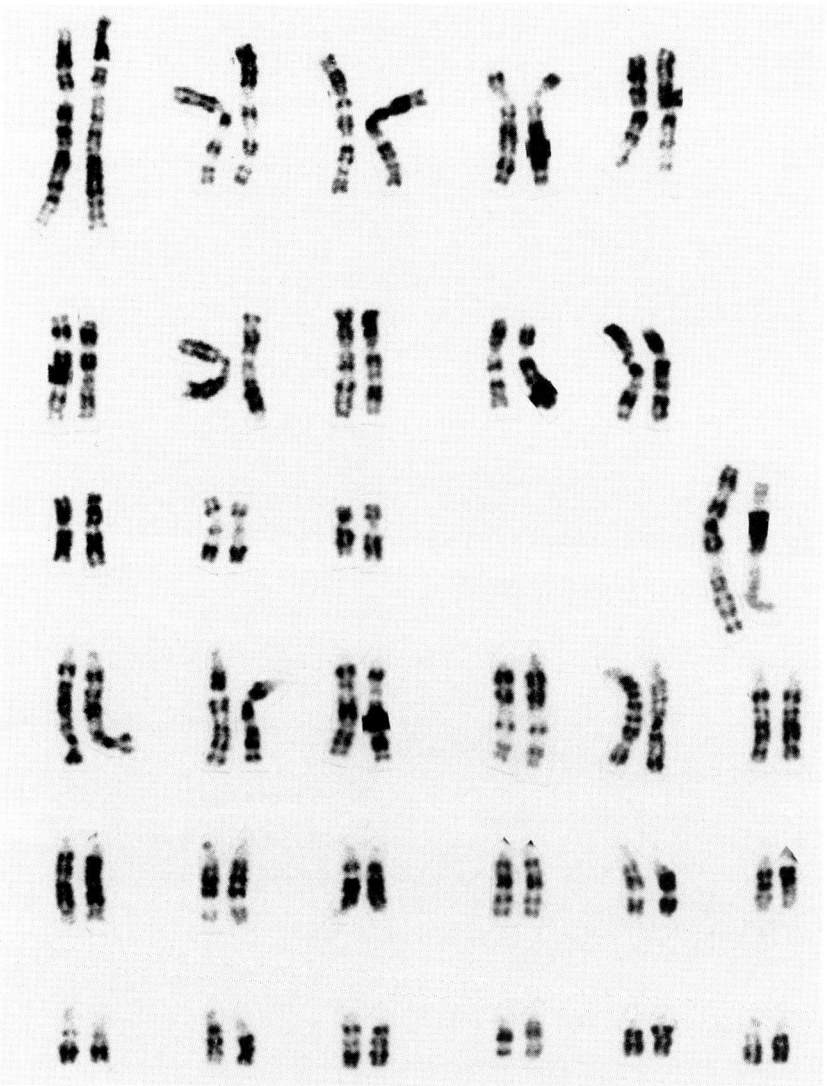

FIG. 4. An RBG-banded normal female karyotype.

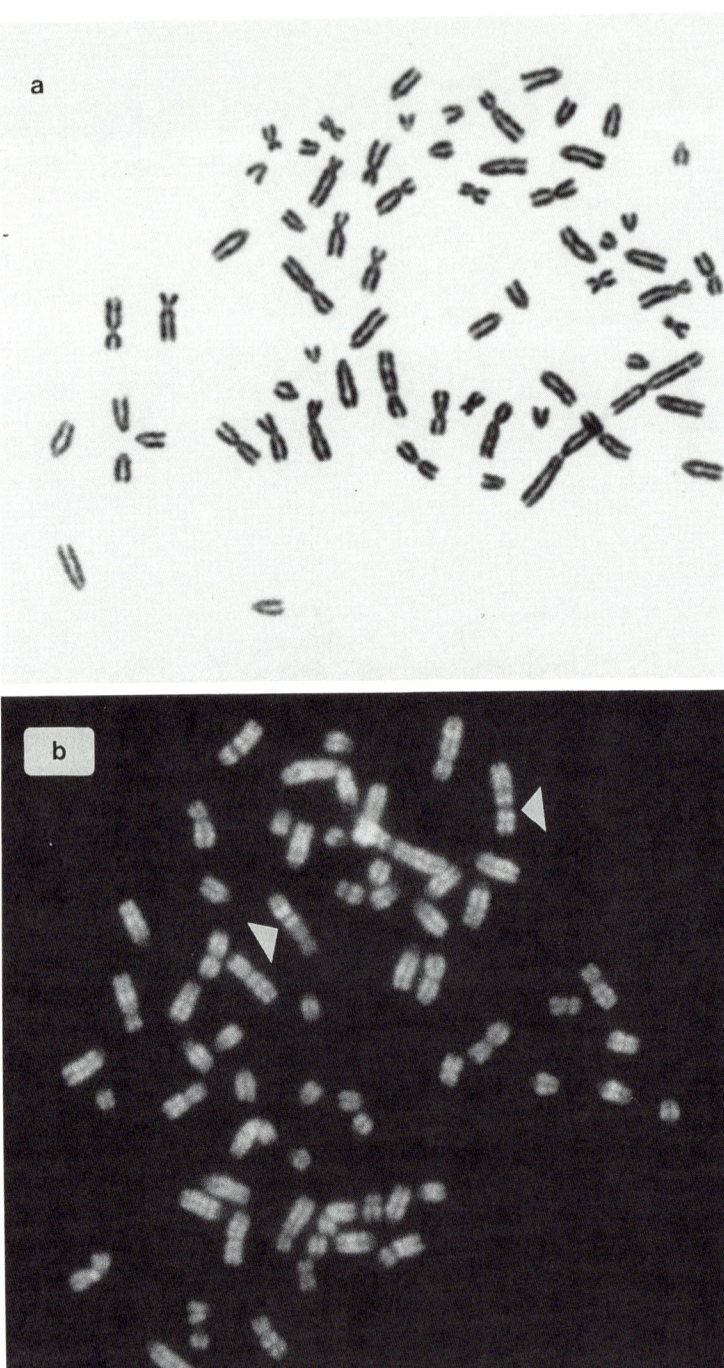

(1976), Buckland et al. (1976), Cribiu and De Giovanni (1978), and Power (1987a). A CBG-banded metaphase is shown in Fig. 6a. The X chromosome is distinctive in having a variably sized interstitial C-band on the long arms. The Y chromosome consists almost entirely of constitutive heterochromatin. Chromosome 1 has small C-bands on the telomeres of the short arms. Chromosome 11 shows virtually no centromeric staining. Chromosome 12 may show an interstitial band on the long arms and both chromosome 12 and 13 may show a considerable variation in C-band size between homologues. A large polymorphism for the amount of centromeric heterochromatin in chromosome 1 has been reported by Haynes and Reisner (1982). Application of C-banding is particularly useful in identifying the sex chromosomes in the horse. However, because the interstitial C-band of the X chromosome may vary by being very small in some cases, caution should be exercised in identifying the X chromosomes solely using a C-banding technique (Power, 1987a; Long, 1988).

5. NOR Banding

Staining of the nucleolar organizer regions (NORs) of the chromosomes of the horse has been reported by Sysa et al. (1977), Wockl et al. (1980), Kopp et al. (1981), Cribiu (1981), and Gadi and Ryder (1983). Kopp et al. (1981), using a consecutive GTG/NOR banding technique, were first to report six chromosomal sites for the NORs on three chromosome pairs. Power (1987a), using consecutive NOR/GTG and NOR/RBG banding techniques, confirmed this finding. Both authors observed that the occurrence of silver-stained NORs varied between four and six per cell (Fig. 6b). Satellite associations are frequently observed between them. According to the Paris Conference (1989) (Richer et al., 1990), the NOR-bearing sites are identified as the telomeric region of the short arms of chromosomes 1 and the secondary constriction region of chromosomes 28 and 31, with the NORs on the chromosome 28 pair being variably expressed.

The staining of NORs in any given metaphase is usually considered to relate to cell activity; that is, the only NORs stained were those that were actively transcribing during the preceding interphase (Miller et al., 1976). The variation in the rate of occurrence of satellite association between the NOR-bearing chromosomes is not thought to be sig-

---

FIG. 5. (a) Giemsa-stained female metaphase spread. (b) An RBH-banded female metaphase with Hoechst 33258 fluorescence showing early and late-replicating (pale-staining) X chromosomes (arrowheads).

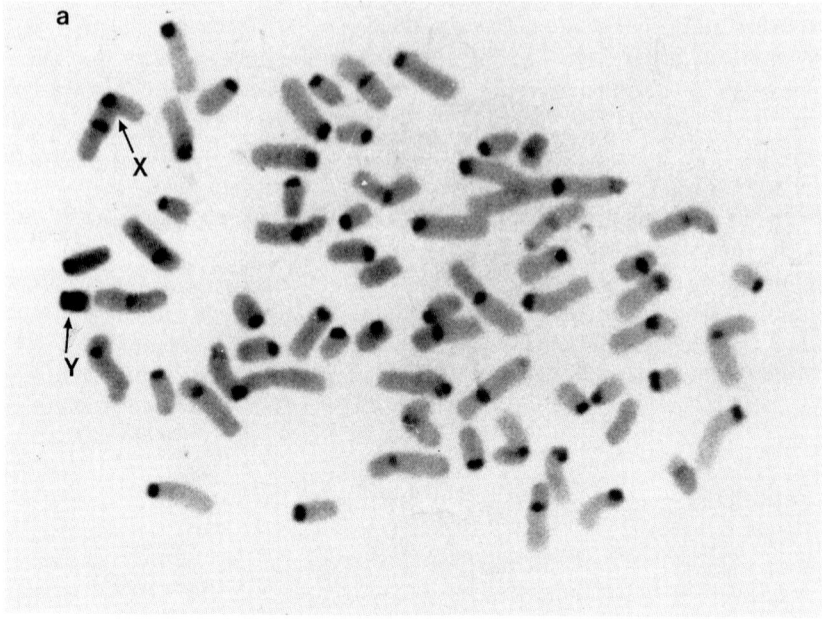

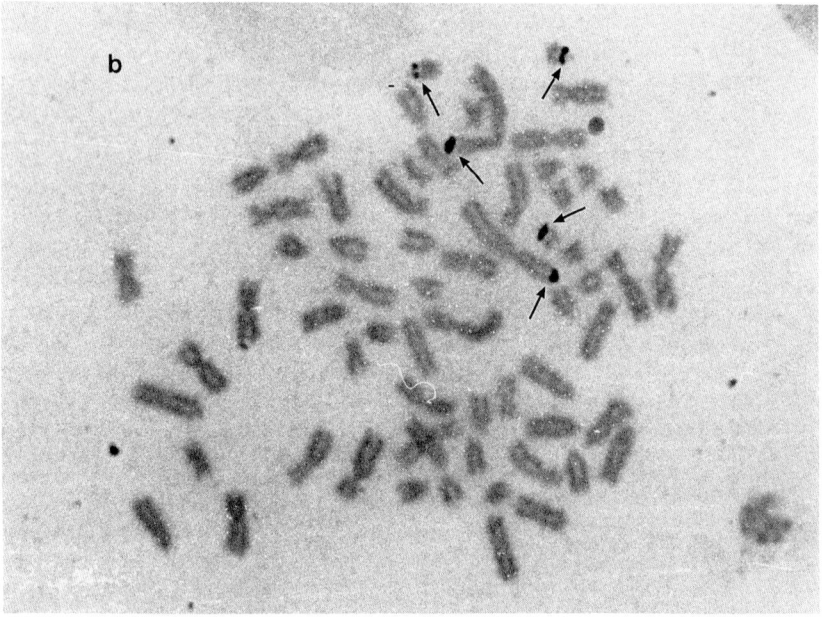

FIG. 6. (a) A CBG-banded male metaphase with X and Y chromosomes. (b) Metaphase showing five positive NOR-banded regions (arrows).

nificant; the satellite associations appear to be no more than remnants of the nucleolus and are possibly influenced by technical procedures for chromosome preparation (Zakharov et al., 1982).

6. *Electron Microscopy*

A method for the banding of horse chromosomes that allows their examination with the electron microscope is described by Richer et al. (1989).

III. The Normal Horse Karyotype

A. Chromosome Morphology

When the 64 chromosomes of the horse are stained by methods that do not produce bands (e.g., Giemsa or orcein stain), they appear as biarmed, metacentric, or submetacentric chromosomes or uniarmed acrocentric chromosomes. The female karyotype has 13 pairs of metacentric or submetacentric autosomes and 18 pairs of acrocentric autosomes plus a large pair of submetacentric X chromosomes. The male has a similar autosomal pattern plus one large submetacentric X and one small acrocentric Y chromosome. None of the chromosomes can be positively identified with this conventional staining method, but some morphological features, such as the satellites on the telomeres of the short arms of the largest chromosome pair and secondary constrictions at the proximal region of two small acrocentric chromosome pairs, can frequently be observed (Fig. 5a). These are the sites of the NORs described in Section II,C,5.

B. Reading Conference (1976)

This was the first conference for the standardization of banded karyotypes of domestic animals (Ford et al., 1980). An international committee decided on a standardized format for the presentation of the G-banded horse karyotype. It retained the term telocentric for acrocentric chromosomes. Although no measurements of total length or centromeric index of individual chromosomes were published, their use was inferred by the placement of chromosomes into metacentric, submetacentric, subtelocentric, or telocentric groups. Of the 31 autosome pairs, 4 were placed in the submetacentric group (1–4); 8, in the metacentric group (5–12); 1, in the subtelocentric group (13); and 18, in the telocentric group (14–31), according to decreasing size. The X chromosome was reported as a large metacentric and the Y as a small telocentric chromosome. The number of bands observable in the karyotype accompanying the report, using the haploid set (31 autosomes, plus X and Y chromosomes) (Harnden and Klinger, 1985), is approximately 215. This report also included a description of the main G-bands and a numbering system for the chromosome pairs.

C. Measurement and Idiograms of Chromosomes

Measurements of unbanded chromosomes were reported by De Giovanni et al. (1979), G-banded chromosomes were reported by Melchior and Hohn (1976) and Stranzinger (1980), and R-banded chromosomes were reported by Molteni et al. (1982). Measurements made on Giemsa-stained chromosomes that had been preidentified with QFQ banding were reported by Hansen (1984a) and Power (1987A). Both of these reports included calculation of the centromeric index according to Levan et al. (1964). These indicated that, on the basis of total length or centromeric index, some chromosomes had been incorrectly described in the Reading Conference report. Such findings, together with a generally expressed wish by those working with and publishing the horse karyotype to try to make it more compact, formed the basis of the changes decided on at the Paris Conference (1989) (Section III,D).

Idiograms of G-banded chromosomes have been reported by Stranzinger (1980), Maciulis et al. (1984), and Power (1987a). R-Banded idiograms have been reported by Molteni et al. (1982), Power (1987a), and Romagnano et al. (1987).

D. Paris Conference (1989)

The karyotypes presented in Figs. 1a–4 are according to the Paris Conference (1989) report (Richer et al., 1990). The committee decided that chromosomes pairs 14–31 should more correctly be described as acrocentric and that their placement should remain as that for the Reading Conference. As measurement of centromeric index showed that chromosome 13 (Reading) was submetacentric and not telocentric, it was decided that it should be placed within the group of biarmed chromosomes (pairs 1–13), which had been shown to be either metacentric or submetacentric. As this entailed a placement and number change for most of the chromosomes within this group it was decided to rearrange all the biarmed chromosomes simply according to decreasing size. These new measurements also showed the X chromosome to be submetacentric and the second largest chromosome in the karyotype. The decision to place the sex chromosome pair on the third line further improved the overall compactness of the karyotype, which had been desired. Measurements were based on consecutive QFQ/Giemsa-stained chromosomes showing approximately 250 bands per haploid set (Harnden and Klinger, 1985). Submissions to the committee of consecutive QFQ/RBG-banded karyotypes also allowed the identification of homologous G- and R-banded chromosomes (Figs. 3 and 4).

Recent improvements in techniques are affording greater definition of the chromosomes of the horse. In Figs. 3 and 4, the G- and R-banded karyotypes show approximately 500 bands, respectively, per haploid set (Harnden and Klinger, 1985).

E. Variants in the Karyotype

1. C-Band and NOR-Band Variants

The C-band and NOR-band variants are discussed in Sections II,C,4 and II,C,5, respectively.

2. Chromosome 12 and 13 Variants

With G- and R-banding, a variation equivalent to the C-band variant may be observed in the pericentromeric region of chromosomes 12 and 13, which may cause considerable size difference within these pairs (Fig. 3).

3. X Chromosome Variants

The interstitial negative G-band on the long arms of the X chromosome, equivalent to the C-band at that site, may also show considerable variation. An XXX female karyotype in Fig. 2a shows two X chromosomes with large negative G-bands and one X chromosome with a small negative G-band.

4. Y Chromosome Length Variation

A possible variation in the length of the Y chromosome was suggested, either from measurement or observation, in reports by Stranzinger (1980), Scott and Long (1980), Murer-Orlando et al. (1982b), and Hansen (1984b). This finding was confirmed in a larger study of 31 animals by Power (1988). The largest Y chromosome was more than twice the length of the smallest Y chromosome measured using a Y:X ratio. The group studied included 20 clinically normal controls and 11 with various clinical abnormalities. Although no clinical significance could be attributed to the length variations observed, a tentative breed association was suggested.

IV. Clinical Application of Cytogenetics in the Horse

A. INTRODUCTION

The most important effects of abnormal karyotypes are their contribution to lowered reproductive performance, either through a decreased ability or complete failure to produce functional gametes, to embryonic death, and to congenital malformation. Of these clinical areas the most extensively studied in the horse to date has been that of primary infertility in the mare. Results show that a remarkable 50–60% of mares with gonadal dysgenesis have an abnormal chromosome pattern (Blue et al., 1978; Bowling et al., 1987). This is analogous to human data in which chromosome abnormality has been detected in 50% of women with a history of primary amenorrhoea (Jacobs et al., 1961).

Many factors make cytogenetic investigation in the horse different and perhaps more difficult than that in other domestic species. The fact that this is a sport animal, usually of high economic value, makes the value judgments of veterinarians and stud farm managers different from those of their counterparts dealing with other species. Cooperation for cytogenetic investigation may not be so readily forthcoming. In cases of possible impairment of fertility or congenital abnormality, owners may be wary that the finding of a chromosome aberration may reflect on the pedigree of the sire or the dam. However, if desired, the acceptance of coded samples should help to overcome this problem.

The reproductive efficiency of horses has commonly been considered to be lower than that of other large domestic animals. Only about two-thirds of mares mated per year produce a live foal (Jeffcott et al., 1982). In some breeds, such as the Thoroughbred, that are monitored carefully, there appears to have been no improvement in the foaling rate in this century, despite many advances in veterinary medicine ("General Stud Book," 1989, and previous volumes). There is also a decrease in foaling rate with increasing maternal age. A study of reproductive performance in the Thoroughbred breed showed that live foaling rates decreased from 84.7% in 2- to 4-year-old mares to 42.6% at 17 years or more (Badi et al., 1981). Platt (1979) also reported an increase in congenital abnormalities in the foals of older mares. Although the exigencies of modern stud practice, including the arbitrary January 1 birthdate for many breeds, may be indicated as limiting the natural mating opportunities and the optimum mating season for the mare, other factors such as chromosome abnormality must also be suspected to contribute to the overall 30–40% reproductive loss in the mare. The diagnosis of a chromosome abnormality early in a mare's reproductive history would save very expensive time spent uselessly at stud.

Subsequent to the production of a live foal, selection for athletic performance increases the wastage substantially in this species. Figures for foaling losses often include those animals euthanatized because it is considered that their congenital abnormalities would affect their eventual athletic performance (Platt, 1979). Jeffcott et al. (1982) has estimated for the Thoroughbred a total wastage from conception until their arrival at the track at 4 years to be 72.2%. This represents an enormous economic loss in this species. The vast majority of cytogenetic investigations to date have been done in mares. As the majority of male horses are gelded, they are unlikely to come under the type of clinical scrutiny that leads to or warrants chromosome analysis. However, those few who are chosen as stallions are selected on the basis of athletic performance and not on fertility. These animals can frequently have tremendously high monetary value and it would seem only a matter of ordinary prudence to establish the chromosome complement of a valuable stallion before putting him to stud.

Sections II,A and II,B outline reports of successful techniques for investigating meiotic chromosomes, the chromosomes of early embryos, abortion material, and perinatal death in the horse. The application of these techniques will hopefully lead to clinical studies in these areas, which have been almost completely uninvestigated to date. The updated standard for the horse karyotype (Paris Conference, 1989) (Section III,D) should also be strictly adhered to in cytogenetic reports.

Table I lists 47 studies that included clinical and cytogenetic reports about the horse between 1968 and 1989. In these studies, 1,377 animals were investigated and 401 were found to be chromosomally abnormal. The latter represented 27 different types of chromosome abnormalities, which are outlined and cross-referenced in Table II. Twenty-four different breeds were represented in this group, of which the vast majority were Thoroughbred or Arabian (Table III).

B. CHROMOSOME ABNORMALITIES REPORTED IN THE HORSE

Only those chromosome abnormalities identified by banding will be discussed. A few further cases of probable translocation, isochromosome or deletion, unidentified by banding, have been included for completeness, in the references in Tables I and II.

TABLE I

SUMMARY OF SOME CLINICAL STUDIES ON ANIMAL CHROMOSOME ABNORMALITIES

Author (year)	Total number of animals studied	Number with chromosome abnormality	Author (year)	Total number of animals studied	Number with chromosome abnormality
(1) Payne et al. (1968)	1	1	(24) Metenier and Cribiu (1980)	157	1
(2) Basrur et al. (1970)	1	1	(25) Blue (1981a)	68	0
(3) Marx et al. (1973)	42	0	(26) Dunn et al. (1981)	2	2
(4) Dunn et al. (1974)	1	1	(27) Cribiu and Losfeld (1982)	2	2
(5) Chandley et al. (1975b)	9	7	(28) Halnan et al. (1982)	17	17
(6) Hughes et al. (1975a)	5	5	(29) Buoen et al. (1983)	146	36
(7) Hughes et al. (1975b)	2	2	(30) Cribiu (1984)	7	7
(8) Taylor and Trommerhausen-Smith (1975)	14	6	(31) Halnan (1985)	24	11
(9) Queinnec et al. (1975)	1	1	(32) Power (1986)	1	1
(10) Gluhovschi et al. (1975)	1	1	(33) Kent et al. (1986)	64	38
			(34) Makinen et al. (1986)	1	1
(11) Kieffer et al. (1976)	1	1	(35) Bowling et al. (1987)	251	124
(12) McIlwraith et al. (1976)	1	1	(36) Power (1987a)	179	6
			(37) Power (1987b)	6	2
(13) Fretz and Hare (1976)	1	1	(38) Gill et al. (1988)	1	1
(14) Hughes and Trommerhausen-Smith (1977)	12	12	(39) Long (1988)	36	3
			(40) Stewart-Scott (1988)	5	5
			(41) Herzog et al. (1988)	1	1
(15) Blue et al. (1978)	1	1	(42) Klunder et al. (1989)	1	1
(16) Bruère et al. (1978)	13	7	(43) Bowling and Millon (1989)	2	2
(17) Trommerhausen-Smith et al. (1979)	28	21	(44) Klunder and McFeely (1989)	130	49
(18) Metenier et al. (1979)	1	1	(45) Long (1989)	17	8
(19) Miyake et al. (1979)	3	3	(46) Moreno-Milan et al. (1989)	1	1
(20) Walker and Bruère (1979)	112	5	(47) Power and Leadon (1990)	1	1
(21) Bielanski et al. (1980)	5	1			
(22) Hohn et al. (1980)	1	1			
(23) Sharp et al. (1980)	1	1			
			Total	1,377	401

1. Translocation

An unbalanced X/autosome translocation, 64,X,−X,+der(X),t(-Xp;15q), was reported in an infertile mare (Power, 1987b) (Fig. 2c). The loss of one short-arm X chromosome and the spread of inactivation into the attached autosomal segment would explain the clinical presentation, which was somewhat similar to the simple X,del(Xp) mares reported by Bowling et al. (1987) (Section IV,B,2). None of the human patients reported with unbalanced X/autosome translocations involving the loss of Xp has been fertile (Keitges and Palmer, 1986).

TABLE II

Types of Chromosome Abnormalities and Number of Cases Reported in Table I Studies

Type of chromosome abnormality	Number of cases reported	Reference number of study from Table I
Translocation	6	(1, 9, 33, 37, 41, 43)
? Isochromosome	4	(29, 41, 43)
Deletion	5	(28, 35)
Autosomal trisomy	4	(37, 42, 43)
Unbalanced X/autosome translocation	1	(37)
X,del(Xp)	4	(35)
63,X	142	(5, 6, 7, 8, 14, 15, 16, 17, 18, 19, 20, 24, 27, 29, 31, 34, 35, 36, 39, 44, 45)
63,X/64,XX	62	(5, 6, 7, 14, 16, 17, 20, 27, 28, 29, 30, 31, 33, 35, 39, 40, 44, 45)
64,[XX/65,XX + fragment 65,XXX]	1	(5)
65,XXX	11	(5, 29, 35, 36, 40, 44, 46)
66,XXXXY	1	(10)
64,XX/65,XXX	1	(38)
63,X/64,XX/65,XXX	1	(45)
63,X/64,XY	13	(14, 17, 26, 28, 33, 35)
64, XX/64XY	11	(12, 26, 29, 31, 44)
64,XX/65,XXY	6	(10, 21, 28, 35)
63,X/65,XYY	1	(22)
63,X/64,X, − Y, + t(YqYq)	1	(41)
63,X/64,XX/64,XY	1	(40)
63,X/64,XY/65,XXY	2	(28, 44)
63,X/64,XX/65,XXY	1	(13)
64,XX/64,XY/65,XXY	1	(4)
64,XX/96,XXY	1	(47)
63,X/64,XX/64,XY/65,XXY	1	(2)
63,X/64,XX/65,XXX/65,XXY/ 66,XXY/66XXYY	1	(44)
64,XY sex reversal	109	(5, 11, 14, 23, 29, 30, 32, 33, 35, 36, 39, 40, 44, 45)

A translocation between two long-arm Y chromosomes was reported as 63,X/64,X, − Y, + t(YqYq) in a pseudohermaphrodite foal (Herzog *et al.*, 1988). The origin of this chromosome rearrangement could also be an isochromosome for the long arms of Y.

An autosomal trisomy resulting from a centric fusion translocation or isochromosome for the long arms of two number 26 chromosomes

TABLE III

Horse Breeds Investigated Cytogenetically in Table I Studies

Breed	Number investigated	Breed	Number investigated
Argentinian Polo Pony	1	Peruvian Paso	1
Appolosso	6	Pony	16
Arabian	193	Quarter Horse	34
Belgian	1	Selle Francais	42
Clydesdale/ Percheron	1	Spanish	1
Connemara Pony	2	Standardbred	14
Falabella	2	Stock Horse	4
Finnish	1	Suffolk Punch	1
French Draught	2	Tennessee Walking Horse	2
French Trotter/Trotter	10	Thoroughbred	459
Morgan	2	Welsh Pony	5
Nonius	1	Breed not stated	574
Paso Fino	2		
		Total	1,377

was reported by Bowling and Millon (1989) (Fig. 2d). This case will be discussed in Section IV,B,3.

2. Deletion

Four mares with a deletion of the short arms of one of the X chromosome pair, 64,X,del(Xp), were reported by Bowling et al. (1987) (Fig. 2b). Two of these mares presented with small stature and poor conformation, similar to that described in the 63,X mares (Section IV,B,4). One showed occasional estrous but never went in foal. At 5 years old, the second mare, after pasture service to a pony, produced a filly foal with the same karyotype as her dam. This report is important in documenting the possibility of both fertility and infertility associated with the del(Xp) condition in the horse.

In 12 human patients the phenotype of Xp deletion ranged from the typical Turner's syndrome, with gonadal dysgenesis and/or short stature, to a normal female phenotype. Three of these patients who were fertile produced both chromosomally normal offspring and those with del(Xp) (Fryns et al., 1981, 1983). Genetic counseling should therefore include consideration of both the possibility of fertility and of having genotypically and phenotypically normal offspring in mares with Xp deletion.

3. Autosomal Trisomy

Autosomal trisomy is well documented in humans. It represents about 50% of chromosomally abnormal abortions (Boue et al., 1975). In fetuses that survive to term, the highest incidence is 1 in 650 births for trisomy 21 (Down's syndrome) and the incidence of all autosomal trisomies seems to be increased with increasing maternal age. At birth, human trisomics invariably have multiple congenital abnormalities and, in those syndromes compatible with survival beyond the neonatal period, physical and mental retardation are consistently observed. It can also be observed that there seems to be a greater viability for those human trisomies that occur in the smaller chromosome groups (Goodman and Gorlin, 1983). This observation has also been made in cattle (Mayr et al., 1985).

The recent description of the first four autosomal trisomies in the horse has indicated that they also may make a significant contribution to congenital malformation in the horse. It is interesting also to note that these viable trisomics have involved the smaller acrocentric chromosomes.

a. Trisomy 23. A 1-year-old Standardbred colt with several developmental defects, including rough hair, failure to thrive, pronounced facial asymmetry, strabismus and small testes, was reported as trisomic for chromosome 23 (65,XY, + 23) (Klunder et al., 1989).

b. Trisomy 26. A Thoroughbred filly born to a 3-year-old mare was assessed at 1 year because of atypical poor conformation and lack of vigor. She had small stature, angular leg deformities, an unusual stiff gait, and was physically inactive. She also appeared mentally dull. Chromosome analysis revealed a *de novo* trisomy for chromosome 26 due either to a centric fusion translocation [64,XX, − 26, + t(26q26q)] or isochromosome formation [i(26q)] (Fig. 2d). At age 5 years she foaled a karyotypically normal colt (Bowling and Millon, 1989).

This first reported case of fertility would indicate that the potential for reproduction in the equine autosomal trisomic may be similar to that of the female Down's syndrome in the human (Masterson et al., 1970).

c. Trisomy 28. A halfbred colt born to a 14-year-old Thoroughbred mare was assessed at 2 years of age because of extremely small stature and cryptorchidism. He showed normal libido but no sperm was observed in the ejaculate. His general behavior was considered to be abnormal. Chromosome analysis showed trisomy for chromosome 28 (65,XY, + 28) (Power, 1987b) (Fig. 1a).

Analysis of semen samples in a number of cases of human male

Down's syndrome have shown azoospermia, and the remaining cases showed subnormal sperm counts (Stearns et al., 1960). Results from conventional meotic studies and synaptonemal complex analysis using electron microscopy on the testes of this trisomy 28 horse demonstrated oligospermy that was due to degenerations at the spermatocyte and spermatid levels. A trivalent was present that in 50% of cells examined showed heterologous pairing between the free axis of the trivalent and the sex bivalent (Power et al., 1990) (Fig. 1b). In other studies it has been proposed that this interference with the sex bivalent prevents the inactivation of the X chromosome, resulting in disturbances of sperm production (Lifschytz and Lindsley, 1972).

d. Trisomy 30. An Arabian filly, born to a 23-year-old mare, was assessed at 1 year because of small stature and atypical poor conformation. She was born prematurely with severe angular deviations and mild polydactyly of the forelimbs. She was mentally alert with no behavioral problems. Chromosome analysis showed trisomy for chromosome 30 (64,XX, +30). The occurrence of this trisomic foal was associated with advanced maternal age (Bowling and Millon, 1989).

4. 63,X (Turner's Syndrome)

Table II includes 142 cases of 63,X; it is the most frequently reported chromosome abnormality in the horse. These mares are frequently small for their age and breed and show either irregular or absent estrus cycles and small gonads lacking follicular development. Poor body conformation has also occasionally been observed. All the mares so far reported have been infertile. In one study, 68% of infertile mares showed sex chromosome abnormality (Blue et al., 1978). In a 12-year study by Bowling et al. (1987), chromosome abnormality was detectable in 98 (54.4%) of 180 mares with gonadal dysgenesis, of which 56 (31%) were 63,X.

The X chromosome monosomy has sporadically been reported in many mammalian species (Johnson et al., 1983). The X monosomy of human Turner's syndrome was first described by Ford et al. (1959) in a female with short stature and gonadal dysgenesis resulting in primary amenorrhoea and infertility. The incidence of pure X monosomy in human liveborn females is about 1 in 9,000, representing half of the genotypes associated with the Turner's syndrome phenotype (Hook and Warburton, 1983). By contrast, it can be estimated that this is the most common chromosome abnormality in man, with an incidence near conception of 1–1.5% and a mortality of 99%. This mortality is almost entirely in the form of early abortion, accounting for 15% of the 50% chromosomally abnormal abortuses (Boue et al., 1975). Ovarian development is normal up to the third month of embryonic development, followed by a high rate of atrasia and dysgenic "streak" gonads by puberty (Polani, 1981). The exceptional cases of fertility in human Turner's syndrome suggest that the number of germ cells that survive into adulthood may vary among individuals or be due to undetected mosaicism.

By contrast, X monosomy mice are fertile, although Burgoyne and Baker (1981) have reported oocyte depletion and a shortened reproductive life in X monosomy mice compared to their XX sibs. The difference in oocyte depletion in human and murine cases may largely be a matter of generation time. Blue et al. (1978) have reported atretic Graffian follicles and apparently functional luteal tissue in the ovary of a 63,X mare. As generation time is shorter in the horse than in man, the finding of an occasional fertile 63,X mare would not be surprising, particularly if breeding occurs at a young age.

The X chromosome monosomy has not yet been shown to be associated with increased prenatal mortality in the horse, as has been described for the human. However, the possible contribution of production and mortality of 63,X embryos to embryonic loss in the horse may be suspected.

5. 63,X/64,XX

Sixty two cases of 63,X/64,XX mosaicism have been reported in 18 different studies, making this the third most frequently reported chromosome anomaly in the horse (Table II). The majority of these X/XX mosaic mares have been reported from groups of phenotypically normal mares with gonadal dysgenesis. Their clinical description frequently closely resembles that of the pure 63,X mare in having normal external genitalia, flaccid cervix, and small inactive ovaries. Some evidence of follicular activity was reported in two cases (Hughes et al., 1975b; Bruère et al., 1978), but none was reported to be fertile. However, of 10 X/XX mosaic mares reported by Halnan (1985), six had been in foal once. The author suggests that these mares may be subfertile at best, as none have so far produced a second foal.

Results from human embryonic and liveborn studies indicate a greater viability for the X/XX embryos than for the X monosomy embryos, and that up to 75% of liveborn mosaics may go undetected because their phenotype is so mild they would not be suspected of having a chromosome abnormality (Hook and Warburton, 1983). The X/XX human patients can span the phenotypic spectrum from complete Turner's syndrome phenotype to clinical normality compatible with normal menarche and repeated childbirth. Kohn et al. (1980) have estimated that 21% of X/XX human females may have spontaneous menses that may, however, be of short duration, terminating in early menopause, and have an increased risk of chromosome abnormality in the progeny. The few cases of X/XX mosaicism so far described in cattle have been infertile (Swartz and Vogt, 1983).

Present data would suggest that the X/XX mosaic horse may have a similar range of clinical expression. Diagnosis of this condition in mares may have an important prognostic value for their reproductive potential.

6. 63,X/64,XY

Thirteen cases of 63,X/64,XY mosaicism have been reported in the horse (Table II). Two of these cases presented as intersex individuals, one with ovotestes (Dunn *et al.*, 1981; Halnan *et al.*, 1982). These are in contrast to three further cases that presented simply as mares with gonadal dysgenesis (Hughes and Trommershausen-Smith, 1977; Trommershausen-Smith *et al.*, 1979). These findings may indicate that, as reported for the human (Hamerton, 1971), X/XY mosaicism may present variably in this species, also from females with gonadal dysgenesis to pseudohermaphroditism in a group of "mixed gonadal dysgenesis."

7. 65,XXX and 64,XX/65,XXX

Eleven cases of trisomy X, 65,XXX, have been reported in the horse (Table II). Very few clinical data are available on most of this group, but it is assumed that they were assessed because of fertility problems and are otherwise clinically unremarkable. In two cases of mares with very small apparently inactive ovaries, no normal cycle was observed, but both produced a follicle on one occasion (Chandley *et al.*, 1975b; Power, 1987a). All cases reported to date have ben infertile. One case of XX/XXX mosaicism apparently cycled normally but was infertile (Gill *et al.*, 1988).

In the human, the incidence of XXX is 1 in 1,000 female births. Although most of this group are merely assessed because of fertility problems, some are found among the subnormal or mentally ill and about one-third have congenital or developmental defects. Ovarian function may range from severe ovarian dysplasia to apparently normal fertility, with the majority in the subfertile range showing delayed menarche to premature menopause. The majority of offspring have been chromosomally normal, but occasional occurrences of sex chromosome trisomies have been reported (Polani, 1981). A similar range of ovarian function has been reported in six cases of XXX cattle (Swartz and Vogt, 1983).

It may be, therefore, that some XXX mares with normal or subfertility do exist but have gone undetected so far in the general population.

8. Intersexuality

Thirty further cases in Table II were sex chromosome mosaics or chimeras reported in various cases of intersexuality or male pseudohermaphroditism in the horse. The occurrence of these mixaploids seems to make a significant contribution to clinical abnormality in the horse. Some bias of ascertainment might be inferred due to the ease with which deviant sexual development can be clinically detected. Most of the reported cases presented as apparent females with varying degrees of virilization of the external genitalia. Other animals presenting initially with cryptorchidism showed varying deficiencies of testicular development.

Some of the 11 XX/XY mosaic cases were reported without clinical details, but two cases were considered to be whole-body chimeras, probably resulting from fusion of male and female embryos. These true hermaphrodites presented as males with cryptorchidism, underdevelopment of the external genitalia, and the presence of ovotestes (McIlwraith *et al.*, 1976; Dunn *et al.*, 1981). By contrast, cytogenetically confirmed XX/XY blood chimeras in equine heterosexual twins indicated that this condition did not affect sexual development of the female co-twin or her subsequent fertility, as has been reported in cattle and sheep (Podliachouk *et al.*, 1974; Greene *et al.*, 1977; Power *et al.*, 1985).

An intersex foal with a normal diploid (64,XX) chromosome pattern in lymphocyte culture and a mosaic diploid/triploid (64,XX/96,XXY) pattern of probable chimeric origin in skin fibroblast culture indicated that it may be important to examine a second cell line in some clinical conditions (Power and Leadon, 1990) (Fig. 1c). Five cases of intersexuality have been reported with a normal 64,XX sex chromosome constitution (Bornstein, 1967; Gerneke and Coubrough, 1970; Miyake *et al.*, 1982). This group may represent a true XX intersex condition in horses, as reported for other species (Lyon *et al.*, 1981). Two further cases of intersexuality that were atypical for their genotypes were reported in a 65,XXX mare (Moreno-Millan *et al.*, 1989) and a 63,X mare (Kent *et al.*, 1989). In the latter case, application of a DNA probe suggested the presence of a Y chromosome fragment that was not detectable cytogenetically.

9. 64,XY Sex Reversal

Table II documents 109 cases of the 64,XY sex reversal syndrome in phenotypic mares with variable clinical presentation. Although this is not a chromosome abnormality per se, the finding of a normal male karyotype, 64,XY, is diagnostic for mares in this group and is generally associated with infertility.

A few cases, analogous to the testicular feminization syndrome in humans, have been reported in the horse. These are infertile mares with masculine behavior, normal external genitalia, a blind-ending vagina, and abdominal testes. A familial pattern of inheritance was observed in one pedigree (Kieffer et al., 1976; Bowling et al., 1987). In the human it has been shown to be caused by an X-linked *Tfm* mutant gene (Meyer et al., 1975).

The phenotypic spectrum of the remaining majority of XY mares ranges from the feminine mare, with an apparently normal reproductive tract, to the greatly virilized mare. The horse is, so far, unique in having even exceptional cases of fertility reported within this group. The progeny of these few mares have been reported as normal XY male, normal XX female, and one XY female (Sharp et al., 1980; Kent, 1989).

Of six pedigrees reported by Kent et al. (1986), five showed an X-linked or autosomal sex-limited dominant transmission through the female, similar to the transmission of XY gonadal dysgenesis in human pedigrees (Polani, 1981). A further pedigree indicated transmission through the sire. These authors suggest that the etiology might be an autosomal sex-limited dominant or a Y chromosome mutation with variable expression. A familial hypothesis was also considered for a stallion siring XY females in another pedigree. These authors considered that one hypothesis to explain the mechanism of the effect would be a translocation of Y chromosome material to an autosome (Bowling et al., 1987). An interesting historical paper by Levens (1911) reports examination of 15 foals, with defectively developed sexual organs, that were sired by the same stallion out of different mares.

Sporadic reports of XY sex reversal throughout the horse population may suggest a *de novo* occurrence in some cases. Cases of XY gonadal dysgenesis, without masculinization, would seem very difficult to distinguish clinically from that of the immature mare or those with 63,X or 65,XXX genotypes. Chromosomes analysis is therefore important not just to determine a cause for infertility but to indicate a possible familial involvement in some cases and aid in the possible elimination of this genetic condition from breeding herds.

V. Horse Breeds and Interspecific Hybrids

A. The Evolution of the Domestic Horse

The taxonomy of the domestic horse, *Equus caballus,* places it in the order Perissodactyla, which are hoofed animals with an uneven number of toes. These include the family Equidae (horses, asses, and zebras), the family Rhinocerotidae (rhinoceroses), and the family Tapiridae (tapirs). The phylogeny of the Equidae is based on a very rich paleontological record. The Eocene epoch saw the emergence of the ancestor of the horse family, the "dawn horse," *Eohippus,* over 50 million years ago, and according to Simpson (1951) the present extant species of the Equidae emerged during the Pleistocene epoch over 3 million years ago. Overall, the Perissodactyla are represented by karyotypes with diploid chromosome numbers ranging from 84 in the black rhinoceros, consisting mainly of acrocentric chromosomes, to 32 in the mountain zebra, with mainly metacentric chromosomes (Hungerford *et al.,* 1967; Benirschke and Malouf, 1967).

The genus *Equus* includes seven living species, *E. caballus* (ECA; domestic horses), *Equus prezwalski* (EPR; Prezwalski's wild horse), *Equus asinus* (EAS; African wild asses and their domestic relatives), *Equus hemionus* (EHE; Asiatic wild asses or onagers), *Equus grevyi* (EGR; Grevy's zebra), *Equus burchelli* (EBU; common zebras), and *Equus zebra* (EZE; mountain zebras). The species acronyms are according to Harnden and Klinger (1985). Matthey (1945) has defined the "nombre fondamental" (NF) as the number of chromosome arms that is constant for a given group. In the Equidae, the diploid chromosome number varies from 66 in EPR to 32 in EZE and the NF varies from 102 in EAS and EHE to 62 in EZE (Ryder *et al.,* 1978). Using such data, Bush *et al.* (1977) have calculated that the Equidae exhibit the fastest rate of karyotype evolution and speciation among the mammals. The extent of the karyotypic diversity in the Equidae suggest that chromosomal changes were at least concomitant with speciation and may have contributed to it (Benirschke and Malouf, 1967).

B. The Domestic Horse Breeds

Horses were first domesticated in Asia about 3,000 BC and probably descended from many local races. There are about 60 recognized breeds in the world today (Simpson, 1951). The studies listed in Table I report cytogenetic investigation of at least one member of 24 different breeds among 1,377 animals (Table III). Apart from recognized variants (Section III,E) and chromosome changes associated with clinical abnormality (Section IV,B), the karyotype appears to be stable in all these breeds and in the Polish primative horse, or tarpan (Rudek, 1981).

One further cytogenetic study has been done on 17 Caspian ponies from the north of Iran. From their conformation, these animals are considered to be minature horses rather than ponies. Eleven animals showed a karyotype similar to that of the domestic horse and six others had a karyotype of a hybrid between the domestic horse and the Prezwalski wild horse. Based on historical and cytogenetic evidence, these animals were considered to be the product of a natural hybridization between these two species. It is interesting, by comparison with fertility reduction associated with centric fusion variants in other species, that despite free access to the stallions the conception rate in the mares of this breed was never more than 40%. Problems of ovulation were noted in the mares and low sperm counts and poor sperm motility were noted in the stallions (Gustavsson, 1971; Hatami-Monazah and Pandit, 1979).

C. Comparative Equine Studies

Prior to the application of banding techniques, equine species with widely divergent karyotypes were found to have a similar DNA content. This, and the ability of the Equidae to produce interspecific hybrids, suggested that the overall genetic content was reasonably constant and that structural rearrangement of the chromosomes must account for the remarkable changes in karyotype and diploid number (Benirschke and Malouf, 1967).

Ryder et al. (1978) complied the first comparative report of G- and C-banded karyotypes in the seven extant equine species. The overall results confirmed a close similarity of the karyotype of EPR and ECA, which mainly differed by just one centric fusion translocation, and of the karyotypes of EBU and EGR. No chromosome was found to be precisely homologous in all seven species. The types of chromosome rearrangement identified were centric fusion/fission and pericentric inversion. A later study in the horse, donkey, and zebra with R-banding indicated some further chromosome homologies that had been rearranged by centric fusion and paracentric and pericentric inversion (Power, 1984). In particular, these studies identified a pericentric inversion differentiating the horse and donkey X chromosome. This difference had formed the basis of the classic experiments using the mule and hinny model to test the hypotheses of the randomness of choice of

X chromosome to be late replicating in mammalian cells (Hamerton and Giannelli, 1970; Power et al., 1982).

D. HYBRIDIZATION IN THE EQUIDAE

An unusual feature of the Equidae is their remarkable ability to produce hybrids among virtually all the member species, regardless of significant chromosomal differences. The types of hybrid crosses that have so far been successfully produced, including a description of their phenotypes and recorded fertility, have been summarized by Gray (1971). The best known of these, due of course to human interest in their production since antiquity, are the mule and the hinny. The mule is the result of a cross between a female horse and a male donkey (ECA × EAS) and the hinny is the result of the reciprocal cross (EAS × ECA) (Harnden and Klinger, 1985). Mules are more frequently bred because of their larger size. The mule and other equine hybrids are of particular interest because of their contribution to our understanding of the taxonomic relationships among the various species and to the study of the notorious infertility of most of these hybrids, or perhaps more importantly how exceptional cases of fertility might occur.

A detailed investigation of testicular meiosis in a mule and hinny has shown abnormalities of chromosome pairing in most germ cells at the pachytene stage of meiotic prophase. Spermatogenesis was almost totally arrested but a few mature spermatozoa were observed in the ejaculate of epididymal flushings of the hinny. The possibility of fertility would probably be excluded in those male interspecific hybrids due to the low number of spermatozoa produced. In contrast, the domestic mare/Prezwalski horse hybrid was fertile and showed normal spermatogenesis (Chandley et al., 1975a; Chandley, 1981).

A histological study of the development of germ cells in the ovaries of fetal, neonatal, and adult mules and hinnies also indicated that most oogonia died early in neonatal life as they entered meiosis. However, an occasional oocyte was observed that could give rise to a Graffian follicle (Taylor and Short, 1973). Recently, two cytogenetically confirmed female mules and one female hinny have been reported to have had foals. One was the product of a female mule and male donkey cross that had a mulelike chromosome complement, suggesting that the mother had donated a haploid set of horse chromosomes (Ryder et al., 1985). This case would fit the theory of "affinity" invoked by Chandley (1981) to explain how fertility might be achieved. However, the two further foals of a female mule and hinny, each mated to a mule donkey, have been reported to have a "mixed" chromosome complement, indicating that affinity of ancestral haploid chromosome sets may not be the only possibility for production of a viable ovum in the female mule (Rong et al., 1988).

The almost limitless hybridization among the Equidae favors their close taxonomic standing. The fact that horses, asses, and zebras hybridize quite easily without abnormalities in the development of the offspring would indicate that the genetic distance between the different species is much smaller than one would expect on the basis of karyotype divergence and that only the technical difficulties at meiosis in hybrids cause sterility.

ACKNOWLEDGMENTS

This work was funded in part by an Eolas Research Grant to M. M. Power. Sincere thanks are due to Ms. Geraldine Barrett for the typing of this manuscript.

REFERENCES

Badi, A. M., O'Byrne, T. M., and Cunningham, E. P. (1981). An analysis of reproductive performance in Thoroughbred mares. *Ir. Vet. J.* **35**, 1–12.

Basrur, K., Kanagawa, H., and Podilachouk, L. (1970). Further studies on the cell populations of an intersex horse. *Can. J. Comp. Med.* **34**, 294–306.

Benirschke, K., and Malouf, N. (1967). Chromosome studies of Equidae. *Equus* **1**, 253–284.

Benirschke, K., Brownhill, L. E., and Beath, M. M. (1962). Somatic chromosomes of the horse, the donkey and their hybrids the mule and the hinny. *J. Reprod. Fertil.* **4**, 319–326.

Bielanski, W., Kleczkowska, A., Tichner, M., and Jagiarz, M. (1980). Comparative cytogenetic examinations of parents and siblings of a colt with a false masculine hermaphroditism. *Med. Weter.* **36**, 492–494.

Blue, M. G. (1981a). Studies of the chromosomes and sex chromatin in the horse. *Theriogenology* **15**, 277–293.

Blue, M. G. (1981b). A cytogenetical study of prenatal loss in the mare. *Theriogenology* **15**, 295–309.

Blue, M. G., Bruère, A. N., and Dewes, H. F. (1978). The significance of the XO syndrome in infertility of the mare. *N. Z. Vet. j.* **26**, 137–141.

Bornstein, S. (1967). The genetic sex of two intersexual horses and some notes on the karyotype of normal horses. *Acta Vet. Scand.* **8**, 291–300.

Boue, J., Boue, A., and Lazar, P. (1975). The epidemiology of human spontaneous abortions. *In* "Aging Gametes" (R. J. Blandau, ed.) pp. 330–348. Karger, London.

Bowling, A. T., and Millon, L. V. (1989). Two autosomal trisomies in the horse: 64,XX,i(26?) and 65,XX,+30. *North Am. Colloq. Cytogenet. Domest. Anim.*, 6th, Purdue, Abstr., p. 12.

Bowling, A. T., Millon, L., and Hughes, J. P. (1987). An update of chromosomal abnormalities in mares. *J. Reprod. Fertil., Suppl.* **35**, 149–155.

Bruère, A. N., Blue, M. G., Jaine, P. M., Walker, K. S., Henderson, L. M., and Chapman

H. M. (1978). Preliminary observations on the occurrence of the equine XO syndrome. *N. Z. Vet. J.* **26,** 145–146.

Buckland, R. A., Fletcher, J. M., and Chandley, A. C. (1976). Characterization of the domestic horse *(Equus caballus)* karyotype using G- and C-banding techniques. *Experientia* **32,** 1146–1149.

Buoen, L. C., Kent, M. G., Madi, J., and Weber, A. F. (1983). Variety of cytogenetic anomalies encountered during a two year period in a veterinary cytogenetics laboratory. *North Am. Symp. Cytogenet. Cell Biol. Domest. Animals, 3rd,* Abstr., p. 246.

Burgoyne, P. S., and Baker, T. G. (1981). Oocyte depletion in XO mice and their XX sibs from 12 to 200 days *post partum. J. Reprod. Fertil.* **61,** 207–212.

Bush, G. L., Case, S. M., Wilson, A. C., and Patton, J. L. (1977). Rapid speciation and chromosomal evolution in mammals. *Proc. Natl. Acad. Sci. U.S.A.* **74,** 3942–3946.

Chandley, A. C. (1981). Does 'affinity' hold the key to fertility in the female mule. *Genet. Res.* **37,** 105–109.

Chandley, A. C., Short, R. V., and Allen, W. R. (1975a). Cytogenetic studies of three equine hybrids. *J. Reprod. Fertil., Suppl.* **23,** 365–370.

Chandley, A. C., Fletcher, J., Rossdale, P. D., Peace, C. K., Ricketts, S. W., McEnery, R. J., Thorne, J. P., Short, R. V., and Allen, W. R. (1975b). Chromosome abnormality as a cause of infertility in mares. *J. Reprod. Fertil., Suppl.* **23,** 377–383.

Chaudhary, B., and Kovacs, A. (1987). Simple lymphocyte cultivation method for horse chromosome studies. *J. Dairy Sci.* **70,** Suppl. 1, 241.

Cribiu, E. P. (1981). Localisation des organisateurs nucléotaires dans les chromosomes du cheval domestique *(Equus caballus). Ann. Genet. Sel. Anim.* **13,** 177–180.

Cribiu, E. P. (1984). Quelques cas de dysgenesie gonadique chez la jument causes par différentes aberrations gonosomiques (monosomie X, mosaique X/XX et caryotype XY). *Genet. Sel. Evol.* **16,** 397–404.

Cribiu, E. P., and De Giovanni, A. (1978). Le Caryotype du cheval domestique *(Equus caballus),* de l'ane *(Equus asinus)* et du mullet par le méthode de bande C. *Ann. Genet. Sel. Anim.* **10,** 161–170.

Cribiu, E. P., and Losfeld, P. (1982). Two further cases of XO and XO/XX chromosome constitution in mares. *Proc. Eur. Colloq. Cytygenet. Domest. Anim., 5th,* Milan, pp. 318–323.

De Giovanni, A., Molteni, G., Succi, G., Castiglioni, M., and Cribiu, E. P. (1979). The idiogram of the domestic horse (*Equus caballus* L.). *Caryologia* **32,** 215–222.

Dunn, H. O., Vaughan, J. T., and McEntee, K. (1974). Bilaterally cryptorchid stallion with female karyotype. *Cornell Vet.* **64,** 265–275.

Dunn, H. O., Smiley, D., Duncan, J R., and McEntee, K. (1981). Two equine true hermaphrodites with 64,XX/64,XY and 63,XO/64,XY chimaerism. *Cornell Vet.* **71,** 123–135.

Ford, C. E., Jones, K. W., Polani, P. E., DeAlmeida, J. C., and Briggs, J. H. (1959). A sex chromosome anomaly in a case of gonadal dysgenesis (Turner's Syndrome). *Lancet* **1,** 711–713.

Ford C. E., Pollock D. L., and Gustavsson I. (1980). Proceedings of the First International Conference for the Standardization of Banded Karyotype of Domestic Animals, University of Reading, Reading, England, 2–6 August. 1976. *Hereditas,* **92,** 145–162.

Fretz, P. B., and Hare, W. C. D. (1976). A male pseudohermaphrodite horse with 63,XO?/64,XX/65,XXY mixaploidy. *Equine Vet. J.* **8,** 130–132.

Fryns, J. P., Petit, P., and Van Den Berghe, H. (1981). The various phenotypes in Xp deletion. Observations in eleven patients. *Hum. Genet.* **57,** 385–387.

Fyrns, J. P., Kleczkowska, A., Petit, P., and Van Den Berghe. H. (1983). Fertility in patients with X-chromosome deletion. *Clin. Genet.* **23,** 212.

Gadi, I. K., and Ryder, O. A. (1983). Distribution of silver-stained nucleolus-organising regions in the chromosomes of the Equidae. *Genetica* **62,** 109–116.

"General Stud Book" (1989). Vol. 41. Weatherbys, Wellingborough, Northants, England.

Gerneke, W. H., and Coubrough, R. I. (1970). Intersexuality in the horse. *Onderstepoort J. Vet. Res.* **37,** 211–216.

Gill, J. J. B., Kempski, H. M., Hallows, B. J., and Warren, A. M. (1988). A 64,XX/65,XXX mosaic mare *(Equus caballus)* and associated infertility. *Equine Vet. J.* **20,** 128–130.

Gluhovschi, N., Bistriceanu, M., and Palicica, R. (1975). Les troubles de la reproduction chez les animaux domestiques dus à des modifications du genome. *Cah. Med. Vet.* **44,** 155–163.

Goodman, R. M., and Gorlin, R. J. (1983). "The Malformed Infant and Child." Oxford Univ. Press, London and New York.

Gray, A. P. (1971). "Mammalian Hybrids." Commonwealth Agricultural Bureau, England.

Greene, W. A., Dunn, H. O., and Foote, R. H. (1977). Sex chromosome ratios in cattle and their relationship to reproductive development in freemartins. *Cytogenet. Cell Genet.* **18,** 97–105.

Gustavsson, I. (1971). Culling rates in daughters of sires with a translocation of centric fusion type. *Hereditas* **67,** 65–74.

Hageltorn, M., and Gustavsson, I. (1974). The application of new banding techniques in the identification of individual chromosome pairs in domestic animals. *Proc. World Congr. Genet. Appl. Livest. Prod., 1st,* Madrid, Part 3, pp. 203–211.

Halnan, C. R. E. (1985). Sex chromosome mosaicism and infertility in mares. *Vet. Rec.* **116,** 542–543.

Halnan, C. R. E., Watson, J. I., and Pryde, L. C. (1982). Detection by G- and C-band karyotyping of gonosome anomalies in horses of different breeds. *J. Reprod. Fertil., Suppl.* **32,** 627–628.

Hamerton, J. L. (1971). "Human Cytogenetics," Vol. 2. Academic Press, London.

Hamerton, J. L., and Giannelli, F. (1970). Non-random inactivation of the X chromosome in the female mule. *Nature (London)* **228,** 1322–1323.

Hansen, K. M. (1984a). The relative length of Q-band/Giemsa stained horse chromosomes. *Proc. Eur. Colloq. Cytogenet. Domest. Anim., 6th,* Zurich, pp. 165–171.

Hansen, K. M. (1984b). Two different lengths of the Y chromosome of the domestic horse *(Equus caballus). Proc Eur. Colloq. Cytogenet. Domest. Anim., 6th,* Zurich, pp. 172–176.

Hare, W. C., and Singh, E. L. (1979). "Cytogenetics in Animal Reproduction." Commonwealth Agricultural Bureaux, England.

Harnden, D. G., and Klinger, H. P. (1985). "An International System for Human Cytogenetic Nomenclature (1985)." Karger, New York.

Hatami-Monazah, H., and Pandit, R. V. (1979). A cytogenetic study of the Caspian pony. *J. Reprod. Fertil.* **57,** 331–333.

Hayes, S. E., and Reisner, A. H. (1982). Cytogenetic and DNA analysis of equine abortion. *Cytogenet. Cell Genet.* **34,** 204–214.

Herzog, A., Hohn, H., and Hecht, W. C. (1988). A 63,XO/64,XYY t(Y;Y) mosaic in a foal. *Proc. Eur. Colloq. Cytogenet. Domest. Anim., 8th,* Bristol, pp. 60–65.

Hohn, H. (1967). Uber die moglichkeiten der karyotypbestimmung post mortem bein kalb. Veterinary Medicine Dissertation, University of Giessen.

Hohn, H., Klug, E., and Rieck, G. W. (1980). A 63,XO/65,XYY mosaic in a case of questionable equine male pseudohermaphroditism. *Proc. Eur. Colloq. Cytogenet. Domest. Anim., 4th,* Uppsala, pp. 82–92.

Hook, E. B., and Warburton, D. (1983). The distribution of chromosomal genotypes associated with Turner's Syndrome: Livebirth prevalence rates and evidence for diminished fetal mortality and severity in genotypes associated with structural X abnormalities or mosaicism. *Hum. Genet.* **64,** 24–27.

Hsu, T. C. (1952). Mammalian chromosomes *in vitro. J. Hered.* **43,** 167–172.

Hughes, J. P., and Trommershausen-Smith, A. (1977). Infertility in the horse associated with chromosomal abnormalities. *Aust. Vet. J.* **53,** 253–257.

Hughes, J. P., Benirschke, K., Kennedy, P. C., and Trommershausen-Smith, A. (1975a). Gonadal dysgenesis in the mare. *J. Reprod. Fertil., Suppl.* **23,** 385–390.

Hughes, J. P., Kennedy, P. C., and Benirschke, K. (1975b). XO-Gonadal dysgenesis in the mare (report of two cases). *Equine Vet. J.* **7,** 109–112.

Hungerford, D. A., Chandra, H. S., and Synder, R. L. (1967). Somatic chromosomes of the black rhinoceros (*Diceros bicornis*, Gray 1821). *Am. Nat.* **101,** 357–358.

Jacobs, P. A., Harnden, D. G., Buckton, K. E., Court-Brown, W. M., king, M. J., McBride, J. A., MacGregor, T. N., and Maclean, N. (1961). Cytogenetic studies in primary amenorrhoea. *Lancet* **i,** 1183–1189.

Jeffcott, L. B. (1977). Clinical haematology in the horse. *In* "Comparative Clinical Haematology" (R. K. Archer and L. B. Jeffcott, eds.), pp. 161–312. Blackwell, Oxford.

Jeffcott, L. B., Rossdale, P. D., Freestone, J., Frank, C. J., and Towers-Clark, P. I. (1982). An assessment of wastage in Thoroughbred racing from conception to 4 years of age. *Equine Vet. J.* **14,** 185–198.

Johnson, S. D., Buoen, L. C., Madl, J. E., Weber, A. F., and Smith, F. C. (1983). X-chromosome monosomy (37,XO) in a burmese cat. *J. Am. Vet. Med. Assoc.* **182,** 986–989.

Keitges, E. A., and Palmer, C. G. (1986). Analysis of spreading of inactivation in eight X autosome translocations utilizing the high resolution RBG technique. *Hum. Genet.* **72,** 231–236.

Kent, M. G. (1989). Fertility among XY sex reversed mares. *North Am. Colloq. Cytogenet. Domest. Anim., 6th,* Purdue, Abstr., p. 16.

Kent, M. G., Shoffner, R. N., Buoen, L., and Weber, A. F. (1986). XY sex-reversal syndrome in the domestic horse. *Cytogenet. Cell Genet.* **42,** 8–18.

Kent, M. G., Schroder, W., and Jones, K. W. (1989). Diagnosis of a Y fragment in an XO mare and fertility in an XO/XX mare: Two case histories. *North Am. Colloq. Cytogenet. Domest. Anim., 6th,* Purdue, Abstr., p. 13.

Kieffer, N. M., Burns, S. J., and Judge, N. G. (1976). Male pseudohermaphroditism of the testicular feminising type in a horse. *Equine Vet. J.* **8,** 38–41.

King, W. A., Bezard, J., Bousquet, J., Palmer, E., and Betteridge, K. J. (1987). The meiotic stage of preovulatory oocytes in the mare. *Genome* **29,** 679–682.

Kirillow, S. (1912). Cited by Painter (1924).

Klunder, L. R., and McFeely, R. A. (1989). Chromosome analysis of 130 equine clinical cases. *North Am. Colloq. Cytogenet. Domest. Anim., 6th,* Purdue p. 8.

Klunder, L. R., McFeely, R. A., Beech, J., McClune, W., and Bilinski, W. F. (1989). Autosomal trisomy in a Standardbred colt. *Equine Vet. J.* **21,** 69–70.

Kohn, G., Yarkoni, S., and Cohen, M. M. (1980). Two conceptions in a 45,X women. *Am. J. Med. Genet.* **5,** 339–343.

Kopp, E., Mayr, B., Czaker, R., and Schleger, W. (1981). Nucleous organiser regions in the chromosomes of the domestic horse. *J. Hered.* **72,** 357–358.

Lear, T. L., Bennett, D. S., Behling, H., Foster, W. R., and Jackson, S. G. (1989). The analysis of metaphase chromosomes from equine amniocytes. *North Am. Colloq. Cytogenet. Domest. Anim., 6th,* Purdue, p. 5.

Levan, A., Fredga, K., and Sandberg, A. A. (1964). Nomenclature for centromeric position on chromosomes. *Hereditas* **52,** 201–220.

Levens, H. (1911). Einige falle vaon pseudohermaphroditismus beim pferd. *Monatsh. Prakt. Tierheilkd.* **22,** 267–273.

Lifschytz, E., and Lindsley, D. L. (1972). The role of X-chromosome inactivation during spermatogenesis. *Hereditas* **94,** 235–240.

Long, S. E. (1988). Chromosome anomalies and infertility in the mare. *Equine Vet. J.* **20,** 89–93.

Long, S. E. (1989). Chromosome analysis and infertility in the horse: Analysis of laboratory results 1985–March 1989. *North Am. Colloq. Cytogenet. Domest. Anim., 6th,* Purdue, p. 7.

Lyon, M. F., Cattanach, B. M., and Charlton, H. M. (1981). Genes affecting sex differentiation in mammals. *In* "Mechanisms of Sex Differentiation in Animal and Man" (C. R. Austin and R. G. Edwards, eds.), pp. 329–386. Academic Press, New York.

Maciulis, A., Bunch, T. D., Shupe, J. L., and Leone, N. C. (1984). Detailed description and nomenclature of high resolution G-banded horse chromosomes. *J. Hered.* **75,** 265–268.

Makinen, A., Katila, T., and Kuokkanen, M. (1986). XO syndrome in the mare. *Nord. Veterinaermed.* **38,** 16–21.

Makino, S. (1942). The chromosomes of the horse *(Equus caballus). Cytologia* **13,** 26–38.

Makino, S., Sofuni, T., and Sasaki, M. S. (1963). A revised study of the chromosomes of the horse, the ass and the mule. *Proc. Jpn. Acad.* **39,** 176–181.

Marx, M. B., Menlyk, J., Persinger, G., Ohno, S., McGee, W., Kaufman, W., Pessin, A., and Gillespie, R. (1973). Cytogenetics of the superhorse. *J. Hered.* **64,** 95–98.

Masterson, J. G., Law, E. M., Power, M. M., Stokes, B. M., and Murphy, D. (1970). Reproduction in two females with Down's Syndrome. *Ann. Genet.* **13,** 38–41.

Masui, K. (1919). Cited by Painter (1924).

Matthey, R. (1945). L'évolution de la formule chromosomiale chez les vertèbres. *Experienta* **1,** 50–56, 78–86.

Mayr, B., Krutzler, H., Auer, H., Schleger, W., Sasshofer, K., and Glawischnig, E. (1985). A viable calf with trisomy 22. *Cytogenet. Cell Genet.* **39,** 77–79.

McIlwraith, C. S., Owen, R. A., and Basrur, P. K. (1976). An equine cryptorchid with testicular and ovarian tissues. *Equine Vet. J.* **8,** 156–160.

Melchior, I., and Hohn, H. (1976). Der Karyotyp des pferdes *(Equus caballus)* dargestellt mit hilfe der G- und C-banden technik. *Giessener Beitr. Erbpathol. Zuchthyg.* **6,** 179–194.

Metenier, L., and Cribiu E. P. (1980). First report on chromosomal examination of racehorses in France. *Proc. Eur. Colloq. Cytogenet. Domest. Anim., 4th,* Uppsala, pp. 390–393.

Metenier, L., Driancourt, M. A., and Cribiu, E. P. (1979). An XO chromosome constitution in a sterile mare. *Ann. Genet. Sel. Anim.* **11,** 161–163.

Meyer, W., Migeon, B. R., and Migeon, C. J. (1975). Focus on X chromosome for dihydrotestosterone receptor and androgen insensitivity. *Proc. Natl. Acad. Sci. U.S.A.* **72,** 1469–1472.

Miller, O. J., Miller, D. A., Dev, V. G., Tanjravahi, R., and Croce, C. M. (1976). Expression of human and supression of mouse nucleolus activity in mouse human somatic cell hybrids. *Proc. Natl. Acad. Sci. U.S.A.* **73,** 4531–4535.

Miyake, Y. I., Ishiwaka, T., and Kawata, K. (1979). Three cases of mare sterility with sex chromosome abnormality (63,X). *Zuchthygiene* **14,** 145–150.

Miyake, Y. I., Inoue, T., Kanagawa, H., Satoh, H., and Ishikawa, T. (1982). Four cases of anomalies of genital organs in horses. Zentralbl. Veterinaermed., Reihe A **29,** 602–608.

Molteni, L., Cribiu, E. P., De Giovanni-Machi, A., Beltrami E., and Succi, G. (1982). Thre R-banded karyotype of the domestic horse. *Proc. Eur. Colloq. Cytogenet. Domest. Anim. 5th,* Milan, pp. 353–367.

Moorhead, P. S., Nowell, P. C., Mellman, W. J., Battips, D. M., and Hungerford, D. A. (1960). Chromosome preparations of leucocytes cultured from human peripheral blood. *Exp. Cell Res.* **20,** 613–616.

Moreno-Millan, M., Delgado Bermejo, J. V., and Lopez Castillo, G. (1989). An intersex horse with X chromosome trisomy. *Vet. Rec.* **124,** 169–170.

Moses, M. J., Counce, S. J., and Paulson, D. F. (1975). Synaptonemal complex complement of man in spreads of spermatocytes with details of the sex chromosome pair. *Science* **187,** 363–365.

Murer-Orlando, M., Richer, C.-L., and Betteridge, K. J. (1982a). Giemsa R-banded chromosomes of the domestic horse. *Proc. Eur. Colloq. Cytogenet. Domest. Anim., 5th,* Milan, pp. 345–352.

Murer-Orlando, M., Betteridge, K. J., and Richer, C.-L. (1982b). Cytogenetic sex determination in cultured cells of pre-attachment horse embryos. *Proc. Eur. Colloq. Cytogenet. Domest. Anim., 5th,* Milan, pp. 372–378.

Painter, T. S. (1924). Studies in mammalian spermatogenesis. *J. Exp. Zool.* **39,** 229–247.

Paul, J. (1975). "Cell and Tissue Culture." Livingstone, Edinburgh.

Payne, H. W., Ellsworth, K., and DeGroot, A. (1968). Aneuploidy in an infertile mare. *J. Am. Vet. Med. Assoc.* **153,** 1293–1299.

Platt, H. (1979). "A Survey of Perinatal Mortality and Disorders in the Thoroughbred." Animal Health Trust, Newmarket, England.

Podliachouk, L., Vandeplassche, M., and Bouters, R. (1974). Gestation gemellaire, chimerisme et freemartinisme chez le cheval. *Acta Zool. Pathol. Antverp.* **58,** 13–28.

Polani, P. E. (1981). Abnormal sex development in man. I. Anomalies of sex determining mechanisms. *In* "Mechanisms of Sex Differentiation in Animals and Man" (C. R. Austin and R. G. Edwards, eds.), pp. 465–547. Academic Press, New York.

Power, M. M. (1984). Comparative R banding in the horse, donkey and zebra. *Proc. Eur. Colloq. Cytogenet. Domest. Anim., 6th,* Zurich, pp. 145–155.

Power M. M. (1986). XY sex reversal in a mare. *Equine Vet. J.* **18,** 233–236.

Power, M. M. (1987a). The chromosomes of the horse. Karyotype definition, clinical applications and comparative interspecies studies. Ph.D. Thesis, National University of Ireland.

Power, M. M. (1987b). Equine half sibs with an unbalanced X;15 translocation or trisomy 28. *Cytogenet. Cell Genet.* **45,** 163 168.

Power, M. M. (1988). Y chromosome length variation and its significance in the horse. *J. Hered.* **79,** 311–313.

Power, M. M., and Leadon, D. P. (1990). Diploid–triploid chimaerism (64,XX/96,XXY) in an intersex foal. *Equine Vet. J.* **22,** 211–214.

Power, M. M., De Arce, M. A., and Masterson J. G. (1982). Reassessment of late replication of the X chromosome in mules and hinnies using bromodeoxyuridine. *Proc. Eur. Colloq. Cytogenet. Domest Anim., 5th,* Milan, pp. 336–344.

Power, M. M., Hanrahan, S., and O'Reilly, P. (1985). Cytogenetic assessment of chimaerism in infertile sheep. *J. Dairy Sci.* **68,** Suppl. I, 250.

Power, M. M., Gustavsson, I., Switonski, M., and Ploen, L. (1990). Synaptonemal complex analysis of an autosomal trisomy in the horse. *Cytogenet. Cell Genet.* (in press).

Queinnec, G., Berland, H. M., Darre, R., and Carlotti, D. (1975). Anomolie chromosomique chez un cheval. *Rev. Med. Vet.* **38,** 323–327.

Richer, C.-L., and Romagnano, A. (1985). Cell synchronization and dynamic G-banding of equine chromosomes by bromodeoxyuridine. *J. Hered.* **76,** 375–376.

Richer, C.-L., Drouin, R., and Messier, P. E. (1989). Banding of horse chromosomes for electron microscopy. *North Am. Colloq. Cytogenet. Domest. Anim., 6th,* Purdue, Abstr., p. 15.

Richer, C. L., Power, M. M., Klunder, L. R., McFeely, R. A., and Kent, M. G. (1990). Standard karyotype of the domestic horse *(Equus caballus). Hereditas,* in press.

Romagnano, A., King, W. A., Richer, C.-L., and Perrone, M. A. (1985). A direct technique for the preparation of chromosomes from early equine embryos. *Can. J. Genet. Cytol.* **27.** 365–369.

Romagnano, A., Richer, C.-L., King, W. A., and Betteridge, K. J. (1986). Analysis of X-chromosome inactivation in pre-attachment equine embryos. *Int. Symp. Equine Reprod., 4th,* Abstr., p. 69.

Romagnano, A., Drouin, R., and Richer, C.-L. (1987). Idiograms of horse chromosomes at prometaphase, early metaphase and midmetaphase after R-banding by BrdU incorporation followed by the fluorochrome–photylysis–Giemsa technique. *Genome* **29,** 674–679.

Rong, R., Chandley, A. C., Song, J., McBeath, S., Tan, P. P., Bai, Q., and Speed, R. M. (1988). A fertile mule and hinny in China. *Cytogenet. Cell Genet.* **47,** 134–139.

Rothfels, K. H., Alexrad, A. A., Siminovitch, L., and McCulloch Parker, R. C. (1959). The origin of altered cell lines from mouse, monkey and man, as indicated by chromosome and transplantation studies. *Proc. Can. Cancer Res. Conf.* **3,** 189–214.

Rudek, Z. (1981). Description of the Polish primative horse *(Equus gmelini, forma silvatica* vet.) karyotype using G- and C-banding techniques. *Folia Biol. (Krakow)* **29,** 59–63.

Ryder, O. A., Epel, N. C., and Benirschke, K. (1978). Chromosome banding studies of the Equidae. *Cytogenet. Cell Genet.* **20,** 323–350.

Ryder, O. A., Chemnick, L. G., Bowling, A. T., and Benirschke, K. (1985). Male mule foal qualifies as the offspring of a female mule and a jack donkey. *J. Hered.* **76,** 379–381.

Scott, I. S., and Long, S. E. (1980). An examination of chromosomes in the stallion *(Equus caballus)* during meiosis. *Cytogenet. Cell Genet.* **26,** 7–13.

Sharp, A. J., Wachtel, S. S., and Benirschke, K. (1980). H-Y antigen in a fertile XY female horse. *J. Reprod. Fertil.* **58,** 157–160.

Simpson, G. G. (1951). "Horses." Oxford Univ. Press, New York.

Stearns, P. E., Droulard, K. E., and Sahhar, F. H. (1960). Studies bearing on fertility of male and female mongoloids. *Am. J. Ment. Defic.* **65,** 37–41.

Stewart-Scott, I. (1988). Infertile mares with chromosome abnormalities. *N. Z. Vet. J.* **36,** 63–65.

Stranzinger, G. (1980). Zytogenetik im dienste der nutztierzucht. *Jahrb. Schweiz. Naturforsch. Ges. Wiss.* **3,** 68–79.

Swartz, H. A., and Vogt, D. W. (1983). Chromosome abnormality as a cause of reproductive inefficiency in heifers. *J. Hered.* **74,** 320–324.

Sysa, P. S., Hohn, H., and Schmidt, I. (1977). Nucleolus organisers in chromosomes of some domestic animals. *Ann. Genet. Sel. Anim.* **9,** 540–541 (abstr.).

Taylor, M. J., and Short, R. V. (1973). Development of the germ cells in the ovary of the mule and the hinny. *J. Reprod. Fertil.* **32,** 441–445.

Taylor, M. J., and Trommershausen-Smith, A. (1975). Equine karyotyping. *Proc. Int. Symp. Equine Hematol., 1st,* pp. 124–131.

Trommershausen-Smith, A., Hughes, J. P., and Neeley, D. P. (1979). Cytogenetic and clinical findings in mares with gonadal dysgenesis. *J. Reprod. Fertil., Suppl.* **27,** 271–276.

Trujillo, J. M., Stenius, C., and Christian, L. C. (1962). Chromosomes of the horse, donkey and the mule. *Chromosoma* **13,** 243–248.

Walker, K. S., and Bruère, A. N. (1979). XO condition in mares. *N. Z. Vet. J.* **27,** 18–19.

Wockl, V. F., and Mayr, B., and Schleger, W. (1980). Moglichkeiten der diagnose von erbfehlern mit hilfe der chromosomenanalyse bei rind, pferd und schwein-eine urbersicht. *Berl. Muench. Tieraerztl. Wochenschr.* **93,** 81–83.

Wodsedalek, J. E. (1914). Cited by Painter (1924).

Zakharov, A. F., Davudov, A. Z., Benjush, V. A., and Egolina, N. A. (1982). Genetic determination of NOR activity in human lymphocytes from twins. *Hum. Genet.* **60,** 24–29.

Chromosomes of Chickens

N. S. FECHHEIMER

Department of Dairy Science, The Ohio State University, Columbus, Ohio

I. Introduction
   A. Historical Survey
   B. Special Features of the Chicken Genome
   C. General Summary of Present Knowledge
II. Methodology
   A. Chick Embryos as a Source of Cells at Metaphase
   B. Preparations from Cultured Cells
   C. Preparations from Meiotic Cells
   D. Microspread Preparations for Synaptonemal Complex Analysis
   E. Staining and Banding Procedures
III. The Mitotic Karyotype
   A. As Revealed in Standard Preparations
   B. As Revealed with Special Staining Procedures
IV. Meiotic Chromosomes and Synaptonemal Complexes
   A. In Primary Spermatocytes
   B. In Secondary Spermatocytes
   C. Synaptonemal Complexes
V. Incidence of Heteroploidy
   A. In Hatched Chicks and Adults
   B. In Embryos
VI. Origins and Etiology of Heteroploidy
   A. Embryos with a Haploid Component
   B. Triploidy
   C. Tetraploidy and Diploid/Tetraploid Mosaicism
   D. Pentaploidy
   E. Diploid/Triploid and Diploid/Diploid Chimeras
   F. Aneuploidy
   G. Diploid/Aneuploid and Aneuploid/Aneuploid Mosaicism
VII. Structural Aberrations
   A. Spontaneously Occurring
   B. Experimentally Produced
VIII. Effects of Structural Aberrations
   A. Pericentric Inversions
   B. Reciprocal Translocations

IX. Concluding Remarks
  A. Extent of Knowledge of Chicken Chromosomes
  B. Advantages of the Chicken as a Model Organism for Cytogenetic Studies
  C. Applicability of Findings to Mammals
  References

I. Introduction

A. Historical Survey

Observations of the chromosomes of the chicken commenced early in the twentieth century with tedious study of sectioned material. Accumulation of reliable information was slow and paralleled similar work with mammals. A review of the early work was presented by Brant (1952), and both Makino (1951) and Romanoff (1960) give extensive lists of citations to the literature. Although almost all workers agreed on the number and morphological characterization of six large chromosomes (macrochromosomes) in the karyotype, one of which was duplicated in males but not in females, the occurrence of large numbers of very small chromosomes (microchromosomes) made it difficult to arrive at accurate counts and many workers thought that the number of elements per cell was not constant. The nature and function of the microchromosomes were therefore matters of controversy until the late 1960s.

In a paper remarkable for its time, Yamashina (1944) reported the constant number of 16 macrochromosomes in males (15 in females) and 62 microchromosomes in both sexes. The $2n$ complement was therefore 78 in males and 77 in females of a number of strains. By inference, the sex-determining apparatus was presumed to be ZZ and ZO. Employing more advanced techniques, including mitosis-arresting agents and hypotonic pretreatment, Newcomer (1957) and Newcomer and Brant (1954) noted allocycly of the microchromosomes, inconstancy in their numbers, and other irregularities that led them to conclude that the microchromosomes were chromosome-like (chromosomoids) but functionally different from regular chromosomes and were probably not carriers of genes. As late as 1965 Shoffner concluded from a review of the literature that no fundamental question of karyology of the fowl had a satisfactory answer. Much useful information was gathered in the next few years, however.

B. Special Features of the Chicken Genome

The DNA content of chicken nuclei equals about 3 pg, roughly half that of man and mouse (Atkin et al., 1965; Bachmann, et al., 1972).

Most if not all of the difference is accounted for by a much lower proportion of the genome in the form of repetitive sequences and fewer large blocks of heterochromatin. Except for the W chromosome, which is composed almost entirely of heterochromatin, and a large terminal C-band on the long arm of the Z chromosome, few consistently occurring segments of heterochromatin appear in the chicken karyotype (Pollock and Fechheimer, 1981). Almost all of the microchromosomes, however, are marked with small C-bands.

Six relatively large chromosomes, comprising 65% of the total length of the entire karyotype, have distinct morphology at metaphase and can be easily identified. A further three or four can be identified in good preparations. The remainder, referred to as microchromosomes, comprise a series of elements of diminishing size, most of which are acrocentric, that are difficult to count accurately and cannot be individually identified. The smallest have a length of less than 1 μm, putting them at the limits of resolution of the light microscope.

The male is homogametic with gonosomic complement ZZ and the female is the heterogametic sex with a complement ZW. The Z chromosome is one of the macrochromosomes, being easily identified as a metacentric element, fifth in order of length. The W chromosome is a small submetacentric element, similar in length to autosomes seven and eight (Owen, 1965). It is late replicating (Schmid, 1962) and largely heterochromatic.

In the chicken there is no dosage compensation to accommodate for the different numbers of the major sex chromosome in the two sexes (Cock, 1964). Accordingly, the two Z chromosomes replicate in synchrony in males, and no sex chromatin, representing the inactive sex chromosome, is seen in interphase nuclei. What was thought to be a sex chromatin-like body in interphase nuclei of females is the heteropycnotic W chromosome (Stefos and Arrighi, 1971).

C. General Summary of Present Knowledge

The slow start of cytogenetics of the chicken relative to that of humans, laboratory mammals, and even mammalian livestock was attributable to difficulties presented by the unique features of the karyotype discussed above, some technical hindrances, and the fact that only a few workers devoted effort to study of chromosomes of this interesting and economically important species. In spite of these hindrances, knowledge has accumulated rapidly so that it is at present at least comparable to what is known of any of the other farm animals.

The normal karyotype has been extensively described and the $2n$ number has been firmly established at 78. The microchromosomes cannot be individually identified, but their function as normal, gene carrying elements is widely recognized. Adaptations of all the commonly used banding methods, including C-, G-, R-, and Q-banding and several others, have been applied to yield useful standards and to extend to 15 or more the number of pairs that can be identified. Banding methods have revealed the ubiquitous occurrence of several variants and provide a basis for cytotaxonomic studies of the chicken relative to other bird taxa.

Meiotic chromosomes at several stages of meiosis I (MI) and metaphase of MII of spermatogenesis can be easily revealed with standard methods. The chromosomes at all stages have been described and the incidence of abnormal occurrence enumerated. Synaptonemal complex analysis has been used to define morphometric attributes of the genome, to identify the pairing regions of Z and W chromosomes in oocytes, and to reveal the nature of several structural aberrations that were experimentally produced. A method has been devised to observe lampbrush chromosomes in oocytes.

More than 20 translocations and several pericentric inversions have been recovered and characterized, and are maintained in special stocks at several locations. They are used to study properties of segregation of multivalents, to produce embryos with duplications and deletions, to map genes, and in the homozygous state to serve as markers in studies of chromosomal abnormalities of embryos.

The relationship between embryo death and chromosome abnormalities has been more extensively studied in the chicken than in any other organism except the mouse. All of the common and many uncommon forms of aneuploidy, euploidy, mosaics, and chimeras have been seen frequently in early embryos and the sites of origin of most of them have been detected. Progress has been made to discover the causal basis of the errors. At present it seems that genetic influences are of utmost importance.

Several aberrant chromosomal complements, including triploidy, trisomy, and some unusual chimerism (e.g., $1n/2n$ and $2n/3n$), are recovered in living birds, enabling observation of their effects on posthatching development and physiological functions. Sex chromosome aneuploidy, on the other hand, is much more rare than it is among mammalian species. It is of great interest to find the reasons for this.

II. Methodology

Most techniques applied to display chicken chromosomes are direct adaptations of those developed primarily for use with human or other mammalian cells. Minor modifications have, in some instances, been found to give more suitable preparations of chicken cells. There has been very little effort devoted to finding optimum conditions for display of the fine structure of chicken chromosomes by the various banding techniques. Such work might well pay large dividends in view of the differences between the chromosomal constituents of birds and mammals. Readers are referred to the several standard works on chromosome methodology (Sharma and Sharma, 1973; Schwarzacher and Wolf, 1974; Verma and Babu, 1989). Shoffner et al. (1967) described methods applicable to the chicken, and Bloom (1978) presented a detailed account of acquiring and preparing chick embryo cells for karyological analysis.

A. CHICK EMBRYOS AS A SOURCE OF CELLS AT METAPHASE

Chicken embryos at all stages of ontogeny are an excellent source of material suitable for many types of chromosomal studies. Fertile eggs can be produced or obtained from commercial sources at low cost, embryos can be treated *in ovo* with colchicine or other suitable agents, and large numbers of embryos can be processed rapidly to produce excellent preparations. For many applications it is most convenient to make cell suspensions of whole embryos or of pieces of tissue that display high mitotic rates at particular stages of embryogenesis.

1. Handling and Incubation of Eggs

Fertile eggs of high quality can be stored at 15°C for 7 days without loss of developmental potential when they are incubated. They are incubated at 37.5°C, 85% humidity, and require 21 days for full development and hatching. From day 3 of incubation, viability of the embryo in an egg can be detected by candling of the egg. Prior to harvest of the embryo for processing, colchicine is administered to the air sac (rounded end of the egg) through a small hole in the shell. For large eggs weighing about 50 g, 0.1 mg colchicine in 0.1 ml of distilled water or saline solution is a suitable dose. Following injection, eggs are returned to the incubator for 1–2 hours, depending on the desired state of contraction of the chromosomes.

2. Processing of Embryonic Tissue

Embryos in eggs incubated for 16–18 hours (overnight) are at the primitive streak stage. When processed at this stage, the yield of analyzable preparations is about 90%. It is the earliest possible stage from which one can get reasonable numbers of cells suitable for analysis at metaphase. Details of a procedure for processing embryos at this stage were given by Fechheimer and Jaffe (1966) and Fechheimer et al. (1968). The entire embryo, located in the central disc of the blastoderm, is lifted from the surface of the yolk on the tip of a scalpel. It is removed from the scalpel in a few drops of Hanks' balanced salt solution (BSS) with a Pasteur pipet and put into a small centrifuge tube containing 2–3 ml of the same solution. A cell suspension is made by aspiration of the contents of the tube. Hypotonic treatment, fixation, and dropping the cells onto cold wet slides are accomplished by the standard methods used for harvest of cultured lymphocytes.

At 2–5 days of incubation, the embryo is growing rapidly and the mitotic rate in several tissues is high. Bloom (1974) has used the allantoic sac and limb buds of embryos at 4 days of incubation with great success. The mitotic activity of various tissues at each stage of chick embryo development has been ascertained (Bloom and Buss, 1968), so an investigator can choose an appropriate tissue from any stage of ontogeny and process it by the method of Fechheimer and Jaffe (1966) or other suitable method [see Bloom (1978), for methods for making squash preparations and other methods for making preparations from solid tissue].

The tissues of late embryos (19–21 days of incubation) and hatched chicks that display remarkably high mitotic indices are bone marrow and bursa of Fabricius. For best results, late embryos are treated with colchicine *in ovo;* newly hatched chicks are injected intraperitoneally. Dose is equivalent to that used for early embryos, given previously. Bone marrow cells can be flushed from the long bones, usually femeri, with 1–2 ml of Hanks' BSS, or the bones can be split longitudinally with a scapel, the marrow scraped out, and a cell suspension prepared in a tube containing Hank's BSS. Cells from the bursa of Fabricius are put in suspension by teasing the extirpated gland with two fine forceps, in a small Petri dish containing 1–2 ml of Hanks' BSS. The gland is easily removed from day-old chicks without harm to them.

Shoffner et al. (1967) have successfully used the pulp of growing feathers from birds of all ages as source of mitotic cells. For best results, it is necessary to administer Colcemid intraperitoneally 2 hours prior to plucking a few growing feathers. The method requires squashing the pulp onto slides. If the bird is to be reared and used for breeding or subsequent experiments, the whole-body treatment with Colcemid renders subsequent observations of heteroploid cells as equivocal.

B. Preparations from Cultured Cells

The standard methods of lymphocyte culture from samples of whole blood or separated lymphocytes require minor modification for successful adaptation to chickens. Whole blood (0.5 ml) cultured for 72 hours in any of a variety of media gives moderately successful results. Growth is never as profuse as that of human or pig cells, but sufficient numbers of cells at metaphase can be found for thorough analysis. The mitogen of choice is pokeweed mitogen; phytohemagglutinin (PHA) is much less satisfactory. Cultures must be incubated at 40–41°C. No growth is achieved at 37°C. Details of procedures have been published (Au et al., 1975; Thorne et al., 1987).

Fibroblasts from biopsies of skin or other tissues are as easily cultured in Petri dishes as are those from mammals, and yield excellent preparations for karyological analysis. Banding procedures on cultured fibroblasts produce results of the highest quality. Ansari et al. (1986) demonstrated the high quality of banded chromosomes prepared from cultured fibroblasts of chickens and other birds.

C. Preparations from Meiotic Cells

All of the methods used for making preparations from mammalian testes can be applied to the chicken without modification. The air-drying method of Evans et al. (1964) has been used to advantage to describe the meiotic and mitotic chromosomes as they appear at various stages of spermatogenesis in chicken (Pollock and Fechheimer, 1978). Spermatogonia at metaphase and spermatocytes at diakinesis and early metaphase I occur in abundance on slides from testes from untreated birds. To increase the number of MII cells at metaphase it is advisable to administer colchicine, vinblastine sulfate, or other mitosis-arresting agents 2 hours prior to obtaining the testis sample. An appropriate dose is 2.5 mg of vinblastine sulfate or 5 mg of colchicine in 2.5 ml of a saline solution, injected intraperitoneally.

No satisfactory procedure has been published to display the meiotic metaphase chromosomes of oocytes, although a dictyotene stage is known to occur in oocytes from late embryonic stages through adult life. Lampbrush chromosomes occur at diplonema and methods for their preparation and study are available (Hutchison, 1987). These structures might well be suited for high-resolution gene mapping by in situ hybridization.

D. Microspread Preparations for Synaptonemal Complex Analysis

Solari (1977) made an extensive detailed analysis of the synaptonemal complexes in oocytes from females either at late stages of incubation or in the first few days after hatching. The method of microspreading enables observation of all axes in single cells either by light or phase-contrast microscopy, or by electron microscopy to resolve more detail. A similar method was used by Kaelbling and Fechheimer (1983a) for observation by electron microscopy of the full complements of synaptonemal complexes of spermatocytes from adult cockerels. Axes of synaptonemal complexes of the microchromosomes are easily resolved and indicate that they possess all of the components possessed by the larger elements, including kinetochores and recombination nodules, and regular pairing behavior.

E. Staining and Banding Procedures

Unstained mitotic metaphase chromosomes can be examined and eight to nine pairs can be unambiguously identified with a phase microscope. Standard staining procedures such as those with Giemsa, acetic orcein, or other commonly used stains are suitable for display of chicken chromosomes.

Of the several methods used for display of differential segments of chromosomes of livestock discussed in detail by Gustavsson (1980), several have been successfully adapted for application to the chicken. Details of a procedure for elucidating C-bands by treatment with BaOH were given by Pollock and Fechheimer (1981), who found the result to be variable, perhaps because most blocks of heterochromatin on autosomes are small compared to those of mammalian chromosomes. After trypsin treatment (Wang and Shoffner, 1974) or a combination of trypsin followed by urea (Stock et al., 1974), G-bands are especially detailed and the method permits identification of nine pairs of microchromosomes as well as six pairs of macrochromosomes. A method for Q-banding with quinacrine mustard that identifies segments of eight pairs of autosomes and the Z chromosome was described by Fritschi and Stranzinger (1985). Bands with highest resolution, which enable identification of smaller segments of chromosomes in rearrangements, are produced by an R-banding method that entails staining with acridine orange after incorporation of bromodeoxyuridine (BrdU) (Carlenius et al., 1981; Olesen, 1987). More elaborate procedures involving sequential staining with distamycin A, chromomycin A_3 (CMA_3), or 4′,6-diamidino-2-phenylindole dihydrochloride (DAPI) and actinomycin D (AMD) (Auer et al., 1987; Fritschi and Stranzinger, 1985) produce karyotypes with many bands that allow identification of as many as 18 pairs of autosomes.

Nucleolus organizing regions (NORs) can be clearly delineated by the silver staining method of Bloom and Bacon (1985). A detailed protocol for showing the differentiation of sister chromatids and the numbers of exchanges between them was given by Bloom (1978).

III. The Mitotic Karyotype

A. As Revealed in Standard Preparations

1. General Description

The normal $2n$ complement is 78 (Pollock and Fechheimer, 1976). The karyotype (Fig. 1) contains seven pairs of relatively large autosomes (each of which can be readily distinguished), 31 pairs of additional autosomes of diminishing size, and the gonosomes. The smallest of the autosomes in metaphase cells is less than 0.5 μm in length, a size near the resolving power of the light microscope. It is very difficult to get an accurate count except from the very best of preparations, but the validity of the $2n$ number has been frequently confirmed from counts of bivalents at MI and more recently from analysis of synaptonemal complexes in spermatogonia and oogonia (Kaelbling and Fechheimer, 1983a; Solari, 1977). The Z is one of the longer elements, number five in order of length, and is metacentric. The W is about the same length as autosomes seven and eight and is submetacentric. It can be difficult to identify in standard preparations because its morphology is similar to two pairs of autosomes of similar length and morphology. The karyotype is usually arranged by ordering the elements by their lengths, but an international standard has not yet been published, so confusion exists regarding the designation of autosomes six to eight and whether or not the Z should be assigned a number (number five) or should be set to the side without numbering, as is the custom with mammalian karyotypes. It seems to be most reasonable to order numbers six to eight not by their lengths, which are very similar, but by morphology, so that number six would be an acrocentric and seven and eight would be the submetacentric elements. Most authors sensibly do not assign a number to the Z or W.

2. Morphometric Attributes

The relative lengths and centromeric indexes of the eight longest pairs of autosomes and the Z are given in Table I and an idiogram constructed from these data is shown in Fig. 2. The total length of the

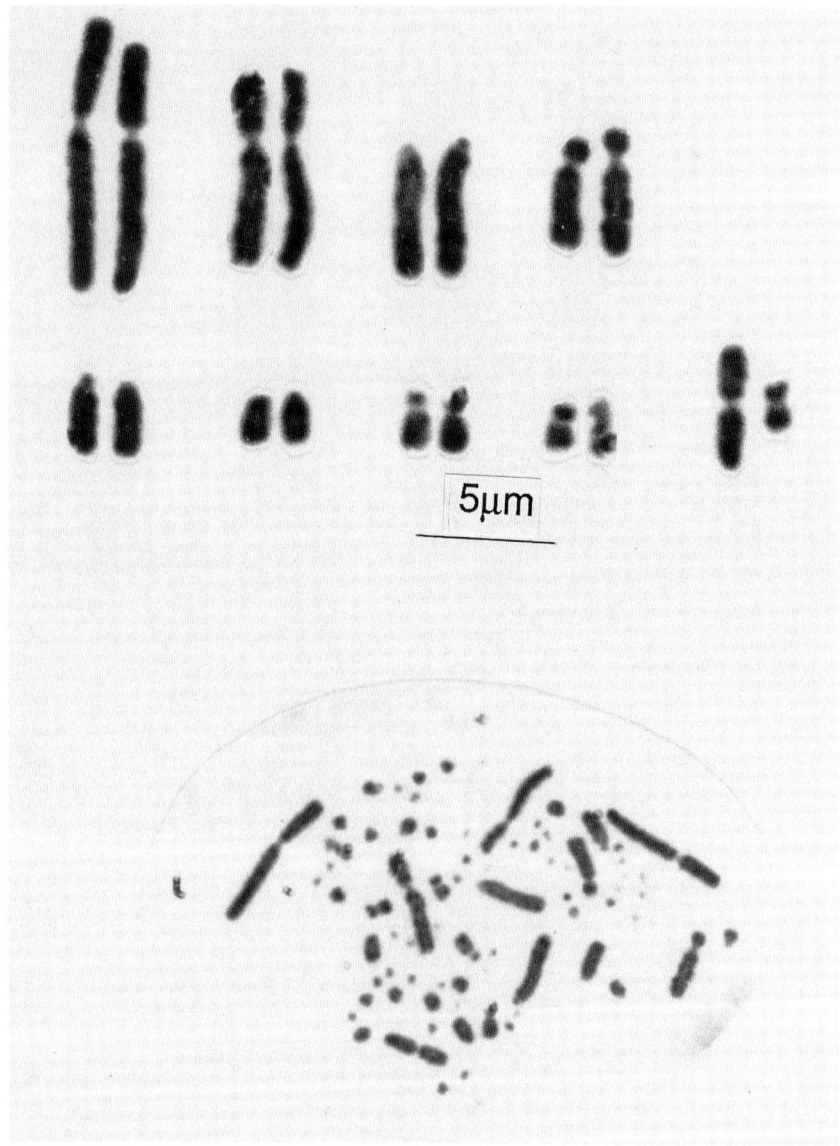

FIG. 1. Partial karyotype of a female (ZW) from a standard preparation, stained with Giemsa stain. (Photomicrograph and karyotype made by K.-H. Lee.)

TABLE I

Relative Lengths and Centromeric Indexes of the Eight Longest Pairs of Autosomes and the Z[a]

Chromosome number	Relative length	Centromeric index[b]
1	0.2418	39.15
2	0.1829	35.96
3	0.1288	5.28
4	0.1131	25.93
5	0.0735	7.66
6	0.0473	5.11
7	0.0536	29.88
8	0.0484	42.90
Z	0.1107	47.80

[a]N = 61. Data from Kaelbling (1980).
[b]Short arm as a proportion of total length of chromosome.

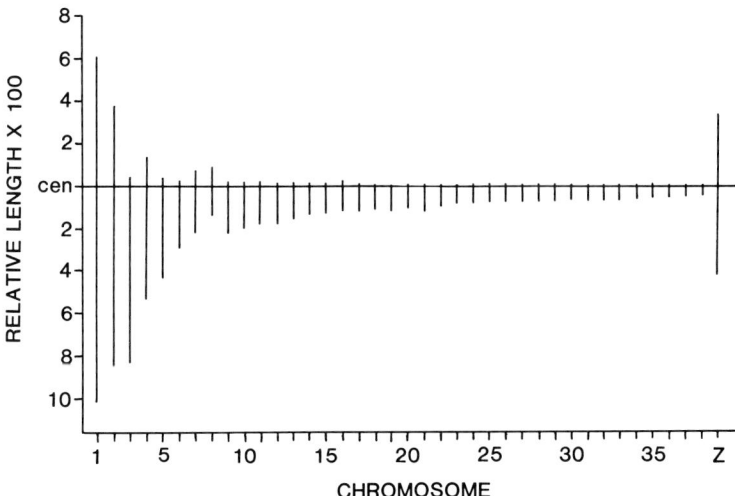

FIG. 2. Idiogram of chicken based on measurements of synaptonemal complexes in spermatocytes. The centromere locations of chromosomes 10–39, shown as acrocentric, are not accurate. (Redrawn from Kaelbling and Fechheimer, 1983a, with permission of S. Karger AG, Basel.)

nine pairs of macrochromosomes comprises 65% of the length of the entire haploid genome containing a Z. The Z is comparable in length to the mammalian X, comprising about 7.6% of an entire haploid genome. The total length of the 30 pairs of microchromosomes sum to about 35% of a haploid genome containing the Z.

B. AS REVEALED WITH SPECIAL STAINING PROCEDURES

1. Q-, G-, and R-Bands

Karyotypes and proposed standards for banding patterns have been published by several workers [e.g., Stahl and Vagner-Capodano (1972), and Fritschi and Stranzinger (1985) for Q-bands; Stock et al. (1974), Wang and Shoffner (1974), and Carlenius et al. (1981) for G-bands; Carlenius et al. (1981) and Olesen (1987) for R-bands]. Representative R- and G-banding karyotypes are shown in Figs. 3 and 4. Results from different laboratories are not in full agreement and no standard banding karyotypes have been agreed upon. It is urgent that such a standard be produced and universally adopted now that the technique of in situ hybridization is being more widely used for gene mapping, and many rearrangements now available require characterization by precise localization of breakpoints (Olsen, 1987). As presently applied, techniques for G- and R-banding and the more elaborate procedures (Auer et al., 1987) (Fig. 5) allow identification of as many as 10 pairs of the microchromosomes, in addition to the 8 pairs of autosomal macrochromosomes and the gonosomes. Ubiquitous and reliable heteromorphisms of banding patterns have not yet been reported, perhaps because only limited numbers of animals have been studied.

2. C-Bands

The autosomal macrochromosomes notably have few prominent C-bands that are reliably and consistently displayed. Small pericentromeric heterochromatic blocks are seen variably on most macrochromosomes, but consistently only on chromosome 6 (Fig. 6). On the other hand, almost all of the microchromosomes display C-bands of such size as to suggest that they possess a disproportionate amount of repetitive DNA. The Z is characterized by a prominent band in the most distal region of the long arm (the long arm is defined as the one bearing the C-band). The region is heteromorphic, appearing in at least three distinct forms (Pollock and Fechheimer, 1981). The W is almost entirely heterochromatic (Stefos and Arrighi, 1971) and therefore stains

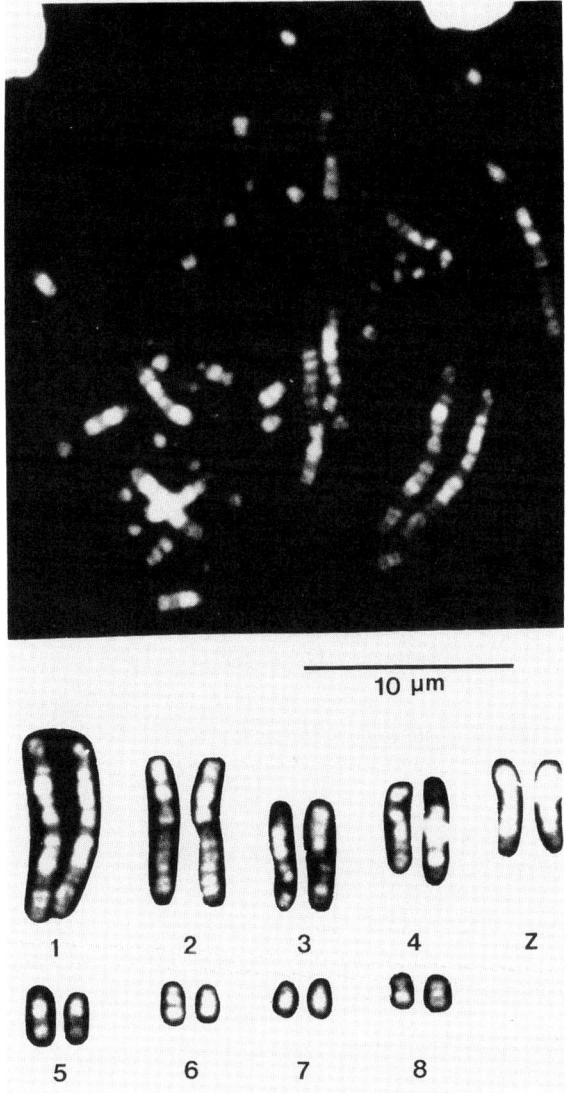

FIG. 3. Partial karyotype of a male exhibiting R-bands produced by BrdU incorporation and stained with acridine orange. (From Olesen, 1987.)

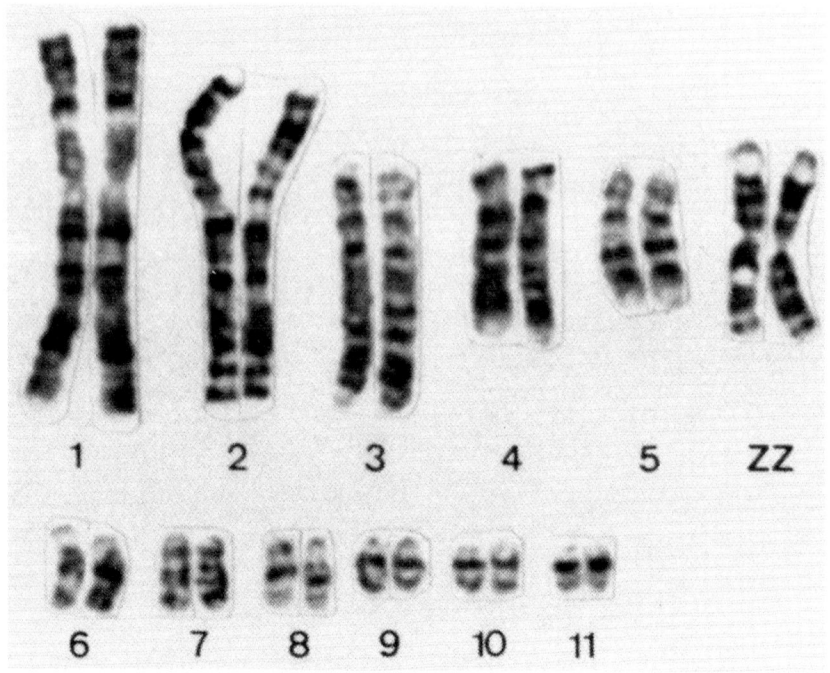

FIG. 4. Partial karyotype exhibiting G-bands produced by treatment with trypsin and urea. (From Stock and Bunch, 1982, with permission of S. Karger AG, Basel.)

almost completely as C-band material. Even in cells at interphase its presence can be detected by the presence of a dense, darkly stained body when C-banding procedures are applied, especially BaOH treatment followed by Giemsa staining, or as a brightly fluorescing body in quinacrine-stained preparations of cells from females. An idiogram depicting both variable and constant C-bands as seen in several cells from many organisms was constructed by Pollock and Fechheimer (1981).

3. NOR Region

A single pair of microchromosomes identified as number 15–18 (Bloom and Bacon, 1985) and as number 17 (Auer *et al.*, 1987) contains the nucleolus organizing region, which is displayed by a silver staining method in metaphase cells, and by fluorescence microscopy of interphase cells stained with acridine orange (Bloom and Bacon, 1985).

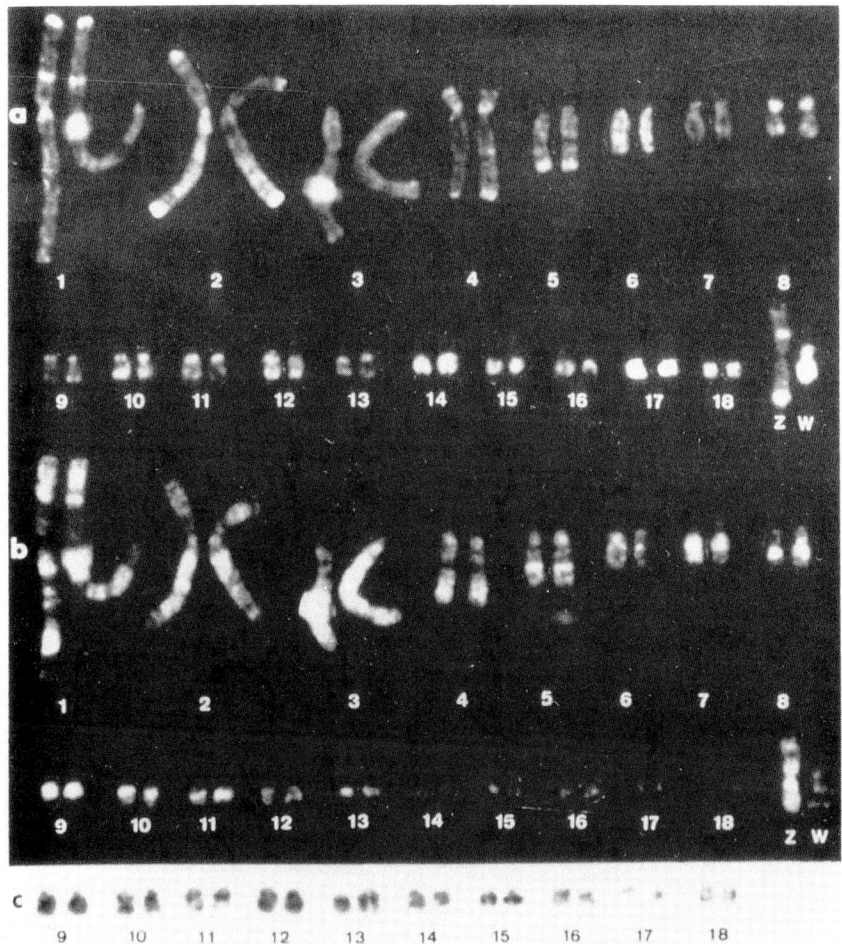

FIG. 5. The chromosomes of a single metaphase cell sequentially stained by (a) CMA_3, (b) DAPI–AMD, and (c) Giemsa staining methods. (From Auer et al., 1987, with permission of S. Karger AG, Basel.)

IV. Meiotic Chromosomes and Synaptonemal Complexes

A. IN PRIMARY SPERMATOCYTES

Descriptive accounts of the various stages of prophase, metaphase, and the events of spermatogenesis are contained in the work of New-

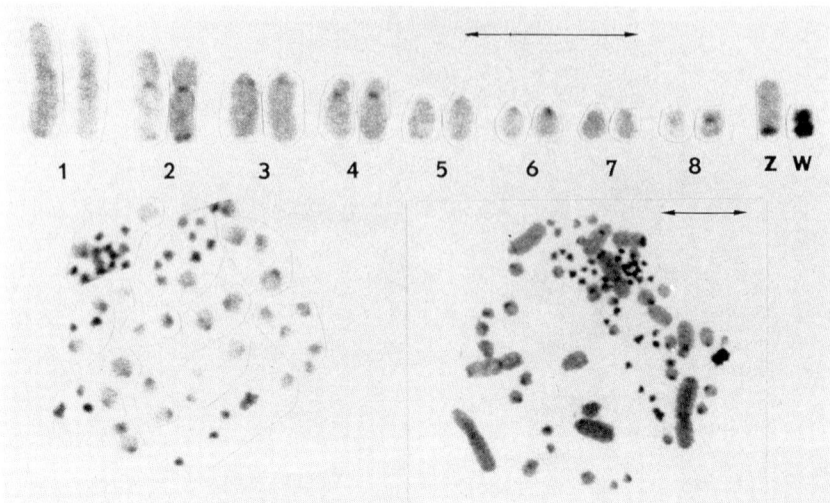

FIG. 6. Partial karyotype exhibiting C-bands produced by treatment with BaOH and stained with Giemsa stain. Bars represent 10 µm. (From Pollock, 1979.)

comer and Brant (1954), Ohno (1961), and Ford and Wollam (1964). In essence, the appearance of the chromatin and the bivalents of MI are similar to what is seen in mammals, with the exception of the occurrence of the microbivalents at diplonema, diakinesis, and metaphase. Because the chromosomes occur as bivalents at these stages, the number of elements is half that at mitotic metaphase and the size of each is larger. It is therefore at these stages that the most accurate counts can be made. The modal number of 39 bivalents was reported in 69% of well-stained, well-spread cells from 10 animals; all other counts were hypomodal (Pollock and Fechheimer, 1978). Only the five largest autosomal, and the Z, bivalents can be identified at diakinesis/metaphase, but number 4 can sometimes be confused with the Z owing to their similar lengths (Fig. 7). Application of C-banding reveals the prominent terminal band on the Z, dispelling any ambiguity of identification (Blazak and Fechheimer, 1980).

At pachynema and early diplonema the microbivalents exhibit a length sufficient that accurate measurements can be made. They also possess a chromomeric structure suggesting that it might well be possible to construct a pachytene map, enabling identification of many microchromosomes. If this were accomplished, the pachytene chromosomes would be useful for gene mapping by *in situ* hybridization.

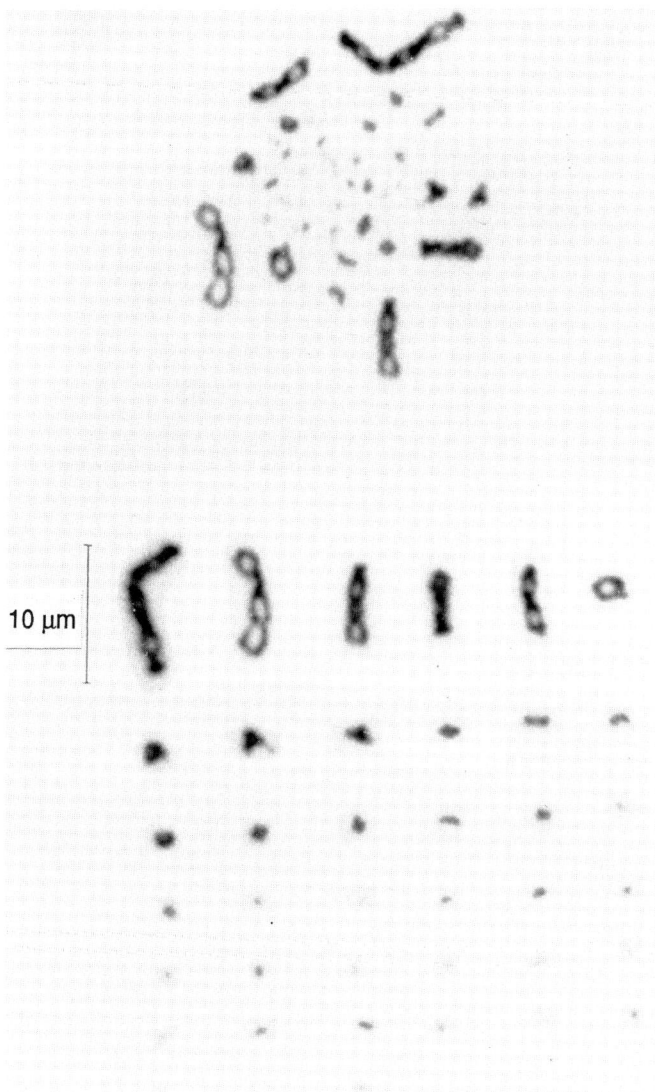

FIG. 7. Karyotype of the 39 bivalents at diakinesis in a spermatocyte. Bivalents 7–39 are arranged in arbitrary order because none can be identified. (Photomicrograph and karyotype made by D. L. Pollock.)

TABLE II

LENGTHS AND CHIASMA COUNTS OF THE SIX MACROBIVALENTS AND THE MICROBIVALENTS AT DIAKINESIS/METAPHASE[a]

Bivalent no.	Approximate length (μm)	Range and mean no. of chiasmata ± SE	Remarks
1	12	6–12	—
		8.1 ± 0.06	—
2	9	5–8	—
		5.9 ± 0.05	—
3	6	3–6	—
		4.6 ± 0.04	—
4	4.5–5	2–5	Difficult to distinguish from Z
		3.6 ± 0.04	
5	2–3	2–3	—
		2.4 ± 0.03	—
Z	4–4.5	2–5	Difficult to distinguish from no. 4 without C-banding
		3.5 ± 0.04	
7–18	±1	1	Star shaped or circular or elliptical
18–39	<0.5	1?	Chiasmata not visible but inferred

[a]Data from Pollock and Fechheimer (1978).

Approximate lengths and chiasmata numbers for the six macrobivalents, assessed from observations of almost 300 cells from 10 males, are shown in Table II. The relative lengths of the macrobivalents are very similar to the relative lengths of the equivalent mitotic chromosomes as shown in Table I. The range of chiasma incidence in the six macrobivalents was 23 to 31 with a mean of 28.1. If it is assumed that each microbivalent contains a minimum of one, the range of numbers of chiasmata per cell is estimated at 56 to 66, with almost half of them appearing in the six largest elements (Pollock and Fechheimer, 1978). Two facets of these observations bear mention. The chiasma frequency in birds is considerably higher than in mammals. Second, the distribution of chiasmata is nonrandom, there being a higher incidence per unit length of microbivalent than in an equivalent length of macrobivalent. Fewer than half of all chiasmata occur in the six largest macrobivalents, which comprise about 60% of the genome length.

B. In Secondary Spermatocytes

Cells at second meiotic metaphase are much less abundant in air-dried preparations of dissociated testis cells than are cells at diakinesis. Their numbers are increased by pretreatment with colchicine or vinblastine sulfate. The distinctive morphology of the six largest elements, including the Z, is maintained at MII so that each can be readily identified (Fig. 8).

Analysis of almost 500 secondary spermatocytes from 10 cockerels revealed 2.1% that were hypoploid (only the six macrobivalents were considered) and 5.8% that were diploid (Pollock and Fechheimer, 1978). It is likely that most, if not all, of the diploid cells are artifacts produced by hypotonic swelling of a dividing spermatocytes before completion of cytokinesis.

C. Synaptonemal Complexes

The synaptonemal complexes (SCs) in microspread preparations of oocytes (Solari, 1977; Rahn and Solari, 1987) and spermatocytes (Kaelbling and Fechheimer, 1983a) have been observed by electron microscopy. The absolute and relative lengths, as well as the centromeric indexes of the longest 10 axes, are very similar in gonocytes from males and females. Their morphometric attributes are also similar to the morphometric attributes of the chromosomes at mitotic metaphase, so that the SC axes representative of each of the macochromosomes can be identified. Most of the microchromosomes appear to be acrocentric, but four or five give indication of being subacrocentric or submetacentric. Recombination nodules (RNs) are clearly delineated in the SCs from cells at pachynema. Their occurrence is thought to indicate sites of chiasma formation. The mean number of RNs per oocyte was 57.5, of which 28.5 were in the 10 longest SCs and 29 were in the microelements, which regularly had one each. The correspondence between numbers of RNs in oocytes and numbers of chiasmata in MI spermatocytes is remarkable.

The Z and W pairing pattern is inferred from observations of SCs in oocytes. There appears to be a short homologous region that is located in the short arm of the W and a terminal segment of the short arm (euchromatic) of the Z, although at late stages of prophase, nonhomologous pairing occurs along the entire W axis. A single RN is invariably present near the paired ZW teleomeres. Thus, the situation is very similar to that in mammals with an XY sex-determining mechanism. The Z contains a short terminal region in which no crossing-over with

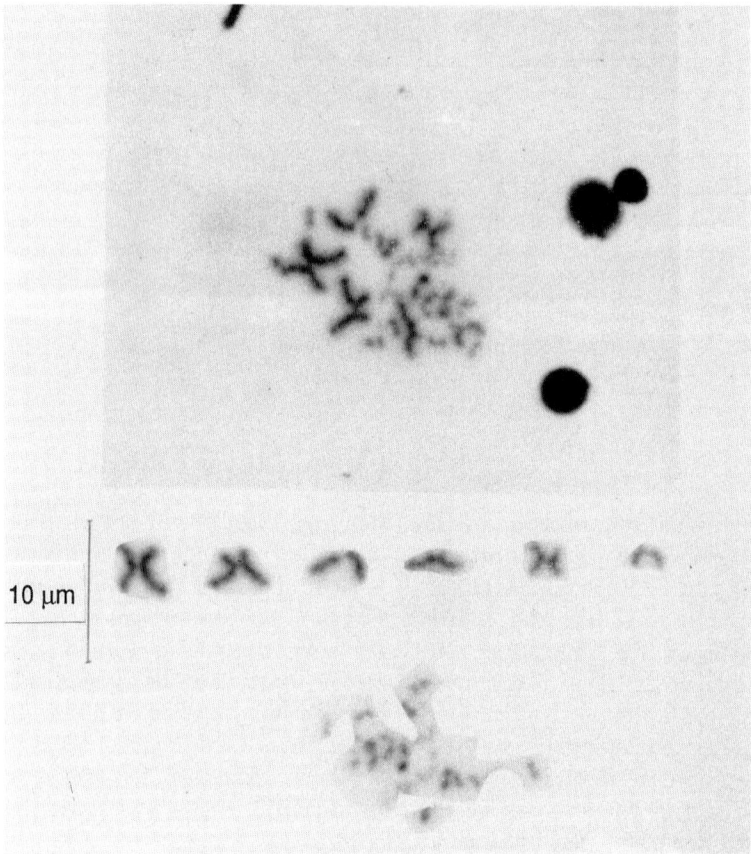

FIG. 8. Karyotype of the chromosomes at MII in a secondary spermatocyte. Only seven macrochromosomes, including the Z, can be identified. (Photomicrograph and karyotype made by D. L. Pollock.)

the W occurs, a pseudoautosomal region; a region about four times the length of the pseudoautosomal region in which crossing-over occurs; and a strictly sex-linked region that comprises all of the long arm and most of the length of the short arm of the Z (Rahn and Solari, 1987; Solari et al., 1988).

SC analysis has been applied to map the breakpoints at which reciprocal translocations occur (Kaelbling and Fechheimer, 1983b), to measure the extent of nonpairing and nonhomologous pairing in translocation multivalents (Solari et al., 1988) and to observe the nature of pairing of homologues, one of which bears a pericentric inversion (Kaelbling and Fechheimer, 1985).

V. Incidence of Heteroploidy

A. IN HATCHED CHICKS AND ADULTS

1. Euploidy

a. Polyploid. Since the first report of a triploid adult intersex chicken (Ohno et al., 1963), several authors have described the regular but low-frequency occurrence of intersex birds that are $3n$.ZZW (Abdel-Hameed and Shoffner, 1971; DeBoer et al., 1984; Miyake et al., 1984). All were diagnosed as females shortly after hatching and began showing secondary sexual characteristics of males at about the time of sexual maturity. They are phenotypically normal. Gonadal development and histology are variable. The gonads are hypoplastic and appear as misshapen testes. Some contain both medullary and cortical regions, but others exhibit only a testis-like structure from the medulla. Vas deferens are absent but reasonably well developed left oviducts are seen.

One juvenile and three advanced embryos with $3n$.ZZZ were all afflicted with anopthalmia and brachygnathia superior (Donner et al., 1969) but another, also ZZZ, was normal (Wang and Shoffner, 1980). Adult $3n$.ZZZ birds appear normal and produce poor-quality semen containing a high proportion of grossly abnormal spermatozoa. No triploids with the sex chromosome complement ZWW have been reported.

Triploid embryos comprise about 1% of samples of early embryos. Clearly, many of these die prior to hatching, including all of those that are ZWW and a high proportion of the ZZW and ZZZ, but those ascertained as adults, although sterile, are otherwise indistinguishable from diploid birds.

b. Euploid Chimeras. Several remarkable birds have been recovered from a line intensely selected for shortened interval between ovipositions, a line that also yields a high frequency of triploidy (20% of embryos). The types found among juvenile and adult animals were 16 haploid/diploid ($1n/2n$), 3 diploid/triploid ($2n/3n$), and 1 haploid/diploid/triploid ($1n/2n/3n$). All of the $1n/2n$ were phenotypically normal and fertile. Those with gonosomic complements Z/ZZ were male and the Z/ZW were female. Of the four $2n/3n$, those with gonosomes ZW/ZZW were also normal fertile females. The single bird with gonosomes ZZ/ZZW was a normal male with a right testis and left ovotestis and vas deferens. One bird with ZW/ZZZ sex reversed from female to male phenotype at 8 weeks and had a left ovotestis, right testis, and a small right oviduct. The single bird that was $1n/2n/3n$ (Z/ZW/ZZW) was a sterile intersex with small left ovary, right ovotestis, and undifferentiated oviducts (Thorne et al., 1987).

2. Autosomal Aneuploidy

A cockerel that displayed three haplotypes at the B blood group locus was found to be trisomic for one of the larger microchromosomes in the range 15–18. The chromosome also contains the only nucleolus organizing region of the entire genome, and can therefore be detected by silver staining. The animal was phenotypically normal and fully fertile, and in matings with disomic hens produced trisomic progeny, but fewer than expected. Matings of trisomic × trisomic yielded some tetrasomic progeny that were smaller than disomic birds but were otherwise normal (Bloom and Bacon, 1985).

Because trisomy for most of the microchromosomes would be difficult to detect without marker genes, attempts have been made to produce chicks with duplications of segments (partial trisomy) of macrochromosomes that are detectable cytologically. The approach is to mate animals heterozygous for reciprocal translocations to karyologically normal birds. It is expected that gametes bearing duplications and deletions will be produced by the heterozygotes (Dinkel et al., 1979; Bonaminio and Fechheimer, 1988). Screenings of several thousand live chicks from such matings have yielded no partial trisomics (N. S. Fechheimer, unpublished data), although embryos with duplications of some segments survive at least to 5 days of incubation (Blazak and Fechheimer, 1981a, and several unpublished studies).

3. Sex Chromosome Aneuploidy

No live chicks with aneuploidy of the sex chromosome have been reported, but early embryos with complements XO and XXY are seen at low frequency in some studies (e.g., Miller et al., 1971).

B. IN EMBRYOS

Interest in chromosome abnormalities of chick embryos was engendered by a report of a $2n/3n$ embryo at 5–7 days of incubation (Bloom and Buss, 1966) and of trisomic and haploid embryos at 1 day (Fech-

TABLE III

FREQUENCIES (PER 1,000) OF CHROMOSOME ABNORMALITIES IN CHICK EMBRYOS

Type of abnormality	Embryos at 16–18 hours incubation ($N = 9,216$)[a]	Embryos at 4–5 days incubation ($N = 6,874$)[b]
Haploidy and haploid chimeras	5.6–20.9[c]	0–50
Triploidy	3.6–19.9	0–33
Tetraploidy	0–1.5	0–3
Pentaploidy	0–1.1	0
Diploid/tetraploid mosaics	0.9–16.3	0
Diploid/diploid chimeras	0–3.1	0
Diploid/triploid chimeras	0–4.2	0
Trisomy	0.4–5.7[d]	0–9
Monosomy	1.7–4.5[e]	0
Diploid/aneuploid mosaics	1.7–2.6	0
Structural	0–0.85	0–10

[a]From Fechheimer (1981), which contained a summary of several studies. Frequencies are for Leghorn and broiler-type chickens and crosses between them.

[b]From Bloom (1974), which summarized observations of 12 strains. Frequencies are ranges for the 12 strains. Sample sizes ranged from 120 to 1,675.

[c]Includes $1n$, $1n/2n$ (majority), $1n/1n$, $1n/1n/2n$, $1n/2n/4n$, $1n/3n$.

[d]Trisomics for all macrochromosomes, including the Z, were recorded, in addition to several double and multiple trisomics.

[e]Monosomics for all macrochromosomes, including the Z, were recorded, in addition to several double and multiple monosomics.

heimer *et al.*, 1968). Extensive subsequent studies in both laboratories surveying several types and strains of chickens established variable frequencies of a great array of different types of heteroploidy. Summaries of this work are in Bloom (1974) and Fechheimer (1981). The latter summary includes data from two experiments in which marker chromosomes were employed to infer the parental source of the genomes in euploid embryos and to estimate the frequency of unusual types of heteroploidy, such as $1n/1n$ and $2n/2n$ chimerism (Fechheimer and Jaap, 1978, 1980).

The frequencies of the several types of abnormalities observed in the two large surveys are shown in Table III. The most prevalent types in meat-type chickens were haploid/diploid chimerism, triploidy, and diploid/tetraploid mosaics, each of which had a frequency greater than 1.6%. Aneuploidy (only the macrochromosomes, about one-quarter of the total number of chromosomes) occurred with a frequency of about 0.5%. Other types had much lower frequencies, none greater than 0.4%

(diploid/triploid chimerism). In the data from Bloom (1974), representing a screening of 12 different strains at 4–5 days of incubation, haploid/diploid chimerism was most prevalent in one strain (3.3%), followed by triploidy (3.3%) and trisomy 0.9% (no monosomics were reported). Differences between the incidences of the various types of heteroploidy in the two studies are attributable to two factors. First, different strains were sampled and it is apparent from both studies that different strains exhibit vastly different frequencies of different abnormalities. Second, embryos were sampled at 1 day of incubation in Fechheimer's (1981) survey and at 4–5 five days in that of Bloom (1974). In both studies the estimates of incidence of abnormalities are low. Particularly, the frequency of aneuploidy is probably grossly underestimated because of the inability to detect the presence or absence of any of the microchromosomes. Chimerism and mosaicism are also undercounted because only limited numbers of cells from each embryo were observed. Therefore, an aberrant cell line present at low frequency would often not be detected.

VI. Origins and Etiology of Heteroploidy

From the relatively large numbers of each type of aberrant embryos, inferences were drawn regarding the site of origin of each type, using the sex chromosome complements as markers (Bloom, 1974; Fechheimer, 1981). Subsequently, the tentative conclusions were confirmed in a series of two experiments in which the male parents of embryos were homozygous for marker chromosomes (Fechheimer and Jaap, 1978, 1980). In one of the experiments, females were inseminated with semen from several males, each of which was homozygous for a different marker, enabling detection of unusual types of aberrant embryos, such as haploid/haploid/-, and diploid/diploid chimeras. Conclusions from several lines of evidence are given in this section. For detailed arguments on which the conclusions are based, readers are referred to the original papers cited.

A. Embryos with a Haploid Component

All haploid embryos ($1n$, $1n/2n$, etc.) and the haploid component of haploid/euploid chimeras are derived from spermatozoa that proliferate by mitosis within the ovum. Pure haploids result when syngamy does not occur and only the sperm undergoes mitosis, while the female pronucleus disintegrates. Much more frequently, one sperm pronucleus engages in syngamy with the female pronucleus, thereby forming a normal $2n$ component, while a second sperm proliferates by mitosis independently, initiating formation of a haploid cell line. In about 10% of cases, two sperm proliferate, yielding embryos with two separate haploid cell lines. In mammals, dispermy ordinarily results in androgenic triploidy, but in the chicken it usually results in $1n/2n$ chimerism.

The incidence of haploidy is much higher in some strains of birds than in others. Furthermore, embryonic progeny of some hens exhibit a much higher incidence than do those from others, i.e., embryos with haploid components are not randomly distributed among progeny from all dams. Sires have no influence (Synder et al., 1975; Bloom, 1974). The genotype of hens apparently is of utmost importance. It is speculated that the cytoplasm of eggs from hens prone to produce haploid embryos contains a factor that promotes mitosis of accessory spermatozoa, or lacks a factor that suppresses their mitotic proliferation.

B. TRIPLOIDY

Triploidy resulting from dispermy or diplospermy is rare in chickens. None of the 20 triploid embryos that were recovered in the experiments in which male gametes were marked by a distinctive autosome contained two sets of paternal chromosomes. Most triploids were derived from eggs that were diploid as a result of the failure to extrude a second polar body. This is known from the proportion of $3n$.ZWW embryos, as diploid eggs with a WW gonosome complement result only from MII suppression. Most of the $3n$.ZZW embryos then are the result of suppression of MI, which yields diploid eggs with ZW gonosomes (see Mong et al., 1974; Fechheimer, 1981, for a full argument).

It was noted by Bloom (1974) and Mong et al. (1974) that hens at the beginning of their laying cycle, when oviposition is erratic, produce a significantly higher frequency of $3n$ embryos than they do later in the cycle when oviposition is more regular. Furthermore, in eggs containing two or more yolks, resulting from multiple ovulations, the incidence of $3n$ embryos is much greater than in eggs with single yolks (Lee et al., 1989). Apparently, eggs from mistimed ovulation containing either premature or senescent ova are prone to failure of the second meiotic division. However, triploidy tends to cluster in embryonic progeny produced by some dams. It does not occur randomly among maternal half-sib families. Just as is the case with haploid/euploid-type abnormalities, the incidence of triploidy is strongly influenced by genotype of the dams of embryos. Its incidence was increased to about

30% in embryos from a line selected for shortened interval between ovipositions, further suggesting an important genetic influence (Thorne et al., 1987). The action of the genes involved might well be to interfere with the timing, or other elements, involved in the initiation or process of MII in hens.

C. Tetraploidy and Diploid/Tetraploid Mosaicism

In every case of $2n/4n$ mosaicism examined, the $4n$ component contained an exact doubling of the $2n$ component. This was true for the sex chromosomes, for marker chromosomes, and for occasional aneuploids. A further manifestation of the same effect was seen in a few $3n/6n$ embryos, and a single $1n/2n$ embryo in which the $2n$ component had the marker represented twice. From such extensive evidence it is clear that the cell line with the doubled genome results from failure of cytokinesis during mitosis of an early cleavage division. Were it to be attributable to cell fusions, one would expect to see a reasonably high incidence of $2n/4n/6n$, the $6n$ component being from a fusion of three $2n$ cells or a $2n$ with a $4n$. The few embryos having only $4n$ cells presumably arise from a failure of cytokinesis at the first cleavage division.

To a greater extent than for any other form of heteroploidy, cases of $2n/4n$ mosaicism are confined to particular families in which they occur with particularly high frequencies. Evidence for genetic control of the error is very strong, the tendency being transmitted to fertilized eggs by both male and female parents (Fechheimer, 1981; Miller et al., 1976).

D. Pentaploidy

The incidence of $5n$ embryos is less than 1 in 1,000. Two were recovered in the experiments involving use of marker chromosomes. In both instances the embryos had only one genome derived from the sire, the remaining four being of maternal origin. The most probable mechanism of origin is that a single spermatozoon fertilizes an egg bearing four sets of chromosomes as a result of the failure of both meiotic divisions.

E. Diploid/Triploid and Diploid/Diploid Chimeras

Chimeric birds with $2n$ and $3n$ components are rare, occurring in 1–2 in 1,000 embryos, primarily in meat-type strains. They are of interest because the condition is not entirely lethal (Thorne et al., 1987) and has been reported in a number of postnatal mammals, including humans (Fechheimer et al., 1983, for review). Several feasible mechanisms of their origin have been proposed. Each has a unique cytological outcome for the array of sex chromosome complements in the two cell lines seen in a sample of embryos. The diploid component can be ZZ or ZW and the triploid component can be ZZZ, ZZW, or ZWW, so six possibilities exist. The sex chromosome complements of all known chick embryos were compared to the expected types from each of six possible mechanisms. Only one of the six proposed mechanisms could have yielded all of the embryos, and it was therefore presumed to have been the mechanism of origin of most, if not all, of them. The mechanism of choice involves the occurrence of binucleated oocytes that undergo meiotic maturation independently. Each of the resulting pronuclei, which might be diploid as a consequence of failure of either MI or MII, is fertilized by one or two sperm. A similar analysis, when applied to a sample of mink embryos, led to the same conclusion (Fechheimer et al., 1983).

Diploid/diploid chimeric embryos are recovered at about the same frequency as diploid/triploid embryos in experiments using marker chromosomes, which allow detection of all cases. A most feasible mechanism for their origin cannot be inferred from analysis similar to that applied to $2n/3n$ chimerism. However, the two types occur in the same strains of chickens and it might be supposed $2n/2n$ chimerism is also derived from binucleated oocytes (Belyaev et al., 1983).

F. Aneuploidy

1. Sex Chromosomes

Not a single case of sex chromosome aneuploidy of posthatched chickens has been reported. Even among samples of early embryos it is seen infrequently. All of the reported cases are of only two types, ZO and ZZW, and these are numbered 6 and 9, respectively. If a single mechanism were involved in the origin of all cases, the most likely would be nondisjunction at MI to yield equal numbers of oocytes with gonosome complements of O and ZW. Fertilization would then produce ZO and ZZW zygotes. All other mechanisms should yield additional types of aneuploidy such as ZZZ or ZWW.

2. Autosomes

Embryos with monosomy or trisomy of each of the macrochromosomes have been reported. Monosomy appears to be lethal at an early stage of development; no embryo was recovered in the sample of more than 6,000 embryos at 4–5 days of development (Bloom, 1974), although in samples of 1-day embryos monosomies are almost as frequent as trisomies.

Because aneuploidy is seen so infrequently, patterns of occurrence are difficult to discern. There are several reports, however, of repeated occurrences within both half-sib and full-sib families. In several of these families three to five embryos aneuploid for the same chromosome were observed (Fechheimer, 1981). Such unlikely occurrences suggest that mutations disrupting the process of normal disjunction at MI or MII of both spermatogenesis or oogenesis occur at low frequencies in some populations of chickens.

G. Diploid/Aneuploid and Aneuploid/Aneuploid Mosaicism

More common than pure aneuploids are aneuploid mosaics that contain two component cell lines, one of which sometimes is $2n$ and the other (or both) being aneuploid ($2n \pm 1$). These abnormalities obviously are derived from errors at mitosis of early cleavage divisions. Nondisjunction at the first cleavage division, which is very rare, yields derivative products that are trisomic and monosomic ($2n + 1/2n - 1$). The same event at a later division results in embryos with three component cell lines, $2n/2n + 1/2n - 1$. Chromosome lagging at anaphase is a mechanism that generates only monosomic cells ($2n - 1$). Its occurrence therefore produces mosaics of the type $2n/2n - 1$. These events occur with different frequencies in some lines of birds (Fechheimer, 1981). In a line of turkeys selected for early growth for 20 generations, the frequency of diploid/hypoploid mosaic embryos was only half as great as among those from a control line. Furthermore, loss of the various chromosomes in the affected embryos was not random (Fechheimer and Nestor, 1989). The reduction in frequency of chromosome lagging at mitosis as a concomitant to intense selection for rapid growth, and the relatively infrequent loss of two chromosomes (number 4 and Z), imply that genetic factors are important causes of such mitotic errors.

VII. Structural Aberrations

A. Spontaneously Occurring

In two large samples of embryos that were screened for chromosome abnormalities, the incidences of structural aberrations were .04 in

1,000 and 0.1 in 1,000 (Fechheimer, 1981; Bloom, 1974). The most frequent type of aberration was an apparent deletion of one of the macrochromosomes. These estimated rates should be considered to be low because deletions or rearrangements among the large numbers of microchromosomes could not have been detected. More than 10,000 hatched chicks surviving to 4–10 weeks of age have been examined and not a single rearrangement was detected (N. S. Fechheimer, unpublished data). Apparently, most of the detectable aberrations afflicting early embryos are lethal.

Testing for the presence of structural aberrations among large samples of sterile and semisterile chickens has not been reported. A single case of a semisterile cock heterozygous for a reciprocal translocation involving segments of chromosomes 2 and 3 was reported by Ryan and Bernier (1968). Another cockerel bearing a reciprocal translocation between segments of chromosomes 1 and 2 was examined by Newcomer (1959), but it is likely that the aberration was the result of X-ray treatment.

B. Experimentally Produced

Reciprocal translocations and pericentric inversions can be readily produced and recovered in hatched chicks. The alkylating agents triethylene melamine (TEM) and ethyl methanesulfonate (EMS) were used by Wang et al. (1982). Mature males were injected intraperitoneally with 400 mg of EMS or 1.2 mg of TEM and subsequently mated to several hens. The resulting eggs were incubated and 314 chicks were hatched, reared, and tested. Of these, 10 were heterozygous for a reciprocal translocation and one for a pericentric inversion of chromosome 1. Wooster et al. (1977) applied 1200 R of X rays to about 2 ml of pooled semen samples. The irradiated semen was used to inseminate hens, the eggs from which were incubated. A total of 204 chicks hatched from 726 eggs. Of the surviving birds, 18 were heterozygous for 19 reciprocal translocations and one pericentric inversion of chromosome 2 (two birds were doubly heterozygous). Breakpoints were located in all of the macrochromosomes, including the Z, and several microchromosomes. The same method was used by Zartman (1973) to produce two translocations involving segments of the long arm of chromosome 1 and the Z.

All of the birds bearing rearrangements derived from the three experiments, whether male or female, were fertile. When mated with karyologically normal birds, heterozygous progeny were recovered roughly in expected proportions (Wooster et al., 1977). Several of the translocations were subsequently obtained in homozygous form from matings of two heterozygotes. A number of reports have served to characterize the aberrations in terms of their appearance at mitotic metaphase and meiosis, affinity to form multivalents at MI, morphometric attributes, and associated phenotypic effects, especially fertility, embryonic survival, growth, and egg production. Several have been used as tools to map the location of genes to specific chromosomal regions (Zartman, 1973; Shoffner, 1981; Telloni et al., 1976; Bitgood et al., 1980).

VIII. Effects of Structural Aberrations

A. Pericentric Inversions

Two pericentric inversions were recovered from the experiments described above, one of chromosome 1, inv(1), and the other of chromosome 2, inv(2). Strains bearing the aberrations were produced for subsequent study and for further characterization. Homozygotes for inv(2) are all afflicted by the absence of tarsometatarsal bones (shankless), but are viable and fertile (Langhorst and Fechheimer, 1985). Homozygotes for inv(1) are not viable past day 2 of incubation (Bitgood et al., 1982).

1. Fertility and Hatchability

Male and female heterozygotes for both inversions are fully fertile. Hatchability of eggs produced by chromosomally normal hens mated to cockerels heterozygous for inv(2), or the reciprocal cross, is not different from matings between normal birds (Dinkel et al., 1979). Eggs from similar matings involving inv(1) have a reduced hatchability attributable to mortality of embryos with duplication or deletion of a portion of chromosome 1.

2. Pairing and Segregation

The two inversions behave differently at MI and as a consequence yield different arrays of genetically balanced and unbalanced gametic products. Examination of bivalents at diakinesis in spermatogonia of males heterozygous for inv(2) reveals a normal-appearing number 2. The chiasma number is slightly less than in normal males. In no instance was any configuration seen that might be interpreted as an inversion loop. However, analysis of synaptonemal complexes revealed some spermatocytes in which small loops were apparent. In most, however, position of the centromeres in the paired axes indicated that nonhomologous pairing at the inverted region was occurring (Kaelbling and Fechheimer, 1985). Accordingly, no crossing-over occurs within the inversion and no unbalanced gametes are produced. Products of segregation bear normal or inverted chromosomes in equal numbers.

In males heterozygous for inv(1), inversion loops are seen at MI; crossing-over within the inverted region occurs, resulting in formation of gametes with a duplication or deletion of a segment of chromosome 1 as well as balanced gametes bearing the normal or the inversion chromosome. From matings between two heterozygotes a few chicks are recovered that bear the deleted and duplicated recombinant chromosomes, which are apparently fully complementary (Bitgood et al., 1982).

B. Reciprocal Translocations

1. Fertility and Hatchability

Extensive data have accumulated regarding the fertility of translocation heterozygotes and survival of their embryonic progeny. Many of the data are from routine recordkeeping when the stocks are annually reproduced and are unpublished. Published data relative to particular translocations are in several reports (Telloni et al., 1977; Dinkel et al., 1979; Blazak and Fechheimer, 1979a,b; Bonaminio and Fechheimer, 1988).

Contrary to findings in mammals, chickens of both sexes heterozygous for all translocations that have been recovered have been fertile and capable of producing progeny bearing the translocation. When compared to chromosomally normal sibs, translocation heterozygotes for most rearrangements display an undiminished level of fertility. Semen characteristics and sperm production likewise are comparable to normal sibs. Even for translocations involving segments of the Z chromosome, there is no detectable effect on reproductive function of heterozygotes (Blazak and Fechheimer, 1979a,b, 1981b).

Eggs produced by, or fertilized by, sperm from heterozygotes exhibit a rate of hatchability about half that of eggs from gametes produced by two normal parents. The observed increase in embryonic mortality is attributable to formation of genetically unbalanced gametes by heterozygous parents. About half of the gametes from heterozygous parents carry balanced genomes and half (resulting from adjacent-1 and less frequently adjacent-2 segregation) are unbalanced (Dinkel et al., 1979; Bonaminio and Fechheimer, 1988).

2. Pairing and Segregation

Synaptonemal complex analysis of gonocytes from animals heterozygous for several translocations has indicated that most usually the four elements engage to form a quadrivalent at MI; the incidence of formation of trivalents plus a univalent is infrequent. Asynapsis in the vicinity of breakpoints is frequently observed, as is nonhomologous pairing for short lengths of the axes of a quadrivalent (Kaelbling and Fechheimer, 1985; Solari et al., 1988).

Analysis at diakinesis–metaphase of MI revealed the regular occurrence of closed quadrivalents (rings), but occasionally an open quadrivalent (chain) is seen in the case of some translocations in which one of the interchanged segments was short. All of the translocations involving the Z chromosome and an autosome form chains in oocytes, because the W chromosome contains only one short terminal region homologous to a segment on the Z chromosome. In males, however, this type of translocation exhibits a high incidence of rings (Blazak and Fechheimer, 1980).

Segregation of the products of translocation quadrivalents has been analyzed by study of secondary spermatocytes at MII (Sussman, 1988; Bonamino and Fechheimer, 1988). Observations indicate that the incidence of alternate segregation, indicated by a balanced genome, is about one-half, i.e., it occurs about as frequently as adjacent-1 and adjacent-2 segregations combined. This result is in accord with theoretical expectation. Adjacent-1 segregation occurs much more frequently than does adjacent-2 for all translocations analyzed. Products of segregation indicating 3 : 1 rather than 2 : 2 segregation are seen infrequently.

Several of the translocations analyzed involved the transposition of a segment of a microchromosome to a terminal position on a broken macrochromosome, and the reciprocal transposition of a long segment of the macrochromosome to the centromere-bearing segment of the microchromosome. Evidence from MII analysis suggests that rearranged chromosomes with the centromere derived from a microchromosome, and having a long segment of a macrochromosome, are prone to lag at anaphase of MI. The result is fewer numbers of cells than expected that contain the rearranged element. Preferential lagging of such elements suggests that the centromeres of microchromosomes are functionally not equivalent to those of the macrochromosomes; they lack the ability regularly to move a long chromosome toward a pole at anaphase of MI.

3. Transmission of Translocated Chromosomes

The array of genetically balanced and unbalanced gametes produced and transmitted to zygotes is delineated by analysis of embryos, one of the parents of which is heterozygous for a particular translocation. A number of such studies have been made (Dinkel *et al.*, 1979; Blazak and Fechheimer, 1979b, 1981a; Bonaminio and Fechheimer, 1988). The result of most of the studies was in accord with expectation. The frequency of embryo having received normal chromosomes or a balanced translocation chromosome from the heterozygous parent was usually about 50%. Of the remainder of embryos, a higher frequency bore products of adjacent-1 than of adjacent-2 segregation. Several embryos in all experiments bore products of 3 : 1 segregation. However, the array of products transmitted by female heterozygous parents was, in several instances, different from that transmitted by male heterozygotes. Either the orientation of quadrivalents and patterns of segregation in oocytes are different than is seen in spermatocytes, or there is differential selection of sperm having different genetic complements sometime between MII and fertilization. Evidence from the work of Bonaminio and Fechheimer (1988) and Dinkel *et al.* (1979) indicates that both phenomena contribute to discrepant frequencies of embryos bearing different products of segregation.

Karyotyping of hatched chicks derived from one normal and one heterozygous parent is done to estimate the proportions bearing the normal and translocated chromosomes. No chicks have been found having an unbalanced genome. The usual finding has been that 50% carry the normal chromosome and 50% carry the balanced translocation, the two gametic products resulting from alternate segregation. In a few instances a deficiency of balanced translocation carriers has been observed.

IX. Concluding Remarks

A. Extent of Knowledge of Chicken Chromosomes

The chromosomes of chicken at mitosis and meiosis have been thoroughly described using standard methods, as well as many of the techniques for revealing features of their structure and organization. Techniques have been developed that permit their observation from many tissues at all stages of the life cycle except in the very early zygote. Extensive observations of embryos have revealed the occurrence of a large number of abnormal chromosome complements at variable frequencies. The origin of most types of heteroploidy has been firmly established, and work to establish the etiological bases is at an advanced stage. Several forms of heteroploidy are not fully lethal and have been observed in juvenile and adult animals.

Many structural rearrangements have been created. Strains bearing the rearranged chromosomes have been put to use to enhance knowledge of their cytological behavior and their effects on reproduction and development. They are also used as chromosome markers in the continuing effort to map genes and to assign linkage groups to chromosomes.

B. Advantages of the Chicken as a Model Organism for Cytogenetic Studies

Despite the presence in the karyotype of large numbers of microchromosomes that cannot be individually identified, the chicken has many attributes suiting it eminently for study of many questions in cytogenetics (Fechheimer, 1990). Among these are the low cost of animals or embryos and of maintaining breeding flocks; the relatively short generation interval; the large numbers of progeny that can be obtained from single female parents; the ready availability of many genetically diverse lines and strains with unique biological properties (Somes, 1978); the immense store of knowledge of the genetics, embryology, and physiology of chickens; the ease with which the karyotype of individuals can be assessed reliably without need of employing banding techniques (Bloom, 1981); the ability to treat embryos *in ovo* under controlled conditions to detect clastogenic or other toxic effects *in vivo* without need for invasive surgery (Bloom, 1978).

C. Applicability of Findings to Mammals

Basic genetic knowledge is universally applicable. Much of what is known in cytogenetics was first revealed in invertebrates, most notably *Drosophila,* and in plants. Certainly knowledge gained from another vertebrate is at least as likely to be applicable to mammals as is that attained from lower forms. Although there are notable differences in mammalian and avian chromosome complements, they are more similar than are those of mammals and insects, or mammals and plants. The types of heteroploidy seen in chick embryos parallel closely those afflicting mammalian embryos and they have similar effects on development. It is likely that the factors of importance in causing the errors are similar. If this is accepted, then the chicken becomes a valuable resource as a pilot organism for the conduct of many experiments that are much more difficult and costly to do with mammals.

The comparative approach to many questions of biological importance has frequently proved to be instructive. Vexing questions of cytogenetics studied comparatively have yielded useful answers. One instance is a search for reasons why mammalian males heterozygous for some types of translocations are sterile. Several of the hypotheses advanced to explain the detrimental effect were negated by the finding that similar aberrations of chickens seldom if ever cause sterility (Blazak and Fechheimer, 1979a,b; 1981b).

The study of cytogenetics of the chicken is at an advanced state. It is providing a substantial amount of useful information that is both directly and indirectly pertinent, not only to fundamental questions of concern to all cytogenetics but also to those relating to applying the knowledge to augment more efficient production of animal products. Except for a few problems, the answers to which are certain to be found in aspects of the reproductive process that are unique to eutherian mammals, the results from cytogenetic research with chickens are bound to be usefully instructive to cytogeneticists working with mammalian farm animals.

REFERENCES

Abdel-Hameed, F., and Shoffner, R. N. (1971). Intersexes and sex determination in chickens. *Science* **172**, 962–964.

Ansari, H. A., Takagi, N., and Sasaki, M. (1986). Interordinal conservatism of chromosome banding patterns in *Gallus domesticus* (Galliformes) and *Melopsittacus undulatus* (Psittaciformes). *Cytogenet. Cell Genet.* **43**, 6–9.

Atkin, N. B., Mattison, G., Becak, W., and Ohno, S. (1965). The comparative DNA content of 19 species of placental mammals, reptiles, and birds. *Chromosoma* **71**, 1–10.

Au, W., Fechheimer, N. S., and Soukup, S. (1975). Identification of the sex chromosomes in the bald-eagle. *Can. J. Genet. Cytol.* **17**, 187–191.

Auer, H., Mayr, B., Lambrou, M., and Schleger, W. (1987). An extended chicken karyotype including the NOR chromosome. *Cytogenet. Cell Genet.* **45**, 218–221.

Bachmann, K., Harrington, B. A., and Craig, J. P. (1972). Genome size in birds. *Chromosoma* **37**, 405–416.

Belyaev, D. K., Isakova, G. K., and Fechheimer, N. S. (1983). Chimerism and twinning in mink and chicken (Title translated from Russian). *Dokl. Akad. Nauk SSSR* **270**, 230–232.

Bitgood, J. J., Shoffner, R. N., Otis, J. S., and Briles, W. E. (1980). Mapping of the genes for pea comb, blue egg, barring, silver, and blood groups A, E, H, and P in the domestic fowl. *Poult. Sci.* **59**, 1686–1693.

Bitgood, J. J., Shoffner, R. N., Otis, J. S., and Wang, N. (1982). Recombinant inversion chromosomes in phenotypically normal chickens. *Science* **215**, 409–411.

Blazak, W. F., and Fechheimer, N. S. (1979a). Gonosome–autosome translocations in the domestic fowl: Their effect upon male fertility and semen characteristics. *Biol. Reprod.* **21**, 575–582.

Blazak, W. F., and Fechheimer, N. S. (1979b). Gonosome–autosome translocations in fowl: Chromosome complements of gametes and viability of embryos derived from singly and doubly heterozygous cockerels. *J. Hered.* **70**, 407–412.

Blazak, W. F., and Fechheimer, N. S. (1980). Gonosome–autosome translocations in fowl: Meiotic configurations and chiasma counts from singly and doubly heterozygous cockerels. *Can. J. Genet. Cytol.* **22,** 343–351.

Blazak, W. F., and Fechheimer, N. S. (1981a). Gonosome–autosome translocations in fowl: The development of chromosomally unbalanced embryos sired by singly and doubly heterozygous cockerels. *Genet. Res.* **37,** 161–171.

Blazak, W. F., and Fechheimer, N. S. (1981b). Testicular sperm reserves in cockerels bearing Z-autosome translocations. *Poult. Sci.* **60,** 2001–2005.

Bloom, S. E. (1974). The origins and phenotypic effects of chromosome abnormalities in avian embryos. *Proc. World's Poult. Congr., 15th, 1974,* pp. 316–320.

Bloom, S. E. (1978). Chick embryos for detecting environmental mutagens. *Chem. Mutagens* **5,** 203–232.

Bloom, S. E. (1981). Detection of normal and aberrant chromosomes in chicken embryos and tumor cells. *Poult. Sci.* **60,** 1355–1361.

Bloom, S. E., and Bacon, L. D. (1985). Linkage of the major histocompatibility (B) complex and the nucleolar organizer in the chicken. *J. Hered.* **76,** 146–154.

Bloom, S. E., and Buss, E. G. (1966). Triploid–diploid mosaic chick embryo. *Science* **153,** 759–760.

Bloom, S. E. and Buss. E. G. (1968). Effect of age and kind of tissue on mitotic activity in chicken embryos. *Poult. Sci.* **47,** 837–838.

Bonaminio, G. A., and Fechheimer, N. S. (1988). Segregation and transmission of chromosomes from a reciprocal translocation in *Gallus domesticus* cockerels. *Cytogenet. Cell Genet.* **48,** 193–197.

Brant, J. W. A. (1952). A review of literature on chromosome studies of the fowl. *Poult. Sci.* **31,** 409–417.

Carlenius, C., Ryttman, H., Tegelstroem, H., and Jansson, H. (1981). R-, G-, and C-banded chromosomes in the domestic fowl *(Gallus domesticus)*. *Hereditas* **94,** 61–66.

Cock, A. G. (1964). Dosage compensation and sex chromatin in nonmammals. *Genet. Res.* **5,** 354–365.

DeBoer, L. E. M., DeGroen, T. A. G., Frankenhuis, M. T., Zonnenveld, A. J., Sallevelt, J., and Belterman, R. H. R. (1984). Triploidy in *Gallus domesticus* embryos, hatchlings, and adult intersex chickens. *Genetica (The Hague)* **65,** 83–87.

Dinkel, B. J., O'Laughlin-Phillips, E. A., Fechheimer, N. S., and Jaap, R. G. (1979). Gametic products transmitted by chickens heterozygous for chromosomal rearrangements. *Cytogenet. Cell Genet.* **23,** 124–136.

Donner, L., Chyle, P., and Sainerova, H. (1969). Malformation syndrome in *Gallus domesticus* associated with triploidy. *J. Hered.* **60,** 113–115.

Evans, E. P., Breckon, G., and Ford, C. E. (1964). An air-drying method for meiotic preparations from mammalian testes. *Cytogenetics* **3,** 289–294.

Fechheimer, N. S. (1981). Origins of heteroploidy in chicken embryos. *Poult. Sci.* **60,** 365–371.

Fechheimer, N. S. (1990). The domestic chicken *(Gallus domesticus)* as an organism for the study of chromosomal aberrations. *In* "Farm Animals in Biomedical Research" (V. Pliska and G. Stranzinger, eds.), pp. 43–54. Parey, Hamburg.

Fechheimer, N. S., and Jaap, R. G. (1978). The parental sources of heteroploidy in chick embryos determined with chromosomally marked gametes. *J. Reprod. Fertil.* **52,** 141–146.

Fechheimer, N. S., and Jaap, R. G. (1980). Origins of euploid chimerism in embryos of *Gallus domesticus. Genetica (The Hague)* **52/53,** 69–72.

Fechheimer, N. S., and Jaffe, W. P. (1966). Method for the display of avian chromosomes. *Nature (London)* **211,** 773.

Fechheimer, N. S., and Nestor, K. E. (1989). Chromosomal abnormalities in turkey embryos from a control line and a line selected for rapid growth. *Proc. Eur. Colloq. Cytogenet. Domest. Anim., 8th,* Bristol, pp. 71–77.

Fechheimer, N. S., Zartman, D. L., and Jaap, R. G. (1968). Trisomic and haploid embryos of the chick *(Gallus domesticus). J. Reprod. Fertil.* **17,** 215–217.

Fechheimer, N. S., Isakova, G. K., and Belyaev, D. K. (1983). Mechanisms involved in the spontaneous occurrence of diploid–triploid chimerism in the mink *(Mustela vision)* and chicken *(Gallus domesticus). Cytogenet. Cell Genet.* **35,** 238–243.

Ford, E. H. R., and Wollam, D. H. M. (1964). Testicular chromosomes of *Gallus domesticus. Chromosoma* **15,** 568–578.

Fritschi, S., and Stranzinger, G. (1985). Fluorescent chromosome banding in inbred chicken: Quinacrine bands, sequential chromomycin and DAPI bands. *Theor. Appl. Genet.* **71,** 408–412.

Gustavsson, I. (1980). Banding techniques in chromosome analysis of domestic animals. *Adv. Vet. Sci. Comp. Med.* **24,** 245–289.

Hutchison, N. (1987). Lampbrush chromosomes of the chicken *Gallus domesticus. J. Cell Biol.* **105,** 1493–1500.

Kaelbling, M. (1980). Synaptonemal complexes in *Gallus domesticus* cockerels. Ph.D. Dissertation, Ohio State University, Columbus.

Kaelbling, M., and Fechheimer, N. S. (1983a). Synaptonemal complexes and the chromosome complement of domestic fowl *Gallus domesticus. Cytogenet. Cell Genet.* **35,** 87–92.

Kaelbling, M., and Fechheimer, N. S. (1983b). Synaptonemal complex analysis of chromosome rearrangements in domestic fowl *Gallus domesticus. Cytogenet. Cell Genet.* **36,** 567–572.

Kaelbling, M., and Fechheimer, N. S. (1985). Synaptonemal complex analysis of a pericentric inversion in chromosome 2 of domestic fowl *(Gallus domesticus). Cytogenet. Cell Genet.* **39,** 82–86.

Langhorst, L. J., and Fechheimer, N. S. (1985). Shankless, a new mutation on chromosome 2 in the chicken. *J. Hered.* **76,** 182–186.

Lee, K.-H., Fechheimer, N. S., and Abplanalp, H. (1990). Euploid chick embryos from eggs containing one, two, or several yolks. *J. Reprod. Fertil.* **89,** 85–90.

Makino, S. (1951). "An Atlas of the Chromosome Numbers in Animals." Iowa State Coll. Press, Ames.

Miller, R. C., Fechheimer, N. S., and Jaap, R. G. (1971). Chromosome abnormalities in 16- to 18-hour chick embryos. *Cytogenetics* **10,** 121–136.

Miller, R. C., Fechheimer, N. S., and Jaap, R. G. (1976). Distribution of karyotype abnormalities in chick embryo sibships. *Biol. Reprod.* **14,** 549–560.

Miyake, Y. I., Syuto, B., and Kanagawa, H. (1984). Gene expression of triploidy in six adult intersexual chickens. *Jpn. J. Vet. Res.* **32,** 143–153.

Mong, S. J., Snyder, M. D., Fechheimer, N. S., and Jaap, R. G. (1974). The origin of triploidy in chick *(Gallus domesticus)* embryos. *Can. J. Genet. Cytol.* **16,** 317–322.

Newcomer, E. H. (1957). The mitotic chromosomes of the domestic fowl. *J. Hered.* **48,** 227–234.

Newcomer, E. H. (1959). Chromosomal translocation in domestic fowl induced by X-rays. *Science* **130,** 390–391.

Newcomer, E. H., and Brant, J. W. A. (1954). Spermatogenesis in the fowl. *J. Hered.* **45,** ⁻79–87.

Ohno, S. (1961). Sex chromosomes and microchromosomes of *Gallus domesticus. Chromosoma* **11,** 484–498.

Ohno, S., Kittrell, W. A., Christian, L. C., Stenius, L. C., and Witt, G. A. (1963). An adult triploid chicken with a left ovotestis. *Cytogenetics* **2,** 42–49.

Olesen, J. B. (1987). Fluorescent R-band patterns on normal and structurally aberrant chromosomes of *Gallus domesticus*. M.Sc. Thesis, Ohio State University, Columbus.

Owen, J. T. T. (1965). Karyotype studies on *Gallus domesticus*. *Chromosoma* **16**, 601–608.

Pollock, B. J. D. (1979). The nature of chromosomal rearrangements in specific lines of *Gallus domesticus:* C-banding and meiotic analysis. Ph.D. dissertation. The Ohio State University, Columbus.

Pollock, B. J., and Fechheimer, N. S. (1981). Variable C-banding pattern and a proposed C-band karyotype in *Gallus domesticus*. *Genetica (The Hague)* **54**, 273–279.

Pollock, D. L., and Fechheimer, N. S. (1976). The chromosome number of *Gallus domesticus*. *Br. Poult. Sci.* **17**, 39–42.

Pollock, D. L., and Fechheimer, N. S. (1978). The chromosomes of cockerels *(Gallus domesticus)* during meiosis. *Cytogenet. Cell Genet.* **21**, 267–281.

Rahn, M. I., and Solari, A. J. (1987). Recombination nodules in the oocytes of the chicken *(Gallus domesticus)*. *Cytogenet. Cell Genet.* **43**, 187–193.

Romanoff, A. L. (1960). "The Avian Embryo." Macmillan, New York.

Ryan, W. C., and Bernier, P. E. (1968). Cytological evidence for a spontaneous chromosome translocation in the domestic fowl. *Experientia* **24**, 623–624.

Schmid, W. (1962). DNA replication patterns of the heterochromosomes in *Gallus domesticus*. *Cytogenetics* **1**, 344–352.

Schwarzacher, H. G., and Wolf, U. (1974). "Methods in Human Cytogenetics." Springer-Verlag, New York.

Sharma, A. K., and Sharma, A. (1973). "Chromosome Techniques—Theory and Practice," 2nd ed. Butterworth, London.

Shoffner, R. N. (1965). Current knowledge about the chromosomes in the domestic fowl. *World's Poult. Sci. J.* **21**, 157–165.

Shoffner, R. N. (1981). Marker chromosomes and G-banding for location of genes in the chicken. *Poult. Sci.* **60**, 1372–1375.

Shoffner, R. N., Krishan, A., Haiden, G. J., Bammi, R. K., and Otis, J. S. (1967). Avian chromosome methodology. *Poult. Sci.* **46**, 333–344.

Snyder, M. D., Fechheimer, N. S., and Jaap, R. G. (1975). Incidence and origin of heteroploidy, especially haploidy, in chick embryos from intraline and interline matings. *Cytogenet. Cell Genet.* **14**, 63–75.

Solari, A. J. (1977). Ultrastructure of the synaptic autosomes and the ZW bivalent in chicken oocytes. *Chromosoma* **64**, 155–165.

Solari, A. J., Fechheimer, N. S., and Bitgood, J. J. (1988). Pairing of ZW gonosomes and the localized recombination nodule in two Z-autosome translocations in *Gallus domesticus*. *Cytogenet. Cell Genet.* **48**, 130–136.

Somes, R. G., Jr. (1978). Registry of poultry genetic stocks. *Bull.—Storrs Agric. Exp. Stn.* **446**.

Stahl, A. M., and Vagner-Capodano, A. M. (1972). Etude des chromosomes du poulet *(Gallus domesticus)* par les techniques de fluorescence. *C. R. Seances Acad. Sci., Ser. D* **275**, 2367–2370.

Stefos, K., and Arrighi, F. E., (1971). The heterochromatic nature of the W chromosome in birds. *Exp. Cell Res.* **68**, 228–231.

Stock, A. D., and Bunch, T. D. (1982). The evolutionary implications of chromosome banding pattern homologies in the bird order Galliformes. *Cytogenet. Cell Genet.* **34**, 136–148.

Stock, A. D., Arrighi, F. E. and Stefos, K. (1974). Chromosome homology in birds: Banding patterns of the chromosomes of the domestic chicken, ring-necked dove, and domestic pigeon. *Cytogenet. Cell Genet.* **13**, 410–418.

Sussman, D. A. (1988). Meiotic behavior of chromosome rearrangements in the domestic fowl. M.Sc. Thesis, Ohio State University, Columbus.

Telloni, R. V., Jaap, R. G., and Fechheimer, N. S. (1976). Cytogenetic and phenotypic effects of a chromosomal rearrangement involving the Z-chromosome and a microchromosome in the chicken. *Poult. Sci.* **55**, 1886–1896.

Telloni, R. V., Jaap, R. G., and Fechheimer, N. S. (1977). Fertility, embryo viability, and hatchability of chickens having 23% of the Z translocated to a micro-chromosome. *Poult. Sci.* **56**, 193–201.

Thorne, M. L., Collins, R. K., and Sheldon, B. L. (1987). Live haploid–diploid and other unusual mosaic chickens *(Gallus domesticus)*. *Cytogenet. Cell Genet.* **45**, 21–25.

Verma, R. S., and Babu, A. (1989). "Human Chromosomes. Manual of Basic Techniques." Pergamon, *New York*.

Wang, N., and Shoffner, R. N. (1974). Trypsin G- and C- banding for interchange analysis and sex identification in the chicken. *Chromosoma* **47**, 61–69.

Wang, N., and Shoffner, R. N. (1980). Induction of heteroploidy in *Gallus domesticus*. *Mutat. Res.* **69**, 263–273.

Wang, N., Shoffner, R. N., Otis, J. S., and Cheng, K. M. (1982). The induction of chromosomal structural changes in male chickens by the alkylating agents: Triethylene melamine and ethyl methanesulfonate. *Mutat. Res.* **96**, 53–66.

Wooster, W. E., Fechheimer, N. S., and Jaap, R. G. (1977). Structural rearrangements of chromosomes in the domestic chicken: Experimental production by X-irradiation of spermatozoa. *Can. J. Genet. Cytol.* **19**, 437–446.

Yamashina, M. Y. (1944). Karyotype studies in birds. I. Comparative morphology of chromosomes in seventeen races of domestic fowl. *Cytologia* **13**, 270–296.

Zartman, D. L. (1973). Location of the pea comb gene. *Poult. Sci.* **52**, 1455–1462.

Chromosomes of Fish

C. LARRY CHRISMAN, KENT H. BLACKLIDGE, AND PENNY K. RIGGS

Cytogenetics Laboratories, Department of Animal Sciences, Purdue University, West Lafayette, Indiana

I. Fish Genetic Research
   A. Karyotypes and Evolution
   B. Animal Models
   C. Sex Determination
   D. Experimental Genetic Manipulation
II. Cytogenetic Tools
   A. Lymphocyte Culture
   B. Short-Term Culture
   C. Chromosome Banding Techniques
   D. Polyploid and Transgenic Fish
III. Summary
   References

I. Fish Genetic Research

The fishes comprise a tremendously diverse group of animals. As evidence of their multifarious nature, the fishes exhibit chromosome complements that range widely in both character and number. Discussion concerning fish chromosomes could easily fill volumes, therefore the scope of this article has been limited to a general overview of fish cytogenetics and its application as a tool for the development of aquaculture and fish biotechnology. This work is not intended as a "cookbook" of chromosome preparation recipes. Fish cytogenetic research has numerous uses in current genetic research, including investigations into the evolutionary history of fishes, environmental toxicology, experimental ploidy manipulation, and production of transgenic fishes. Such research will be described, and specific methodology will be briefly reviewed.

A. KARYOTYPES AND EVOLUTION

The elucidation of karyotypes has progressed more slowly for fishes than for mammals. Techniques previously applied to mammalian systems, especially human, have been employed with limited success in cytogenetic investigations of fishes.

Chromosome complements ($2n$) in fishes range in number from 16 to 174, and individual chromosome lengths range from less than 1 to about 30 μm (Denton, 1973). These sets include autosomes and heteromorphic pairs that may or may not be sex chromosomes. Sex in some species of fish is controlled by polygenic factors, which will be presented later in this discussion. Most fishes have between 40 and 60 chromosomes, with 48 a generally accepted number for some common ancestral fish.

The evolution of the fishes, including the generation of new species, has principally involved the mechanisms of chromosome rearrangement and chromosome duplication. The most primitive fishes generally have large numbers of acrocentric chromosomes. Inversions, deletions, duplications, and translocations have all contributed to the evolution of fish species. The most common translocation in fishes is the Robertsonian type, wherein the centromeres of two nonhomologous chromosomes join to produce one metacentric chromosome. Aneuploidy is rarely observed in fishes. Diploid numbers are most common, but triploidy and tetraploidy are possible. Haploids, pentaploids, or greater orders of polyploidy are not known to occur in nature, but have been experimentally induced.

Ohno and Atkin (1966) and Ohno et al. (1967, 1968, 1969) did considerable research that examined the relationship of DNA quantity to chromosome number in fishes. Differences in DNA values of fishes have been interpreted to represent changes brought about by gene duplication. Ohno hypothesized that the most primitive fish karyotype consisted of 48 acrocentric chromosomes, with DNA content equal to approximately 20% of the DNA value of mammals. [Despite great variation in diploid chromosome number, DNA content is fairly constant across placental mammal species (Ohno, 1970a,b).] Mechanisms for change in the amount of DNA are thought to be unequal exchange between sister chromatids during mitosis, unequal crossing-over between two homologues during meiosis, regional redundant duplication of DNA molecules in specific chromosomes, and increase in ploidy level due to duplication of whole chromosomes.

Earlier studies by Goin and Goin (1968) compared amounts of DNA per nucleus for different animals and concluded that massive increases of nuclear DNA occurred before the beginning of pisces evolution. Within teleosts, or bony fishes, DNA quantities are highest for the more primitive forms and are lowest for the most advanced ones. Unless additional chromosome duplication events occur, the norm is for more advanced fish species to have less DNA and fewer chromosomes than do primitive species. Deletions and translocations are the mechanisms for these reductions; therefore, fishes with low amounts of DNA appear to be near the ends of evolutionary lines. The Salmonidae, with chromosomes numbering between 55 and 80, likely have experienced such an additional duplication event. Gradual diploidization, a process of natural selection that eliminates irregularities such as multivalents and bridges, typically follows chromosome duplication occurrences. Evidence of this process is seen in the Salmonidae family.

The evolution of the Salmonidae karyotype has been the subject of research and discussion for decades. In 1945, Svardson (referenced in Denton, 1973) suggested that the chromosome number of all fishes originated from a common ancestor having $n = 10$ chromosomes. If this hypothesis is valid, polyploidization could explain the numbers of chromosomes in most fish species. Early in the 1970s, however, Ohno and collaborators presented evidence that the hypothesis developed by Svardson did not accurately explain the numbers of chromosomes found in salmonids. Rather, the occurrence of a single tetraploid event in a common ancestor of salmonids between 25 and 100 million years ago was suggested. This ancestor would have possessed a karyotype of 48 acrocentric chromosomes. Ohno has proposed more widely that this ancestral karyotype is common to teleost fishes (Ohno, in Hartley, 1987).

The first salmonid would have possessed some 96 acrocentric chromosomes, according to Ohno. This conclusion is based on studies involving a comparison of chromosome arm number with that in other species, DNA content, the number of duplicated gene loci, and the presence of multivalents at meiosis. Furthermore, Ohno suggested that salmonids are presently undergoing diploidization. Hartley (1987) established strong evidence for considerable structural rearrangements via pericentric inversions and Robertsonian translocations during the evolution of modern salmonid karyotypes. He proposed a scheme (Fig. 1) wherein the evolution of salmonid karyotypes proceeded from either a tetraploid ancestor with 96 acrocentric chromosomes (Fig. 1, Route B) or a tetraploid ancestor in which some rearrangement of the diploid ancestral karyotype had taken place before tetraploidy (Route A). Hartley's scheme suggests that centric fusions have played a more important role in salmonid karyotype evolution than have pericentric inversions.

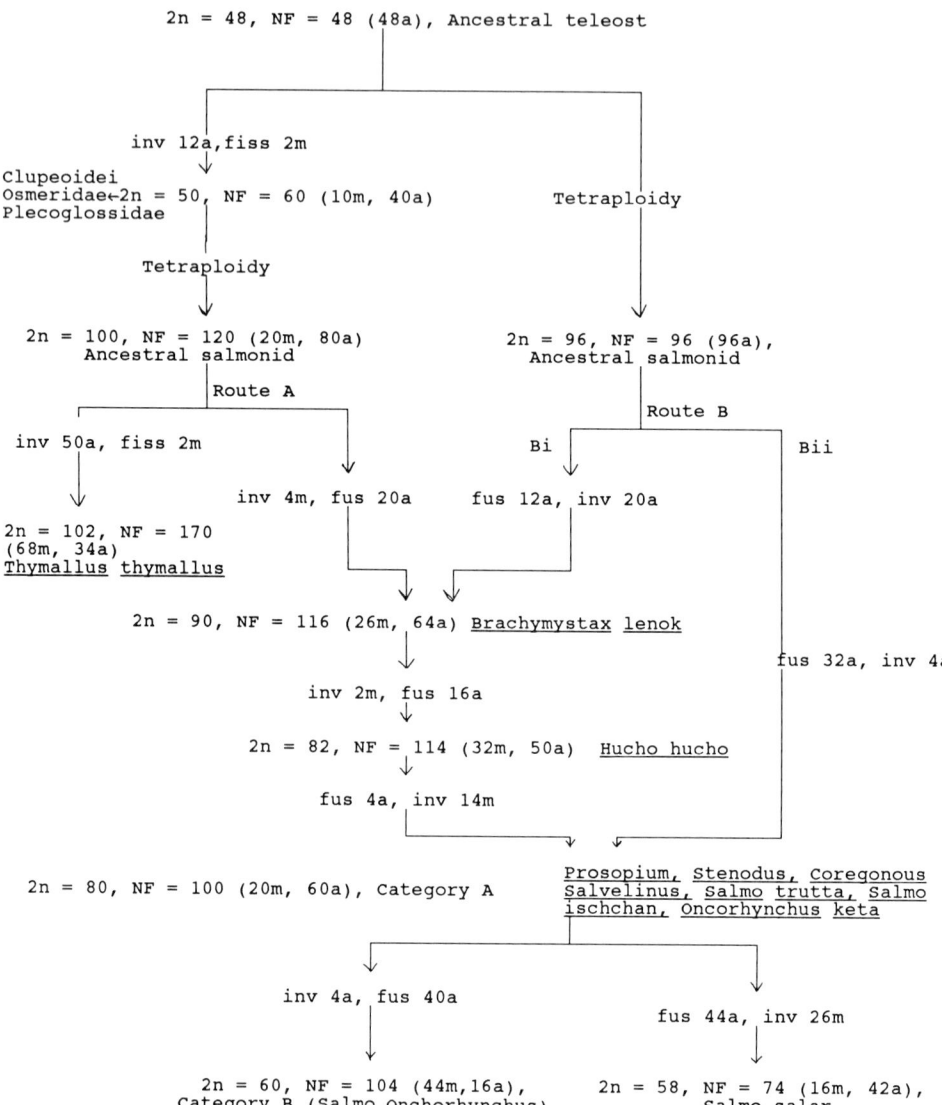

FIG. 1. Scheme for the evolution of salmonid karyotypes from an ancestral teleost containing $2n = 48$, NF = 48. Abbreviations: a, acrocentric (one-armed) chromosomes; inv, inversions; fiss, centric fissions; m, metacentric (two-armed) chromosomes; fus, centric fusions. The steps from one karyotype to the next involve inversions and fusions or fissions, e.g., from *Brachymystax lenok*, $2n = 90$, NF = 116 (26 metacentrics, 64 acrocentrics) to *Hucho hucho*, $2n = 82$, NF = 114 (32 metacentrics, 50 acrocentrics) requires pericentric inversions in two metacentric chromosomes and centric fusion of 16 acrocentric chromosomes. (After Hartley, 1987. © 1987 by the Cambridge Philosophical Society. Reprinted with the permission of Cambridge University Press.)

Data from studies of nucleolar organizing regions (NORs) have also been useful in determining evolution patterns in salmonids. The quantities and chromosomal locations of NORs in five North American species of *Salvelinus*, for example, by Phillips *et al.* (1989) and Phillips and Ihssen (1985), support the grouping of *Salvelinus malma* with *Salvelinus alpinus*, *Salvelinus fontinalis* with *Salvelinus namaycush*, and *Salvelinus confluentus* alone. Stock-specific differences also lend themselves to NOR studies (Phillips *et al.*, 1988). Phillips and colleagues conclude that differences in chromosome locations of NORs in different stocks combined with other cytologic and molecular methods will likely be helpful in delineating genetic relationships among allopatric and sympatric stocks.

B. Animal Models

The potential of fishes as models for medical and environmental cytogenetic studies is great. Of the more than 20,000 fish species that comprise 44 orders and 550 families, only about 20 species have been examined in detail. The biology of the Salmonidae and Ictaluridae families has been most clearly elucidated. Selected others from various families have been studied when used in specific genetic research efforts. In North America, these include members of the Catostomidae, Centrarchidae, Cichlidae, Esocidae, Percidae, and Umbridae families.

Fishes as *in vivo* models are already being used as systems for screening the toxic effects of a variety of environmental pollutants. A great deal of research has gone into the effort to define quantitative chemical structure versus biological activity relationships for pollutants in an aquatic environment. Typically, biological activity has most often been measured as the lethal concentration to a portion of the test population, the level of some behavioral variable, the change in some biochemical product or intermediate, or the degree of reproductive success. Little has been done concerning toxicological effects upon chromosomes. However, beginning in the mid-1970s, some studies involving the incidence level of sister chromatid exchange have been reported. These investigations were undertaken to determine the appropriateness of using fishes as biological monitors of mutagens in polluted waters. Such correlations were established using the central mudminnow *(Umbra limi)* as the bioassay organism (Kligerman *et al.*, 1975; Kligerman and Bloom, 1976; Kligerman, 1979; Alink *et al.*, 1980).

Certainly, as cytogenetic techniques become more available to the field of aquatic toxicology, expanded studies of the effects of pollutants upon chromosomes are expected. Perhaps, comprehensive quantitative structure–activity relationship (QSAR) models involving chromosome morphology will be developed. These studies may correlate genetic changes with deleterious events earlier and at a more sensitive stage than is presently possible.

The search is underway to determine which fish species are most useful as models in cytogenetic research. One candidate is the central mudminnow, which is easily obtained in the United States and has only 22 chromosomes. The chromosomes of the mudminnow are large, and the fish is relatively small (about 7 cm), which permits keeping large numbers in captivity.

Current United States federal requirements for aquatic toxicological studies for new compounds commonly involve bluegill *(Lepomis macrochirus)*, bass *(Micropterus salmoides)*, and fathead minnows *(Pimephales promulus)* as well as invertebrates. However, mammals remain the most accepted models for evaluating the toxic potential of chemicals to human beings.

Oncological and mutation research are additional areas for cytogenetic exploration in fishes. Investigators of the metabolism of contaminants have shown that fishes share similar pathways with mammals for the detoxification of xenobiotics. As with mammals, many of the intermediates formed during detoxification are carcinogenic and have produced tumor formation in fishes. Melanoma formation has been investigated in the Xiphophorin fish, which possess characteristic macromelanophore spot patterns (Anders *et al.*, 1973).

Teleosts were first used as models for mutation research by Samokhvalova (1938). She found a presumed dominant mutation of the gene complex "Bimaculatus" in the guppy, *Lebistes reticulates,* following 750-R dosages of X rays to spermatozoa. Subsequent to Samakhvalova's work, many other mutations have been noted in a variety of fishes following irradiation. These include congenital malformations, inheritance of radiation-induced spinal curvatures, exchange between the sex chromosomes, synergistic action of newly induced recessive mutations, formation of premelanomas, sex reversal, changes of behavioral traits, and gynogenesis (Purdom and Woodhead, 1973).

Mutation research in fishes is important both theoretically and practically. In aquaculture, it plays a role in the search for disease resistance, tolerance to crowding, stress reduction, increased growth rates, and other important characteristics. The understanding of the role of new mutant genes associated with the formation of melanomas and premelanomas in fishes has obvious implications for understanding carcinogenesis in general. Greater understanding of the effects of ionizing radiation has already been realized. Studies involving chemical mutagens offer additional research opportunities. More sophisticated methods of detecting chromosome aberrations are needed to screen for the mutagenic effects of a myriad of compounds to be used in medicine or in the environment. Mutation research on fishes may also direct understanding of the questions of the evolution of vertebrates.

Opportunities to develop new models for cancer research, environmental toxicology, and evolution are likely to become more numerous as the biology of fishes unfolds. However, an immediate opportunity for research requiring the cooperation of cytogeneticists and molecular biologists is in the rapidly emerging aquaculture industry. Exploring the use of genetic manipulation to enhance the growth characteristics of fishes in commercial culture settings is one of the most important challenges facing this industry. The goals of genetic enhancement of fish species are to increase growth rates, feed conversion efficiency, and processing yields. These goals may be reached through a combination of technologies that have been demonstrated in various species. These technologies include sex reversal through hormone treatment; polyploidization through heat, cold, or pressure shock to produce triploids and tetraploids; and gene insertion to produce transgenic animals with improved growth characteristics.

C. Sex Determination

Fishes exhibit nearly every type of genetic determination of sexual phenotype described for vertebrates (Yamamoto, 1969). Although the majority of species are gonochoristic, hermaphroditism is also represented with a wide range of expression.

Sex in fishes is generally believed to be determined by polygenic rather than chromosomal factors (Kosswig, 1964; Yamamoto, 1969; Denton, 1973; Kallman, 1984). The sex chromosomes are designated as those that possess the genes that play a major role in affecting primary sex characteristics. Additional genes that also influence sex determination are located on various autosomes. In some cases, certain combinations of these autosomal genes may override the primary sex-determining gene(s).

Most fishes do not possess heteromorphic sex chromosomes, so discussion of X, Y, W, or Z chromosomes is often based upon the results of genetic crosses. The most extensive genetic studies involve the species *Xiphophorus* (reviewed by Kallman, 1984). For the most part, members of this species have male heterogamety, with the female designated XX and the male designated XY. The medaka, *Oryzias latipes*, and the goldfish, *Carassius auratus*, have also been identified as having an XX/XY system. Wolters et al. (1982a) observed a 1:1 male to female sex ratio in their triploid channel catfish *(Ictalurus punctatus)* production studies. This ratio is expected if sex determination is controlled by the XX/XY system, although heteromorphic chromosomes have not been observed in catfish. Inheritance of melanistic spotting patterns in eastern mosquitofish *(Gambusia affinis holbrooki)* indicates this species also conforms to an XX/XY sex-determining mechanism (Angus, 1989).

Exceptions to the XX/XY system have been identified in the platyfish, *Xiphophorus maculatus,* and in *Tilapia hornorum.* The sex-determining mechanism of *X. maculatus* apparently involves three sex chromosomes, W, X, and Y. The combinations WY, WX, and XX result in female differentiation, while XY and YY produce males (Kallman, 1965, 1973). Previous studies by several authors in 1926 suggested the platyfish was better described by a WZ female/ZZ male system and some disagreement about terminology may still exist (Yamamoto, 1969). A mechanism similar to that found in *X. maculatus* was proposed by Chen (1969) to explain sex determination in *T. hornorum* (now named *Sarotherodon hornorum*), although the three sex chromosomes alone were insufficient for explaining some irregularities in sex ratios of offspring in some of the breeding studies. This fish is still poorly understood, but Avtalion and Hammerman (1978) suggested that like *X. maculatus, T. hornorum* utilizes a three-gonosome system (X, Y, and W) wherein a given individual has two sex chromosomes as well as a pair of influencing autosomes that determine sex. By including the influence of autosomal sex-determinant genes, Avtalion and Hammerman were able to explain the results of Chen's breeding studies.

Although infrequently cited in the fish cytogenetics literature, heteromorphic sex chromosomes were observed by Ebeling and Chen (1970) in males in 12 of 25 species of deep-sea fishes representing the Bathylagidae, Myctophidae, and Sternoptychidae families. The fishes studied were presumed to be XY males with the exception of two cases, wherein the males were considered to have an XO chromosome constitution *(Sternoptyx diaphana* and *Lampanyctus ritteri).* In contrast, Ebeling and Chen observed heteromorphic sex chromosomes in only 5 of 30 shallow-water fishes. In the western mosquitofish *(Gambusia affinis affinis)* and one stickleback *(Apeltes quadracus),* females possess the heteromorphic chromosomes and presumably a WZ/ZZ sex-determining system. The remaining fishes *(Fundulus diaphinus, Fundulus parvipinnis,* and *Gasterosteus wheatlandi)* exhibited heteromorphic chromosomes in males (XX/XY).

In summary, sex determination in fishes is complicated and not well understood. As might be expected in such a diverse group of organisms, multiple mechanisms appear to operate in various combinations to influence sexual differentiation. Perhaps, the mechanistic diversity is indicative of the fishes' evolutionary station, intermediate between invertebrates and mammals.

The lack of clear-cut deterministic mechanisms has been exploited, however, to accomplish *phenotypic* sex reversal in fish by treatment with appropriate hormones, including 17-α-methyl testosterone and 17-β-estradiol. Phenotypic sex reversal of genetic females has been accomplished in numerous species, including salmonids, tilapia, medaka, carp (Yamamoto, 1958; Yamazaki, 1983;), and yellow perch (Malison *et al.*, 1986). When sex-reversed, genetic females become fully functional phenotypic males that may be used in breeding schemes wherein all female progeny are desired. Likewise, sex reversal has been carried out in genetic males in many of the same species (Donaldson and Hunter, 1982; Yamamoto, 1965). This reversal is used to produce XY phenotypic females. XY females bred to normal XY males produce F_1 progeny consisting of XY males, XX females, and YY males (Yamamoto, 1965; 1975). Subsequently, YY males may be used in breeding schemes wherein all male progeny are desired.

D. Experimental Genetic Manipulation

Ploidy manipulation in fish has been the subject of attention of numerous researchers interested in fishes (Thorgaard, 1986). Experimentally enhanced ploidy levels have been produced in species such as trout (Chourrout and Happe, 1986), carp (Cassani and Caton, 1985), and walleye (Baumgartner *et al.*, 1986). Extensive ploidy manipulation with channel catfish has been carried out by C. L. Chrisman and G. S. Libey (Wolters *et al.*, 1981a; 1982a; Chrisman *et al.*, 1983; Bidwell, 1984; Bidwell *et al.*, 1985; Lucker, 1987).

In catfish, significant improvements in feed conversion and rates of weight gain were seen in triploid versus normal diploid animals (Wolters *et al.*, 1982a). At 8 months, triploid catfish showed a nearly complete lack of gonadal development compared to full sibling normal diploids. Production of second-generation triploid trout by mating tetraploid males and diploid females has been shown by Chourrout and Happe (1986). Preliminary experiments have been successful in producing tetraploid channel catfish that showed normal gonadal development (Bidwell *et al.*, 1985).

The introduction of genes into the germ lines of various fishes is the subject of intense interest (Maclean et al., 1987). Dunham et al. (1987) have demonstrated the transfer of the metallothionein–human growth hormone gene into channel catfish. Maclean et al. (1987) described successful gene transfer in rainbow trout, goldfish, common carp, mirror carp, mud carp, silver crucian, loach, and Wuchang fish. Ozato et al. (1986) have produced transgenic medaka (O. latipes) by microinjecting a chicken δ-crystallin gene into eggs. Gene constructs consisting of various promoter sequences fused with human growth hormone gene have been successfully introduced into the medaka (Lu et al., 1989). This research with medaka has demonstrated the ability to pass favorable characteristics to progeny via insertion of a transgene into a founder fish.

To date the majority of transgenic fish research has focused on the integration of growth hormone fusion gene constructs. The isolation and integration of additional gene constructs, especially those containing tissue-specific promoter sequences, will significantly affect the aquaculture industry. For example, the inclusion of genes for disease resistance, stress reduction, resistance to cold water temperatures, or the production of ω-3 fatty acids could improve cultured stocks, thus enhancing the development of aquatic species as agricultural crops.

II. Cytogenetic Tools

Fish cytogenetics has progressed more slowly than chromosome studies of many mammalian species. As noted earlier in this discussion, complete karyotypes have been established for only about 2–3% of the more than 20,000 fish species (Gold, 1979), although chromosome number has been identified in many additional species (reviewed by Gold et al., 1980; Sola et al., 1981). At present, a variety of both short-term and long-term culture techniques and the development of some banding methods have significantly improved the cytogeneticist's ability to obtain metaphase chromosomes in good condition. However, reliable high-resolution banding techniques have yet to be developed for fish chromosomes. As fish genetic and biotechnology research rapidly progresses, cytogenetics will likely become essential as a diagnostic tool.

Several authors have reviewed chromosome preparation techniques in great detail (Denton, 1973; Blaxhall, 1975; Ojima, 1978; Hartley and Horne, 1985; Zhuo, 1988). These references should be consulted for specific instruction concerning methodology.

A. Lymphocyte Culture

Lymphocyte culture is an effective method for obtaining chromosomes from larger fish, as removal of a small blood sample causes little or no harm to the animal. The culture procedure is similar, although not identical, to mammalian lymphocyte cultures. In most cases, 3-day cultures are maintained at 27–30°C. During harvest, hypotonic action is accomplished with 0.4% potassium chloride. Lymphocyte cultures have been successfully employed to provide metaphase figures from several species, including carp and goldfish (Labat et al., 1967; Ojima et al., 1970; Heckman and Brubaker, 1971), trout (Heckman et al., 1971; Thorgaard, 1976), Japanese eel (Kang and Park, 1975), salmon (Grammeltvedt, 1975), and catfish (Wolters et al., 1981b).

B. Short-Term Culture

Short-term culture, or direct preparation of solid tissues (gill epithelium, scale, kidney, and intestine), is useful for preparing chromosomes if the fish can be sacrificed. This method may be necessary with small fish because blood volume is limited. Short-term cultures have furnished metaphase chromosomes from fishes after *in vivo* treatment with colchicine (Kligerman and Bloom, 1977b). Hollenbeck and Chrisman (1981) treated the hematopoietic kidney tissue from catfish with colchicine *in vitro* to allow better dosage control and prevent overconstriction of chromosomes. Direct preparations from early embryo tissue have also been successful (Thorgaard et al., 1981; Phillips and Zajicek, 1982). Harvest procedures are similar to those for lymphocyte cultures, although Chourrout and Happe (1986) harvested short-term kidney and embryo cultures using 0.8% trisodium citrate as the hypotonic agent rather than conventional potassium chloride treatment.

Long-term fibroblast or epithelial cell cultures derived from various tissues, particularly scale or fin, have been used to allow chromosome analysis from small fishes without requiring sacrifice of the animal (Wolf and Quimby, 1969; Ojima, 1978; Zhuo, 1988). This method is advantageous for determining ploidy of young fishes, or for obtaining chromosomes for *in situ* DNA hybridization analysis in young transgenic fishes. However, long-term culture necessitates karyotyping of early passages of the culture because some changes may occur over time as the cells are maintained *in vitro*.

C. CHROMOSOME BANDING TECHNIQUES

Banding techniques that have found the most widespread use for analysis of fish chromosomes include C-banding and silver or chromomycin A_3 (CMA_3) staining to detect NORs. Standard C-banding methods that include treatment with sodium hydroxide (NaOH) or barium hydroxide (BaOH) followed by incubation in standard saline citrate (SSC) have been modified for fish chromosomes (Zenzes and Voiculescu, 1975; Thorgaard, 1976; Kligerman and Bloom, 1977a). Fish chromosomes seem to require a shorter NaOH or BaOH treatment time than most mammalian C-band preparations.

Silver staining or CMA_3 staining has been used to identify NORs in fish chromosomes (Kligerman and Bloom, 1977a; Howell and Black, 1979; Phillips and Ihssen, 1985). Silver staining identifies NORs that were active at the last interphase, whereas treatment with CMA_3 identifies NORs in fishes regardless of activity. C-Banding and NOR localization have been useful for studying phylogenetic relationships of various fish species, as well as identifying stock-specific differences within a species (Phillips and Kapuscinski, 1987, 1988).

G-Banding, although frequently utilized in mammalian chromosome studies, has not found favor with fish cytogeneticists. Most attempts at G-banding have been reported as unsuccessful (Thorgaard, 1976; Kligerman and Bloom, 1977b; Uwa and Ojima, 1981). Successful reports failed to demonstrate bands of good resolution or definitive, repeatable patterns useful for chromosome identification purposes (Rishi, 1979; Blaxhall, 1983).

Other approaches to obtaining chromosome bands include Q-banding (Kligerman and Bloom, 1977a), the use of restriction endonucleases (Lloyd and Thorgaard, 1988), and incorporation of 5-bromodeoxyuridine (BrdU) to produce replication banding patterns (Delaney and Bloom, 1984; Hong and Zhou, 1985; Zhuo, 1988). Q-Band polymorphisms have been studied in several species (Phillips and Ihssen, 1986; Pleyte *et al.*, 1989), but these banding techniques have not yet been developed as useful methods for routine karyotype analysis of fishes. The difficulty in banding fish chromosomes has not been explained, although a number of hypotheses have been proposed (reviewed in Hartley and Horne, 1985; Lloyd and Thorgaard, 1988). Possibly, procedures attempted to date have not produced sufficiently elongated chromosomes to allow banding of adequate resolution. Zhuo (1988) found that untreated midmetaphase chromosomes of channel catfish average 1.3–1.5 μm in length. (In comparison, the smallest human chromosome is about 1.5 μm at midmetaphase.) Incorporation of BrdU increased overall chromosome length by about 70%, indicating that BrdU incorporation and synchronization of cell cultures may allow a more reliable banding technique to be developed.

D. POLYPLOID AND TRANSGENIC FISH

In addition to traditional chromosome analysis (metaphase chromosome preparations and banding techniques), other molecular and cytological methods are important for identifying triploid, tetraploid, and/or transgenic fish.

As ploidy level increases, the change in total DNA content and chromosome number is reflected by an increase in nuclear size. One may take advantage of the nucleated erythrocytes of fish to determine ploidy by a number of methods. Flow cytometry, Coulter counter analysis, or simply microscopic measurement of erythrocyte nuclei can be used to identify ploidy of individual fish.

Frequently, ploidy levels have been determined for various fish species by erythrocyte measurements obtained by using an eyepiece micrometer (reviewed by Wolters *et al.*, 1982b). In some cases, measurement of nuclear volume alone was variable in its effectiveness for correctly identifying ploidy because of overlapping distributions. However, Wolters and his colleagues found that individual channel catfish can be correctly classified according to mean major axis measurements with a probability of about 92% accuracy.

A Coulter counter (or similar device), which automates the process of estimating nuclear volume, can allow the processing of large numbers of fish cells over a fairly short period of time. Wattendorf (1986) showed that use of the Coulter counter was perfectly correlated to manual erythrocyte nuclear volume measurements for diploid and triploid grass carp *(Ctenopharyngodon idella)*. Fishes whose modal nucleus size fell into an area of overlap between the diploids and triploids were correctly classified when cell sample size was increased from 100 to 1,000. The Coulter counter procedure has also been used to identify ploidy levels in Atlantic salmon *(Salmo salar;* Benfey *et al.*, 1984).

Flow cytometry, another rapid and automated technique, quantitates fluorescently labeled DNA within the cell. Propidium iodide, a DNA intercalator, is a commonly used staining agent. Cells in suspension are passed through the cytometer in which a laser beam excites the intercalated stain. Fluorescence levels, proportional to DNA quantity, are compared to standards and 2n controls. Thousands of cells may be analyzed for ploidy level in a matter of minutes. This technique has been utilized by Thorgaard et al. (1982), Allen (1983), Allen and Stanley (1983), Utter et al. (1983), Solar et al. (1984), and Lucker (1987).

Another method of ploidy determination involves an application of the silver staining technique to identify NORs. Microscope slides of cells from gill tissue are prepared and treated in a manner similar to the NOR staining procedures previously described. Ploidy can then be easily determined by counting silver-stained nucleoli. Many species possess only one chromosome with an NOR per haploid genome (Phillips et al., 1986, 1989). In studies involving three salmonid species (rainbow trout, *Salmo gairdneri;* chinook salmon, *Oncorhynchus tshawytscha;* and coho salmon, *Oncorhynchus kisutch*), haploid individuals had one nucleolus per cell; diploids had one or two nucleoli per cell; and triploids had one, two, or three nucleoli per cell. The results allowed positive identification of triploids because no haploid or diploid individuals possessed cells containing three nucleoli. This technique can provide a simple screening system for ascertaining ploidy, but is not particularly useful for *Salvelinus* species such as lake trout *(S. namaycush)* and brook trout *(S. fontinalus)*, which carry multiple chromosome pairs with NORs.

Transgenic fish are initially identified by DNA analyses described in numerous molecular biology textbooks. However, *in situ* DNA hybridization allows cytogenetic analysis of these animals. A radioactive probe for the foreign gene (transgene) is hybridized to metaphase chromosomes and the microscope slide is coated with photographic emulsion (Naylor et al., 1987). Following development and staining, a developed silver grain will be found at the chromosomal location of the transgene. Knowledge of transgene insertion sites may prove useful as biotechnological research progresses. It should be noted, however, that *in situ* hybridization must be carried out with high-quality chromosome preparations in order to provide meaningful results.

III. Summary

The future for cytogenetic research in fishes appears bright. Technical difficulties in working with fish chromosomes are being overcome through application of techniques currently employed for other phyla, as well as through development of new techniques. As aquaculture and biotechnology involving both fresh and marine species develop, cytogenetic and molecular techniques will likely be integrated as essential research tools.

REFERENCES

Alink, G. M., Frederix-Wolters, E. M. H., Vandergaag, M. A., van de Kerkhoff, J. F. L., and Poels, C. L. M. (1980). Induction of sister-chromatid exchanges in fish exposed to Rhine water. *Mutat. Res.* **78,** 369–374.

Allen, S. K. (1983). Flow cytometry: Assaying experimental polyploid fish and shell fish. *Aquaculture* **33,** 317–328.

Allen, S. K., and Stanley, J. G. (1983). Ploidy of hybrid grass carp and bighead carp determined by flow cytometry. *Trans. Am. Fish. Soc.* **112,** 431–435.

Anders, A., Anders, F., and Klinke, K. (1973). Regulation of gene expression in the Gordon-Kosswig melanoma system. I. The distribution of the controlling genes in the genome of the xiphophorin fish, *Platypoecilus maculatus* and *Platypoecilus variatus.* In "Genetics and Mutagenesis of Fish." (J. H. Schroder, ed.), pp. 33–52. Springer-Verlag, New York.

Angus, R. A. (1989). Inheritance of melanistic pigmentation in the eastern mosquitofish. *J. Hered.* **80,** 387–392.

Avtalion, R. R., and Hammerman, I. S. (1978). Sex determination in sartherodon *(Tilapia)* I. Introduction to a theory of autosomal influence. *Bamidgeh* **30,** 110–115.

Baumgartner, A. P., Chrisman, C. L., Libey, G. S., Lucker, D. B., and Woolcott, B. L. (1986). Standard karyotype of the wallyeye (*Stizostedion vitreum:* $2n = 48$): Induction of polyploidy by heat shock. *Midwest Fish Wildl. Conf., 48th,* Omaha pp. 39–40.

Benfey, T. J., Sutterlin, A. M., and Thompson, R. J. (1984). Use of erythrocyte measurements to identify triploid salmonids. *Can. J. Fish. Aquat. Sci.* **41,** 980–984.

Bidwell, C. A. (1984). Induced spawning and heat shock induced tetraploidy in channel catfish. MS Thesis, Purdue University, West Lafayette, Indiana.

Bidwell C. A., Chrisman, C. L., and Libey, G. S. (1985). Polyploidy induced by heat shock in channel catfish. *Aquaculture* **51,** 25–32.

Blaxhall, P. C. (1975). Fish chromosome techniques—A review of selected literature. *J. Fish Biol.* **7,** 315–320

Blaxhall, P. C. (1983). Chromosome karyotyping of fish using conventional and G-banding methods. *J. Fish Biol.* **22,** 417–424.

Cassani, J. R., and Caton, W. E. (1985). Induced triploidy in grass carp, *Ctenopharyngodon idella val. Aquaculture* **46,** 37–44

Chen, F. Y. (1969). Preliminary studies on the sex determining mechanism of *Tilapia mossambica* Peters and *T. hornorum* Trewavas. *Verh.—Int. Ver. Theor. Angew. Limnol.* **17,** 719–724.

Chourrout, D., and Happe, A. (1986). Improved methods of direct chromosome preparation in rainbow trout, *Salmo gairdneri. Aquaculture* **52,** 255–261.

Chrisman, C. L., Wolters, W. R., and Libey, G. S. (1983). Triploidy in channel catfish. *J. World Maric. Soc.* **14,** 279–293.

Delany, M. E., and Bloom, S. E. (1984). Replication banding patterns in the chromosomes of the rainbow trout. *J. Hered.* **75,** 431–434.

Denton, T. E. (1973). "Fish Chromosome Methodology." Thomas, Springfield, Illinois.

Donaldson, E. M., and Hunter, G. A. (1982). Sex control in fish with particular reference to salmonids. *Can. J. Fish. Aquat. Sci.* **39,** 99–110.

Dunham, R. A., Eash, J., Askins, J., and Townes, T. M. (1987). Transfer of the metallothionein–human growth hormone fusion gene into channel catfish. *Trans. Am. Fish. Soc.* **116**, 87–91.

Ebeling, A. W., and Chen, T. R. (1970). Heterogamety in teleostean fishes. *Trans. Am. Fish. Soc.* **99**, 131–138

Goin, O. B., and Goin, C. J. (1968). DNA and the evolution of the vertebrate. *Am. Midl. Nat.* **80**, 289–298.

Gold, J. R. (1979). Cytogenetics. *In* "Fish Physiology" (W. S. Hoar and D. J. Randall, eds.), Vol. 8, pp. 353–405. Academic Press, New York.

Gold, J. R., Karel, W. J., and Strand, M. R. (1980). Chromosome formulae of North American fishes. *Prog. Fish.-Cult.* **42**, 10–23.

Grammeltvedt, A. (1975). Chromosomes of salmon *(Salmo salar)* by leukocyte culture. *Aquaculture* **5**, 205–209.

Hartley, S. E. (1987). The chromosomes of salmonid fishes. *Biol. Rev. Cambridge Philos. Soc.* **62**, 197–214.

Hartley, S. E., and Horne, M. T. (1985). Cytogenetic techniques in fish genetics. *J. Fish Biol.* **26**, 575–582.

Heckman, J. R., and Brubaker, P. E. (1971). Chromosome preparation from fish blood leukocytes. *Prog. Fish.-Cult.* **32**, 206–208.

Heckman, J. R., Allendorf, F. W., and Wright, J. E. (1971). Trout leukocytes: Growth in oxygenated cultures. *Science* **173**, 246–247.

Hollenbeck, P. J., and Chrisman, C. L. (1981). Kidney preparations for chromosomal analyses of *Ictaluridae*. *Copeia*, pp. 216–217.

Hong, Y., and Zhou, T. (1985). Chromosome banding in fishes I. An improved BrdU–Hoechst–Giemsa method for revealing DNA-replication bands in fish chromosomes. *Acta Genet. Sin.* **12**, 67–71.

Howell, W. M., and Black, D. A. (1979). Location of the nucleolus organizer regions on the sex chromosomes of the banded killifish, *Fundulus diaphanus*. *Copeia*, pp. 544–546.

Kallman, K. D. (1965). Genetics and geography of sex determination in the poeciliid fish, *Xiphophorus maculatus*. *Zoologica (N.Y.)* **50**, 151–190.

Kallman, K. D. (1973). The sex-determining mechanism of the platyfish, *Xiphophorus maculatus*. *In* "Genetics and Mutagenesis of Fish" (J. H. Schröder, ed.), pp. 19–28. Springer-Verlag, New York.

Kallman, K. D. (1984). A new look at sex determination in poeciliid fishes. *In* "Evolutionary Genetics of Fishes" (B. J. Turner, ed.), pp. 95–172. Plenum, New York.

Kang, K. Y., and Park, E. H. (1975). Leucocyte culture of the eel without autologous serum. *Jpn. J. Genet.* **50**, 159–161.

Kligerman, A. D. (1979). Induction of sister-chromatid exchanges in the central mudminnow following *in vivo* exposure to mutagenic agents. *Mutat. Res.* **64**, 205–217.

Kligerman, A. D., and Bloom, S. E. (1976). Sister chromatid differentiation and exchanges in adult mudminnows *(Umbra limi)* after *in vivo* exposure to 5-bromodeoxyuridine. *Chromosoma* **56**, 101–109.

Kligerman, A. D., and Bloom, S. E. (1977a). Distribution of F-bodies, heterochromatin, and nucleolar organizers in the genome of the central mudminnow, *Umbra limi*. *Cytogenet. Cell Genet.* **18**, 182–196.

Kligerman, A. D., and Bloom, S. E. (1977b). Rapid chromosome preparations from solid tissues of fishes. *J. Fish. Res. Board Can.* **34**, 266–269.

Kligerman, A. D., Bloom, S. E., and Howell, W. M. (1975). *Umbra limi:* A model for the study of chromosome aberrations in fishes. *Mutat. Res.* **31**, 225–233.

Kosswig, C. (1964). Polygenic sex determination. *Experientia* **20**, 190–199.

Labat, R., Larrouy, G., and Malaspin, L. (1967). Technique de culture des leukocytes de *Cyprinus carpio* L. *C. R. Hebd. Seances Acad. Sci.* **264**, 2473–2474.

Lloyd, M. A., and Thorgaard, G. H. (1988). Restriction endonuclease banding of rainbow trout chromosomes. *Chromosoma* **96**, 171–177.

Lu, J. K., Andrisani, O. M., Pease, K., Dixon, J. E., and Chrisman, C. L. (1990). Germ line transmission and performance of Japanese medaka transgenic for the human growth hormone gene. *J. Reprod. Fertil. Suppl.* **41** (in press).

Lucker, D. L. B. (1987). Induction of autopolyploidy and allopolyploidy in catfish determined by flow cytometry. MS Thesis, Purdue University, West Lafayette, Indiana.

Maclean, N., Penman, D., and Zhu, Z. (1987). Introduction of novel genes into fish. *Bio/Technology* **5**, 257–261.

Malison, J. A., Kayes, T. B., Best, C. D., Amundson, C. H., and Wentworth, B. C. (1986). Sexual differentiation and use of hormones to control sex in yellow perch *(Perca flavescens)*. *Can. J. Fish. Aquat. Sci.* **43**, 26–35.

Naylor, S. L., McGill, J. R., and Zabel, B. U. (1987). *In situ* DNA hybridization of metaphase and prometaphase chromosomes. *In* "Methods in *Enzymology*" (M. M. Gottesman, ed.), Vol. 151, pp. 279–292. Academic Press, San Diego, California.

Ohno, S. (1970a). "Evolution by Gene Duplication." Springer-Verlag, New York.

Ohno, S. (1970b). The enormous diversity in genome sizes of fish as a reflection of nature's extensive experiments with gene duplication. *Trans. Am. Fish. Soc.* **99**, 120–130.

Ohno, S., and Atkin, N. B. (1966). Comparative DNA values and chromosome complements of eight species of fishes. *Chromosoma* **18**, 455–466.

Ohno, S., Buramoto, J., and Christian, L. (1967). Diploid–tetraploid relationship among old-world members of the fish family, Cyprinidae. *Chromosoma* **23**, 1–9.

Ohno, S., Wolf, U., and Atkin, N. (1968). Evolution from fish to mammals by gene duplication. *Hereditas* **59**, 169–187.

Ohno, S., Muramoto, J., and Christian, S. L. (1969). Microchromosomes in holocephalian, chondrostean, and holostean fishes. *Chromosoma* **26**, 35–40.

Ojima, Y. (1978). Preparation of cell-cultures for chromosome studies of fishes. *Proc. Jpn. Acad., Ser. B* **54**, 116–120.

Ojima, Y., Hitotsumachi, S., and Hayashi, M. (1970). A blood culture method for fish chromosomes. *Jpn. J. Genet.* **45**, 161–162.

Ozato, K., Kondoh, H., Inohara, H., Iwamatsu, T., Wakamatsu, Y., and Okada, T. S. (1986). Production of transgenic fish: Introduction and expression of chicken delta-crystallin gene in medaka embryos. *Cell Differ.* **19**, 237–244.

Phillips, R. B., and Ihssen, P. E. (1985). Identification of sex chromosomes in lake trout *(Salvelinus namaycush)*. *Cytogenet. Cell Genet.* **39**, 14–18.

Phillips, R. B., and Ihssen, P. E. (1986). Inheritance of Q-band chromosomal polymorphisms in lake trout. *J. Hered.* **77**, 93–97.

Phillips, R. B., and Kapuscinski, A. R. (1987). A Robertsonian polymorphism in pink salmon *(Oncorhynchus gorbuscha)* involving the nucleolar organizer region. *Cytogenet. Cell Genet.* **44**, 148–152.

Phillips, R. B., and Kapuscinski, A. R. (1988). High frequency of translocation heterozygotes in odd year populations of pink salmon *(Oncorhynchus gorbuscha)*. *Cytogenet. Cell Genet.* **48**, 178–182.

Phillips, R. B., and Zajicek, K. D. (1982). Q-band chromosomal banding polymorphisms in lake trout *(Salvelinus namaycush)*. *Genetics* **191**, 222–234.

Phillips, R. B., Zajicek, K. D., Ihssen, P. E., and Johnson, O. (1986). Application of silver staining to the identification of triploid fish cells. *Aquaculture* **54**, 313–319.

Phillips, R. B., Pleyte, K. A., and Hartley, S. E. (1988). Stock-specific differences in the number and chromosome positions of the nucleolar organizer regions in arctic char *(Salvelinus alpinus)*. *Cytogenet. Cell Genet.* **48,** 9–12.

Phillips, R. B., Pleyte, K. A., and Ihssen, P. E. (1989). Patterns of chromosomal nucleolar organizer region (NOR) variation in fishes of the genus *Salvelinus*. *Copeia*, pp. 47–53.

Pleyte, K. A., Phillips, R. B., and Hartley, S. E. (1989). Q-band chromosomal polymorphisms in arctic char *(Salvelinus alpinus)*. *Genome* **32,** 129–133.

Purdom, C. E., and Woodhead, D. S. (1973). Radiation damage in fish. *In* "Genetics and Mutagenesis of Fish" (J. H. Schröder, ed.), pp. 68–73. Springer-Verlag, New York.

Rishi, K. K. (1979). Somatic G-banded chromosomes of *Colisa fasciatus* (Perciformes: Belontidae) and confirmation of female heterogamety. *Copeia*, pp. 146–149.

Samokhvalova, G. V. (1938). Effect of X-rays on fishes *(Lebistes reticulatus, xiphophorus hellerii,* and *carassius vulgaris)*. *Biol. Zh.* **7,** 1023–1034.

Sola, L., Cataudella, S., and Capanna, E. (1981). New developments in vertebrate cytotaxonomy. III. Karyology of bony fishes: A review. *Genetica* **54,** 285–328.

Solar, I. I., Donaldson, E. M., and Hunter, G. A. (1984). Induction of triploidy in rainbow trout *(Salmo gairdneri)* by heat shock, and investigation of early growth. *Aquaculture* **42,** 57–67.

Svardson, G. (1945). Chromosome studies on Salmonidae. *Medd. Undersokn.- Forsoksanst. Sotvattensfisket (Stockholm)* **23,** 1.

Thorgaard, G. H. (1976). Robertsonian polymorphism and constitutive heterochromatin distribution in chromosomes of the rainbow trout *(Salmo gairdneri)*. *Cytogenet. Cell Genet.* **17,** 174–184.

Thorgaard, G. H. (1986). Ploidy manipulation and performance. *Aquaculture* **57,** 57–64.

Thorgaard, G. H., Jazwin, M. E., and Stier, A. R. (1981). Polyploidy induced by heat shock in the rainbow trout. *Trans. Am. Fish. Soc.* **110,** 546–550.

Thorgaard, G. H., Rabinovitch, P. S., Shen, M. W., Gall, G. A. E., Propp, J., and Utter, F. M. (1982). Triploid rainbow trout identified by flow cytometry. *Aquaculture* **29,** 305–309.

Utter, F. M., Johnson, O. W., Thorgaard, G. H., and Rabinovitch, P. S. (1983). Measurement and potential applications of induced triploidy in Pacific salmon. *Aquaculture* **35,** 125–135.

Uwa, H., and Ojima, Y. (1981). Detailed and banding karyotype analysis of the medaka, *Oryzias latipes,* in cultured cells. *Proc. Jpn. Acad., Ser. B* **57,** 39–43.

Wattendorf, R. J. (1986). Rapid analysis of ploidy via a Coulter Counter with channelyzer. *Prog. Fish.-Cult.* **48,** 125–132.

Wolf, K., and Quimby, M. C. (1969). Fish cell and tissue culture. *In* "Fish Physiology" (W. S. Hoar and D. J. Randall, eds.), Vol. 3, pp. 253–305. Academic Press, New York.

Wolters, W. R., Libey, G. S., and Chrisman, C. L. (1981a). Induction of triploidy in channel catfish. *Trans. Am. Fish. Soc.* **110,** 310–312.

Wolters, W. R., Chrisman, C. L., and Libey, G. S. (1981b). Lymphocyte culture for chromosomal analyses of channel catfish, *Ictalurus punctatus*. *Copeia*, pp. 503–504.

Wolters, W. R., Libey, G. S., and Chrisman, C. L. (1982a). Effect of triploidy on growth and gonadal development of channel catfish. *Trans. Am. Fish. Soc.* **111,** 102–105.

Wolters, W. R., Chrisman, C. L., and Libey, G. S. (1982b). Erythrocyte nuclear measurements of diploid and triploid channel catfish, *Ictalurus punctatus (Rafinesque)*. *J. Fish. Biol.* **20,** 253–258.

Yamamoto, T. (1958). Artificial induction of functional sex-reversal in genotypic females of the medaka *(Oryzias latipes)*. *J. Exp. Zool.* **137,** 227–264.

Yamamoto, T. (1965). Estriol-induced XY females of the medaka *(Oryzias latipes)* and their progenies. *Gen. Comp. Endocrinol.* **5,** 527–533.

Yamamoto, T. (1969). Sex differentiation. *In* "Fish Physiology" (W. S. Hoar and D. J. Randall, eds.), Vol. 3, pp. 117–173. Academic Press, New York.

Yamamoto, T. (1975). A YY male goldfish from mating estrone-induced XY female and normal male. *J. Hered.* **66,** 2–4.

Yamazaki, F. (1983). Sex control and manipulation in fish. *Aquaculture* **33,** 329–354.

Zenzes, M. T., and Voiculescu, I. (1975). C-banding patterns in *Salmo trutta,* a species of tetraploid origin. *Genetica (The Hague)* **45,** 531–536.

Zhuo, L. (1988). Elongated fish chromosomes prepared from fin tissue culture. MS Thesis, Purdue University, West Lafayette, Indiana.

Chromosome Abnormalities and Pregnancy Failure in Domestic Animals

W. ALLAN KING

Biomedical Sciences, Ontario Veterinary College, University of Guelph, Guelph, Ontario N1G 2W1, Canada

I. Introduction
II. Cytogenetic Study of Germ Cells and Embryos
III. Germ Cells
IV. Embryos
V. Effects of Chromosome Abnormalities
VI. Embryonic and Fetal Loss
VII. Conclusions
    References

I. Introduction

Prenatal loss of fertilized ova is encountered in most mammals, although the incidence varies among species. For example, the female elephant shrew ovulates 50–150 oocytes and the majority are fertilized, yet only two develop to term (Tripp, 1970), whereas black wildebeest and hartebeest have a remarkably low rate of embryonic mortality (Skinner et al., 1974). Embryonic and fetal losses are broadly attributed to environmental and genetic factors, including chromosome abnormalities. The classical work of Snell et al. (1934) on translocation heterozygous mice laid the foundation for the concept that structurally abnormal chromosomes behave as dominant lethals in mammals, and that sterility or semisterility in males is indicative of chromosomal rearrangements in germ cells. However, the most compelling evidence for the association between pregnancy failure and chromosome abnormalities in mammals comes from our own species. Since the 1967 publication of D. H. Carr's abstract entitled "Chromosome Abnormalities as a Cause of Spontaneous Abortion," it has been established that fully half of human spontaneous abortuses during the first and second trimesters of pregnancy are chromosomally abnormal (Jacobs, 1982).

Chromosome abnormalities responsible for embryonic mortality fall into one of two categories, according to their origin. Those of the first type are hereditary, because they are found in the gametes and embryos of chromosomally abnormal individuals and occur during gametogenesis as a direct consequence of the abnormality; abnormalities of the second type occur spontaneously during gemetogenesis, at fertilization, or during embryo development and are not related to the chromosomal make up of the sire or dam.

In this article the incidence, origin, and effect of chromosome abnormalities in the embryos of domestic animals will be reviewed. Domestic animals will be discussed together rather than as individual species.

II. Cytogenetic Study of Germ Cells and Embryos

The development of techniques for the study of chromosomes during gametogenesis and in the developing embryo and fetus has generated a wealth of knowledge in a number of species. For example, the phenotypic expression and developmental effects of genetic imbalance in the mouse due to duplication and deficiency of specific segments of translocated chromosomes have been established. In other species the incidence of spontaneous and induced chromosome abnormalities in germ cells and embryos has been calculated.

Even though there have been a number of studies in domestic animals, relatively little is known about the incidence or effect of chromosome abnormalities in gametes and embryos. There are a number of limitations that interfere with the design of experiments on domestic animal embryos. For example, the high cost of maintaining large domestic animals with a relatively long gestation period and generation interval is prohibitive. As a result, species that ovulate one or few oocytes each estrus cycle are usually administered exogenous gonadotropins to maximize the production of ova and embryos. This treatment serves to stimulate additional oocyte maturation, including resumption of meiosis and progression to the second meiotic metaphase stage and ovulation. Because it is known that the ability to resume meiosis, fertilize, and develop is acquired after the treatment, it is difficult to rule out an effect of gonadatropins on chromosome segregation. While there are some observations that suggest that superovulation in domestic animals increases the incidence of chromosomal abnormalities in gametes and embryos (Williams and Long, 1980), other studies suggest the reverse (Murray et al., 1986b). It has, however, been shown in rats that retarded or abnormal embryos are frequently recovered after such treatment (Miller and Armstrong, 1981) and that there is consistent reduction of implantation (Miller and Armstrong, 1982). It is hoped that advances in *in vitro* oocyte maturation and fertilization and in the zona-free hamster oocyte penetration assay will lead to an affordable means of investigating chromosomal aspects of development in domestic animals. Technical difficulties related to the preparation, number, and morphology of chromosomes and low mitotic index due to a poor understanding of the cell cycle of early embryos provide challenges for future research.

III. Germ Cells

Early observations of the chromosomes of domestic animals were carried out on gonadal tissue (Makino and Nishimura, 1952). At present, the conventional study of the postsynaptic stages of meiosis is used to obtain an estimate of irregular segregation and conformation and gives a preview of the chromosomal composition of embryos that might result from such germ cells. Chromosome analysis of germ cells during the first meiotic division provides information about the premeiotic or gonial divisions. Analysis of the second meiotic metaphase indicates the combined gonial and first meiotic incidence of abnormalities. In this regard, examination of the zygotic pronuclei provides a more complete picture of meiosis in males or females, because it reflects the combined results of gonial and meiotic divisions. Although it is widely hypothesized that there is no prefertilization selection of gamete types (Ford, 1975), it must be remembered that a certain amount of discrepancy can be expected when extrapolating from partially completed meiosis to the zygote. However, when used to interpret the chromosome complement of embryos, the study of germ cells allows the differentiation between meiotic and postmeiotic abnormalities.

In males, meiosis is a continuous process throughout most of adult life, and testicles are amenable to direct preparation of chromosomes for the study of meiosis. In contrast, meiosis in the female begins in the fetal ovary and is arrested at the prophase of the first meiotic division until the follicle containing the oocyte responds to luteinizing hor-

TABLE I

INCIDENCE OF ANEUPLOID AND DIPLOID SECONDARY SPERMATOCYTES AND OOCYTES IN NORMAL AND TRANSLOCATION HETEROZYGOUS DOMESTIC ANIMALS

Species	Karyotype	Aneuploid (%)	Diploid (%)	Reference
Cattle	60,XY	19.0[a]	7.7	Gustavsson (1969)
	60,XY	2.8	—	Logue and Harvey (1978)
	60,XX	0	2.9	Jagiello et al. (1974)
	60,XX	0	2.4	King et al. (1986)
	59,XY,t(1;29)	51.6[a]	7.2	Gustavsson (1969)
	59,XY,t(1;29)	6.4	—	Logue and Harvey (1978)
	59,XY,t(1;29)	54.6[a]	—	Popescu (1978)
Sheep	54,XY	6.8	—	Logue (1977)
	54,XY	2.0	—	Long (1978)
	54,XY	0	—	Bruère et al. (1981)
	54,XY,t1	6.1	—	Long (1978)
	54,XY,t1	5.6	—	Chapman and Bruère (1975)
	54,XY,t2	4.5	—	Chapman and Bruère (1975)
	54,XY,t3	9.2	—	Chapman and Bruère (1975)
Horse	64,XY	3.4	—	Scott and Long (1980)
	64,XX	5.5	2.7	W. A. King et al. (1990)
Pig	38,XX	3.4	12.2	McGaughey and Polge (1971)

[a]Data not adjusted to compensate for possible artifactual loss of chromosomes.

mone in adult life or until the oocyte is removed from the follicle. Meiosis is then blocked at the second meiotic metaphase (MII) and is completed only on fertilization or activation. Advances in recovery and culture techniques for oocytes have provided new access to the study of meiosis in females. As a result, oocytes from individual females or populations of females can be analyzed.

The rates of nondisjunction during male and female meiosis leading to aneuploid MII spreads in individuals with a normal or presumed normal karyotype in a number of species are summarized in Table I. Four basic MII chromosome configurations have been reported, haploid (Fig. 1a), hypohaploid, hyperhaploid (Fig.1b), and diploid (Fig. 1c). De novo structural rearrangements have not been reported. There is an interspecies variation in the overall rate of nondisjunction, although the base line for karyotypically normal individuals of the domestic species studied so far is between 2 and 7%. The within-species variation noted among studies may reflect differences among livestock populations or laboratories.

Heterozygosity for structural alterations of chromosomes is usually associated with reduced fertility or litter size. Study of the secondary spermatocytes from such individuals (Table I) shows higher incidence of aneuploid MII configurations than is seen in normal animals. In sheep heterozygous for Robertsonian translocations, the incidence of aneuploid secondary spermatocytes can be as high as 9% above that of normal controls. In cattle, the 1/29 translocation was shown to lead to an increased incidence of aneuploidy of 3.6%. In the pig, a number of reciprocal translocations have been reported (see Gustavsson, this volume). Although extensive studies of conventional postsynaptic meiosis have not been reported, a few examples of unbalanced MII spreads such as the one shown in Fig. 1d have been observed.

In some species there are very few systematic studies on meiosis in the male owing to difficulties in obtaining chromosome preparations from secondary spermatocytes. One such species is the pig. Recently, Creighton and Houghton (1987) reported the first observations on pig sperm chromosomes by *in vitro* penetration of zona-free hamster ova. An incidence of 5% (1/20) nondisjunction was reported. It is hoped that as more information on the chromosome complement of sperm is added to that on preliminary studies in pigs (Creighton and Houghton, 1987) and cattle (Tateno and Mikamo, 1987; Kovacs and Foote, 1989) and other species, it will be possible to determine the incidence of spontaneous abnormalities from a sample of spermatozoa.

It should be noted that one of the technical drawbacks of the methods for chromosome preparation from both oocytes and spermatocytes is chromosome loss during fixation and slide preparation. Nondisjunction during the first meiotic division is expected to lead to equal portions of hyperhaploid and hypohaploid germ cells. Some investigations compensate for potential false bias toward hypohaploidy by expressing the incidence of nondisjunction as twice the incidence of hyperhaploid MII spreads. Although this method of calculation may not be a true representation of meiotic nondisjunction, it is a conservative estimate that errs in favor of normal meiosis. The fact that others do not make this distinction may be seen as comparatively higher nondisjunction rates. However, there is some evidence that supports the suggestion that there is a preference for hypohaploidy during female meiosis (Martin, 1984).

It is tantalizing to speculate that there may be a higher rate of abnormal meiosis in females (2.4–15.6%) than males (0–6.8%). Unfortunately, there is too little information on the chromosomal complement of secondary oocytes for comparison with the secondary spermatocytes. Indeed, observations on the chromosome complement of human sperm and oocytes suggest a substantially higher incidence of abnormalities

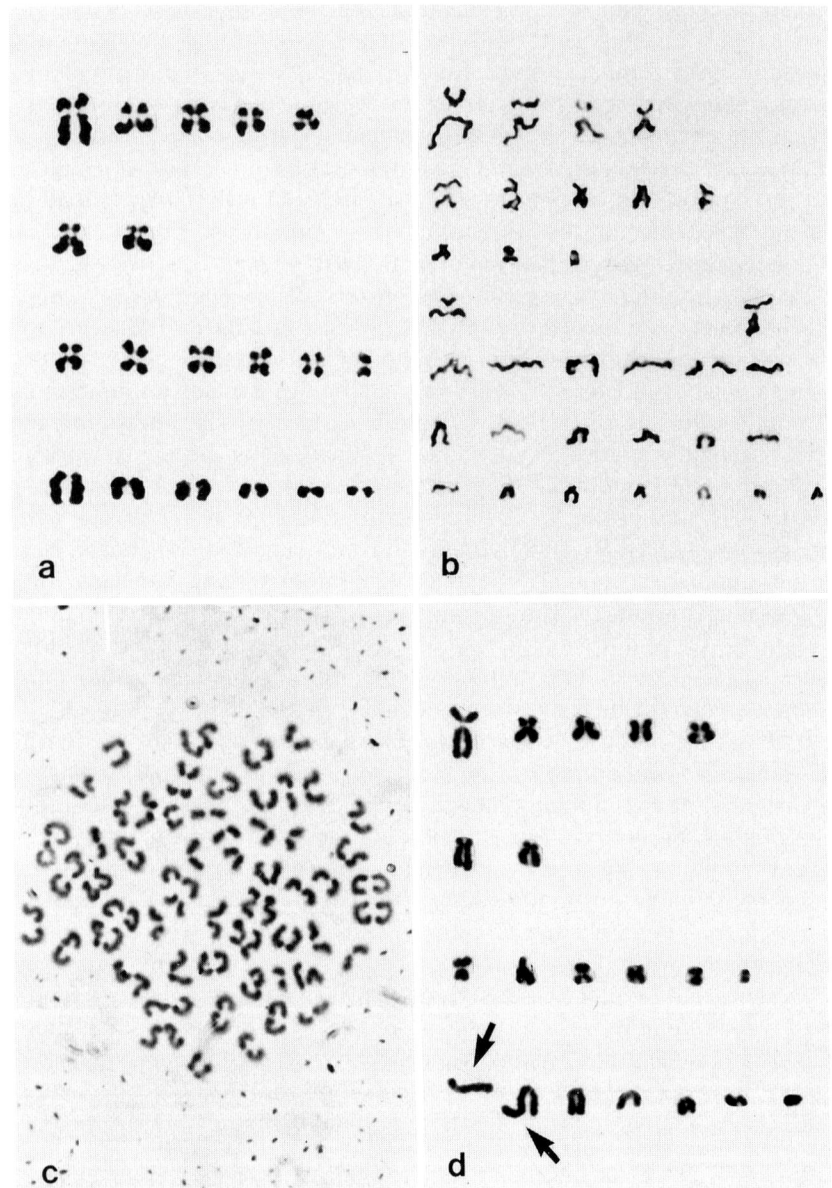

in females (23.3%; Ma *et al.*, 1989) than in males (12.1%; Martin, 1989). Notably, the incidence of aneuploidy in males and females was observed to be 11.1 and 21.3%, respectively. However, the observations on oocytes are confounded by the fact that some were cultured for extended periods of time while others had been exposed to sperm in an attempt to fertilize *in vitro* before subsequent fixation. Recent studies on the morphological and physiological features of developing human embryos have shown remarkable similarities to embryos of domestic ruminants such as sheep and cattle (Tesarik, 1988). The information gained from the study of meiosis in domestic animals may increase the understanding of chromosomal abnormalities in our own species.

IV. Embryos

Since the publication of the first observations of the chromosomes of pig embryos by McFeely in 1966, studies on embryos of a number of domestic animals have been reported. These investigations can generally be separated into two categories: studies of the gametic products of chromosomal rearrangements are investigated in the embryos of carrier animals, and studies of spontaneously occurring abnormalities in the embryos of karyotypically normal or presumed normal individuals are investigated.

The first structural abnormalities of chromosomes to be reported in domestic animals were a Robertsonian translocation in cattle (Gustavsson and Rockborn, 1964) and a reciprocal translocation in pigs (Henricson and Backström, 1964). Since then, embryos produced by heterozygotes for these and other rearrangements in cattle, sheep, and pigs have been studied. Table II summarizes these studies

Embryos with unbalanced karyotypes were observed in all studies with the exception of the one involving Massey I translocation heterzygotes. In pigs, the effect of reciprocal translocations is a drastic reduction in litter size (see Gustavsson, this volume). All studies of embryos produced by such animals revealed a high incidence of embryos with

---

FIG. 1. Oocyte karyotypes. (a) Haploid second meiotic metaphase from a pig oocyte. Note that there are 19 chromosomes. (b) Hyperhaploid second meiotic metaphase from a horse oocyte. Note that due to an extra acrocentric chromosome there are 33 chromosomes instead of 32. (c) Diploid second meiotic metaphase from a cow oocyte. Note that there are 60 chromosomes. (d) Second meiotic metaphase from an oocyte collected from a pig heterozygous for the rcp(13;14) translocation. Note the asymmetrical chromatids indicated by the arrows.

TABLE II

FREQUENCY DISTRIBUTIONS OF EMBRYOS WITH NORMAL, BALANCED, OR UNBALANCED KARYOTYPE THAT PRODUCED HETEROZYGOTES FOR A STRUCTURAL REARRANGEMENT

Species	Sire or dam abnormality	Age (days)	Embryo karyotypes			Reference
			Total	Normal/balanced[a]	Unbalanced[a]	
Cattle	t(1;29)	1–7	52	50 (96.2)	2 (3.8)	Popescu (1980)
Cattle	t(1;29)	13	38	36 (94.7)	2 (5.6)	King et al. (1981a)
Cattle	ins(16)	1–56	13	11 (84.6)	2 (15.4)	Moraes and Mattevi (1983)
Sheep	Massey I	10–18	75	75 (100)	0 (0)	Long (1977)
Pigs	rcp(11;15)	10–88	113	101 (89.3)	12 (10.6)	Åkesson and Henricson (1972)
	rcp(13;14)	1–16	69	49 (71.0)	20 (28.8)	King et al. (1981b)
	rcpl(4;14)	9–10	27	16 (59.3)	11 (40.7)	Popescu and Boscher (1982)
	rcpl(7;11)	21	27	21 (77.8)	6 (27.2)	Gustavsson et al. (1983)

[a]Values in parentheses are percentages.

unbalanced chromosomal complements. Systematic study of the embryos produced by 13/14 translocation heterozygotes showed unbalanced karyotypes (Fig. 2a) only during the preimplantation stages. Unbalanced embryos produced by the 11/15 translocation heterozygotes were observed during the preimplantation and postimplantation stages. This suggests that the time of loss of the embryos is related to the chromosome segments involved in the rearrangement. Among embryos sired by 1/29 translocation heterozygotes, the 3.8–5.6%incidence of trisomy 1 closely parallels the increase in both rate of nondisjunction (3.6%; Logue and Harvey, 1978) and return to service (3–6%; Gustavsson, 1979). In the case of the Massey I translocation, no embryos with unbalanced karyotypes were found in spite of the 6% increase in the rate of aneuploid MII. It has been suggested that there is a prefertilization selection of gametes in favor of normal chromosome complements, thereby maintaining normal fertility (Bruère, 1975). The fact that no embryos with aneuploid karyotypes were observed at days 10–18 would seem to support this hypothesis. However, spontaneously occurring aneuploid embryos at days 2–3 (Williams and Long, 1980), similar in makeup to what might be expected as a result of nondisjunction due to the translocation, seem to suggest early loss of aneuploid embryos.

As it became known that spontaneously occurring chromosomal imbalance was associated with embryonic loss in humans (Carr, 1967) and pigs (McFeely, 1967), investigators began to examine the embryos of a number of domestic species. Table III summarizes 19 published studies involving 3,724 embryos produced by cattle, sheep, pigs, and horses with normal or presumed normal karyotypes, of which 1,802 (48.4%) could be karyotyped, revealing abnormalities in 131, or 7.3%, of those karyotyped. All embryos in these studies were produced by fertilization *in vivo*, but many of the females were superovulated. Of the 683 cattle embryos, 606 sheep embryos, 421 pig embryos, and 92 horse embryos that the authors were able to determine the karyotype with some degree of certainty, 71, 40, 20, and 0 embryos, respectively, were considered to be chromosomally abnormal. The chromosomally abnormal embryos listed in Table III, which were described in sufficient detail in the original articles, are summarized in Table IV according to the chromosomal complement.

Aneuploid embryos such as the one presented in Fig. 2d account for more than 21% (8 hypodiploid, 15 hyperdiploid, and 2 with multiple anomalies) of abnormal embryos. As mentioned earlier, the potential loss of chromosomes during fixation adds confusion to the interpretation of results. The higher incidence of hyperdiploidy than hypodip-

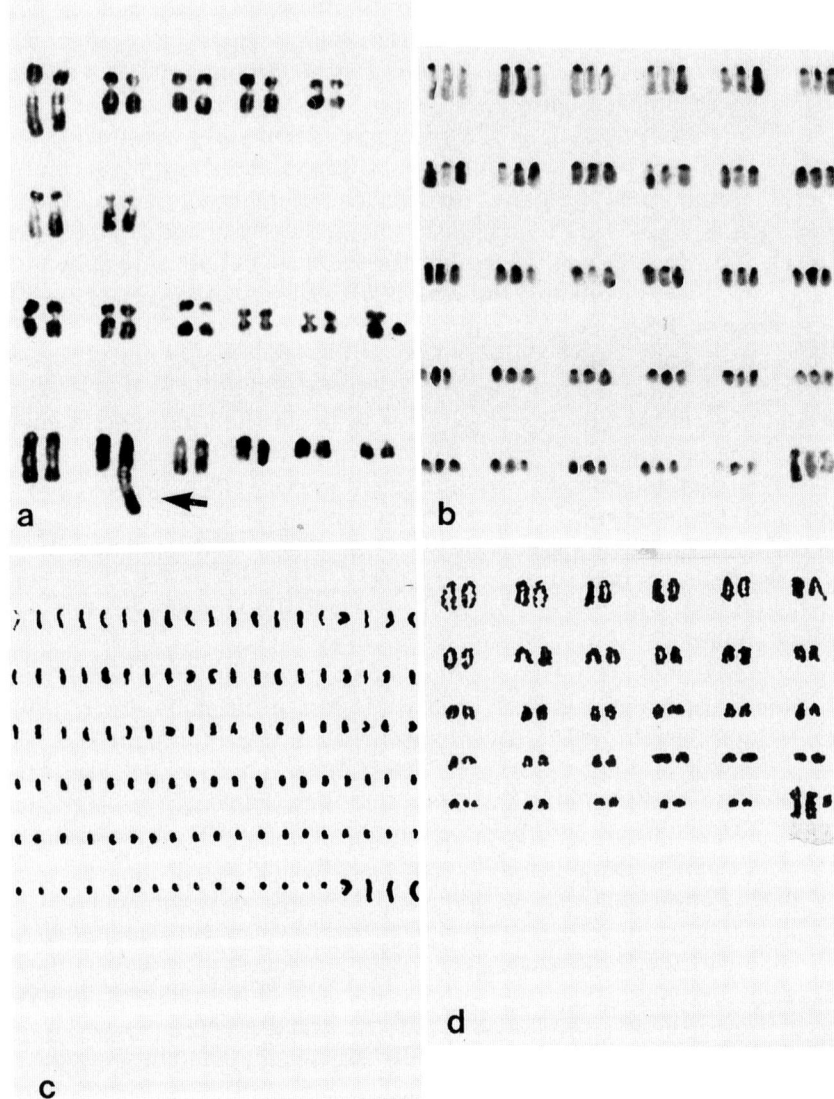

FIG. 2. (a) The karyotype of a day-10 pig embryo produced by a heterozygote for the rcp(13;14) translocation. The embryo may have arisen by fertilization of an oocyte such the one in Fig. 1d. The arrow indicates partial duplication of chromosome 13. (b) The karyotype of a two-cell-stage bovine embryo with 90,XXX chromosome complement. (c) The karyotype of an eight-cell-stage bovine embryo with near tetraploid (114,XXXX) chromosome complement. (d) The karyotype of a day-7 bovine embryo with 61,XXY chromosome complement.

TABLE III

Summary of Chromosomal Analysis of Embryos Produced by Animals with Normal or Presumed Normal Karyotypes

Species	Age (days)	Number of embryos			References
		Total	Analyzed	Abnormal[a]	
Cattle	2–4	145	47	8 (17.0)	Verini Supplizi et al. (1988)
	2–4	134	34	4 (11.8)	Murray et al. (1985)
	3–7	548	265	19 (7.1)	Gayerie de Abreu et al. (1984)
	5–7	24	11	4 (36.3)	King and Picard (1985)
	7[b]	163	39	14 (35.8)	Benevides-Filho and Pinhero (1988)
	7[c]	103	96	16 (16.6)	King et al. (1987)
	7	23	23	0 (0)	King et al. (1987)
	12–15	198	159	3 (1.9)	Hare et al. (1980)
	12–16	12	12	0 (0)	McFeely and Rajakoski (1968)
	Total	1,350	683 (51%)	71 (10.4)	
Sheep	2–3	435	91	21 (23.1)	Williams and Long (1980)
	2–3	376	89	5 (5.6)	Long and Williams (1982)
	2–3	177	73	8 (10.9)	Murray et al. (1985)
	2–7	290	48	3 (6.3)	Murray et al. (1986a)
	12–14	146	103	2 (1.9)	Murray et al. (1986b)
	20	218	86	1 (1.2)	Williams and Long (1980)
	24–32	125	116	0 (0)	Murray et al. (1986b)
	Total	1,767	606	40 (6.6)	
Pigs	3–4	115	82	6 (7.3)	van der Hoeven et al. (1985)
	10	88	85	8 (9.4)	McFeely (1967)
	10	170	169	0 (0)	Dolch and Chrisman (1981)
	10	71	70	2 (2.9)	Long and Williams (1982)
	10	41	15	4 (26.6)	Moon et al. (1975)
	Total	485	421 (87%)	20 (5%)	
Horses	6–28	122	92	0	Romagnano et al. (1987)
	Total	3,724	1,802 (48.4%)	131 (7.3%)	

[a] Values in parentheses are percentage abnormal of number analyzed.
[b] Some embryos were morphologically abnormal.
[c] All embryos were morphologically abnormal.

loidy probably reflects the degree of caution with which the results were interpreted. The aneuploids could arise as a result of nondisjunction during the first or second meiotic division in formation of the ovum or spermatozoon or during mitosis in the zygote. The incidence of nondisjunction based on observations of embryos exceed the 2–6.8%

TABLE IV

Distribution of the Abnormal Embryos from Table III According to Species and Type of Abnormality

Karyotype	Species			Total (%)
	Cattle	Sheep	Pigs	
Haploid	3	4	1	8 (7.3)
Hypodiploid	7	1	—	8 (7.3)
Hyperdiploid	6	9	—	15 (13.8)
Triploid	4	4	6	14 (12.8)
Tetraploid	2	1	4	7 (6.4)
Haploid/diploid	6	17	—	23 (21.1)
Diploid/triploid	4	—	1	5 (4.6)
Diploid/tetraploid	6	1	4	11 (10.1)
Diploid/hexaploid	7	—	2	9 (8.3)
Diploid/$\geqslant$, octoploid	2	—	2	4 (3.7)
Other	2	3	—	5 (4.6)
Total	**49**	**40**	**20**	**109** (100.0)

that might be projected from MII stage in males. This suggests a number of possible explanations for which supporting data are lacking. First, there could be a high incidence of nondisjunction at the second meiotic division or during the first cleavage. Second, there could be a higher incidence of nondisjunction during meiosis in the female than in the male. Third, superovulation of the donors (all studies involving cattle and two in sheep) might have increased the incidence of nondisjunction. Finally, there could be populations of cattle and sheep that are prone to high rates of nondisjunction.

Haploidy (n) and haploid/diploid $(n/2n)$ mixoploids account for 28.4% of the abnormalities recorded. The haploid embryos arise from zygotes with a single pronucleus of either spermatozoon or oocyte origin. The observation of a Y chromosome in some of these confirms the male origin either through monospermic fertilization and subsequent loss of the female pronucleus or in the case of mixoploids through polyspermic fertilization with syngamy involving only two of the three pronuclei (King and Picard, 1985). Mitotic activity of a polar body or fertilization of an activated oocyte with two pronuclei without subsequent fusion of the nuclei could also account for $n/2n$ mixoploids.

The 14 (12.8%) triploid $(3n)$ embryos such as the one depicted in Fig 2b, were undoubtedly formed by dispermy or by retention of all MII chromosomes in the fertilized oocyte (digyny). It has been suggested that aging of gametes increases the incidence of triploidy through failure of the block to polyspermia or failure of polar body extrusion (Austin, 1978). The 2–12% incidence of diploid secondary oocytes confirms that failure of polar body extrusion is possible, particularly because oocytes were cultured *in vitro* and might have inadvertently been aged. However, recent studies on the effect of delaying insemination in superovulated heifers by as much as 36 hours did not show a higher incidence of $3n$ embryos. The rate of fertilization did, however, decline as the interval between ovulation and insemination increased (Diop *et al.*, 1988).

The 7 (6.4%) tetraploid embryos (Fig. 2c) may have originated by polyandry, a combination of polyandry and polygyny, or by endoreduplication at the zygote stage. Examples of these three mechanisms have been reported in domestic animals (polyandry or combination; King *et al.*, 1981; Murray *et al.*, 1985; endoreduplication, King *et al.*, 1988).

The haploid/diploid and diploid/polyploid mixoploids (Fig. 3a and b) observed in 57 embryos account for 52.4% of all abnormalities. The origin of the haploid cells in mixoploids has been discussed above. The triploid cells in diploid/triploid mixoploids could have arisen by fusion of a diploid and haploid cell. Similarly, the tetraploid, hexaploid, and high order polyploids may have arisen by fusion of two or more cells. Alternatively, endoreduplication has been noted as one of the mechanisms leading to polyploid cells in the mouse trophoblast (Ilgren, 1981) and bovine parthenogenotes (King *et al.*, 1988). The postzygotic origin of the diploid/polyploid mixoploids is supported by their exclusive observation in cleaved embryos. In cattle, the incidence was higher in day-7 embryos that were morphologically disorganized and had a low cell number (King *et al.*, 1987).

The development of techniques for the *in vitro* maturation of oocytes collected from slaughtered females with subsequent fertilization and development *in vitro* provides new opportunities for the study of the chromosomal composition of embryos (King, 1985; King *et al.*, 1988; Iwasaki *et al.*, 1988). Recently, the incidence of chromosomal abnormalities was reported in 1,005 early embryos derived from *in vitro* fertilization (Iwasaki *et al.*, 1989). The incidence reported was 1.4% haploid, 0.2% hypodiploid, 0.6% hyperdiploid, 10.0% triploid, 1.2% tetraploid, 0.2% diploid/triploid mixoploids, and 0.1% diploid/tetraploid mosaics. Because the types of abnormalities and overall frequencies parallel those observed *in vivo*, it is anticipated that controlled studies will add to our understanding of the mechanisms leading to chromosomal aberrations. In addition, the study of the chromosomes

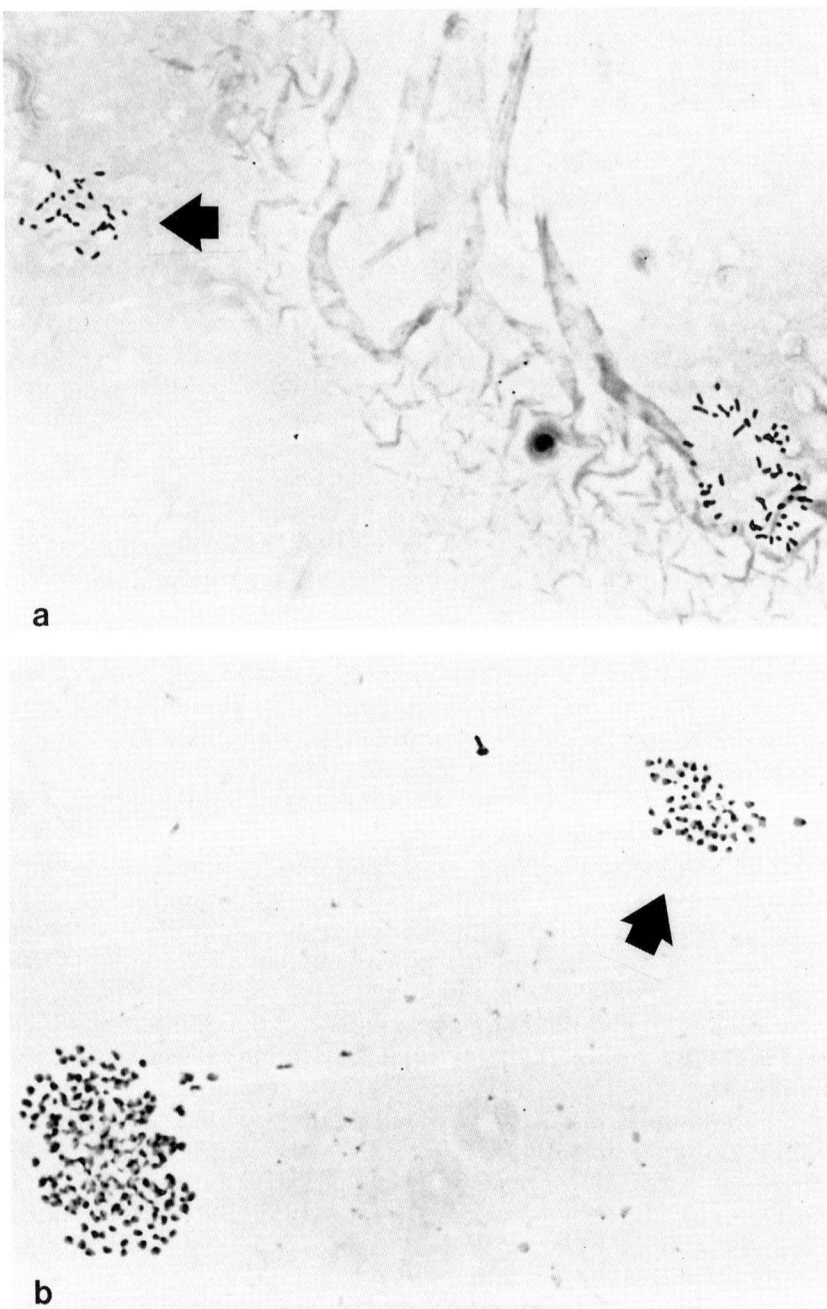

at the pronucleus stage will allow the study of the segregation of the gametic products of heterozygotes for structural rearrangements.

V. Effects of Chromosome Abnormalities

The fact that a number of chromosomally unbalanced embryos have been observed in most species, with very few subsequent liveborn animals with unbalanced chromosomal composition being noted, leaves little doubt that chromosome anomalies are a source of prenatal loss. The decline in the frequency of abnormalities in older embryos examined in most species implies progressive loss of abnormal embryos at specific stages of development. The sharp drop in frequency after morula and blastocyst stages suggests that the periods of transition from maternal to embryonic control of development and organization into cell lineages are particularly sensitive stages of development that cannot tolerate gross alterations of the genome.

Aneuploidy is not necessarily incompatible with development to term. Several liveborn and adult individuals with autosomal trisomy or sex chromosome monosomy and trisomy have been observed. In general terms, though, those with autosomal trisomy have been congenitally malformed, whereas those with aneuploidy involving the sex chromosome have been sterile (Hare and Singh, 1979). Most embryos with duplications and/or deletions of chromosome segments as a result of meiosis in translocation heterozygotes are lost during the first month of development (Åkesson and Henricson, 1972; King et al., 1981b; Popescu and Boscher, 1982; Gustavsson et al., 1983). In species such as cattle, this is usually noted as an increased interval between parturition events for carrier females and a lowered nonreturn rate for carrier bulls (Gustavsson, 1969; Refsdal, 1976; Kovacs and Csukly, 1980). In litter-bearing species the loss of such unbalanced embryos leads to a reduction of litter size.

Mixoploids are the most frequently observed abnormalities in embryos. Haploid/diploids are observed in both two-cell and day 5–7 cattle embryos, but not in older embryos or in liveborn calves. Similarly, mixoploids in sheep seen at day 2 are not seen at day 20. Because some of the mixoploids originate from at least three gametes, blood chime-

---

FIG. 3. (a) Chromosome preparation from a two-cell-stage haploid/diploid mixoploid bovine embryo. The arrow indicates the haploid cell. (b) Chromosome preparation from a day-7 diploid/polyploid mixoploid bovine embryo. The arrow indicates the diploid cell.

rism might be expected. However, unexplained cases of chimerism in single-born calves have not been observed (G. J. Kraay, personal communication). This suggests that either there is loss of the embryo, only one of the cell lines contributes to the embryo proper, or one of the cell lines becomes quiescent. Diploid/polyploid mixoploidy is observed in the trophoblast of most domestic species as the trophoblast is elongating during the second week of development. This is considered a normal feature of the trophoblast cells. It is not known if this type of mosaicism observed in day 5–7 embryos is compatible with further development. However, it is known that diploid/polyploid mixoploidy is observed more frequently in morphologically abnormal cattle embryos than in normal ones (King et al., 1988).

Pure triploid ($3n$) cattle embryos have been observed at the two-cell stage, the blastocyst stage, and at days 12–13 (Verini Supplizi et al., 1988; Hare et al., 1980). It is not known if they can survive beyond this period, although no triploid offspring have been observed. Interestingly, three cases of triploid/diploid mixoploidy have been described in cattle (Hare and Singh, 1979), suggesting that there are instances in which triploid cells can survive the developmental process.

VI. Embryonic and Fetal Loss

For many species, embryonic and/or fetal mortality are essential for maintaining an adequate interval between births to allow survival of newborn and suckling young. In the case of the rabbit, postpartum fertilization will lead to viable embryos; however, if the doe is in poor condition and/or suckling more than three or four young, all new embryos will die at the blastocyst stage (Short, 1984). Embryonic mortality also serves as a means of eliminating genetically aberrant embryos before birth. Once again, it is our own species that dramatically illustrates this point. Extensive global data suggest that 25% of all human pregnancies are lost by spontaneous abortion during the first and second trimester of clinically recognized pregnancies, with fully half of them being chromosomally abnormal. The incidence of chromosomally abnormal embryos at, or shortly after, fertilization is not known, although some estimates place it much higher. The subsequent incidence of chromosomally abnormal infants at birth is around 0.2%, suggesting that embryonic and fetal mortality are effective means of reducing the incidence of chromosomally abnormal products of fertilization. From an agricultural point of view, embryonic mortality among domestic animals also serves to eliminate developmentally inferior embryos that would reduce the efficiency of livestock production should abnormal individuals result. However, the initial production of abnormal embryos adds to the overall reduction in reproductive efficiency and leads to economic loss.

Mortality and resorption or expulsion of the fertilized ovum, embryo, or early fetus from the female genital tract often goes undetected. There are, however, a number of ways to determine the incidence of embryonic loss in domestic animals. These fall into three broad categories: (1) use of breeding records to determine return to estrus, interval between parturitions, and litter size; (2) assay of pregnancy-related products such as platelet-activating factor or progesterone in blood, milk, or urine; and (3) physical detection of the embryo by transrectal palpation, ultrasound examination, or observation of the reproductive tract following surgery or at slaughter. Using these methods of study, the incidence of reproductive wastage in domestic animals has been well established (for reviews, see Ayalon, 1981; Boyd, 1965; Ball, 1988; Edey, 1969; Scofield, 1976). Roughly, the difference between the number of ova shed and the number of liveborns indicates losses of 45–65% in cattle, 30–50% in pigs, 20–30% in sheep, and 15–20% in horses. Fertilization failure can vary depending on the reproductive status of the sire and dam; however, when both are genitally sound, 90% or more of the ova become fertilized.

The slaughter of inseminated cattle and subsequent examination of their reproductive tracts revealed that the greatest losses occur within 18 days of fertilization (Diskin and Sreenan, 1980; Maurer and Chenault, 1983). Similar observations have been made in pigs (Scofield, 1976), sheep (Edey, 1969) and horses (Ball, 1988). This critical period corresponds to the stages of development shown to have the highest incidence of chromosome abnormalities.

VII. Conclusions

Up to 50% of all fertilized ova are lost during the embryonic and fetal stages of development in domestic animals. Chromosome abnormalities contribute to this loss. The overall incidence of chromosome abnormalities, based on the combined studies in each species (Table III), could account for approximately 20% of the total embryonic and fetal loss for each species. However, the estimates are based on pooled observations from several stages of development in each species and probably underestimate the actual incidence of chromosome abnormalities, because embryonic loss may have occurred prior to examination. In the case of translocation heterozygotes, a substantial portion of the increased reproductive loss can also be attributed to loss of embryos, with unbalanced combinations of the chromosomes involved in the translocation.

The incidence of chromosomally abnormal embryos generally exceeds what might be projected from observation of MII. This suggests that the abnormalities originate at two times, during gametogenesis and during or subsequent to fertilization. The relative incidence of abnormalities according to origin can be evaluated if the following two broad assumptions are made: (1) the majority of aneuploids result from disturbances in gametogenesis and (2) the majority of haploids, polyploids, and mixoploids occur during or subsequent to fertilization. Partitioning the observations summarized in Table IV in this manner suggests that about one-quarter of the abnormalities can be attributed to errors in meiosis and the remaining three-quarters occur around the time of fertilization. This emphasizes the critical nature of the fertilization process. It seems likely that as our understanding of the factors controlling the events surrounding fertilization expands, we should be able to reduce the incidence of chromosomally abnormal embryos and fetuses in domestic animals and thereby reduce the incidence of embryonic loss.

ACKNOWLEDGMENT

I thank NSERC Canada for financial support.

REFERENCES

Åkesson, A., and Henricson, B. (1972). Embryonic death in pigs caused by unbalanced karyotype. *Acta Vet. Scand.* **13**, 151–160.
Austin, C. R. (1978). Patterns in metazoan fertilization. *Curr. Top. Dev.* **12**, 1–9.
Ayalon, N. (1981). Embryonic mortality in cattle. *Zuchthygiene* **16**, 97–109.
Ball, B. A. (1988). Embryonic loss in mares. Incidence, possible causes, and diagnostic considerations. *Vet. Clin. North Am.: Equine Pract.* **4**,(2) 263–290.
Benevides-Filho, I. M., and Pinheiro, L. E. L. (1988). Cytogenetic analysis of 39 bovine embryos obtained from superovulated females. *Rev. Bras. Genet.* **11**, 661–670.
Boyd, H. (1965). Embryonic death in cattle, sheep and pigs. *Vet. Bull. (London)* **36**, 251–266.
Bruère, A. N. (1975). Further evidence of normal fertility and formation of balanced gametes in sheep with one or more different Robertsonian translocations. *J. Reprod. Fertil.* **45**, 323–331.
Bruère, A. N., Scott, I., and Henderson, L. M. (1981). Aneuploid spermatocyte frequency in domestic sheep heterozygous for three Robertsonian translocations. *J. Reprod. Fertil.* **63**, 61–66.

Carr, D. H. (1967). Chromosome abnormalities as a cause of spontaneous abortion. *Am. J. Obstet. Gynecol.* **97,** 283.

Chapman, H. M., and Bruère, A. N. (1975). The frequency of aneuploidy in the secondary spermatocytes of normal and Robertsonian carrying rams. *J. Reprod. Fertil.* **45,** 333–342.

Creighton, P., and Houghton, J. A. (1987). Visualization of pig sperm chromosomes by *in vitro* penetration of zona-free hamster ova. *J. Reprod. Fertil.* **80,** 619–622.

Diop, P. E. H., King, W. A., and Bousquet, D. (1988). The influence of the time of insemination and fertilization in superovulated heifers. *Proc.—Int. Congr. Anim. Reprod. Artif. Insemin.* **11** (2), 157–159.

Diskin, M. G., and Sreenan, J. M. (1980). Fertilization and embryonic mortality rates in beef heifers after artificial insemination. *J. Reprod. Fertil.* **59,** 463–468.

Dolch, K. M., and Chrisman, C. L. (1981). Cytogenetic analysis of preimplantation blastocysts from prepuberal gilts treated with gonadotropins. *Am. J. Vet. Res.* **41**(2), 344–346.

Edey, T. N. (1969). Prenatal mortality in sheep; a review. *Anim. Breed Abstr.* **37,** 43–58.

Ford, C. E. (1975). The time in development at which gross genome unbalance is expressed. *In* "The Early Development of Mammals" (M. Balls and A. E. Wild, eds.), pp. 285–304. Cambridge Univ. Press, London and New York.

Gayerie de Abreu, F., Lamming, G. E., and Shaw, R. C. (1984). A cytogenetic study of early stage bovine embryos—Relation with embryo mortality. *Proc.—Int. Congr. Anim. Reprod. Artif. Insemin.* **10**(2), 82.

Gustavsson, I. (1969). Cytogenetics, distribution and phenotypic effects of a translocation in Swedish cattle. *Hereditas* **63,** 68–169.

Gustavsson, I. (1979). Distribution and effects of the 1/29 Robertsonian translocation. *J. Dairy Sci.* **62,** 825–835.

Gustavsson, I., and Rockborn, G. (1964). Chromosome abnormalities in three cases of lymphatic leukaemia in cattle. *Nature (London)* **203,** 990.

Gustavsson, I., Settergren, I., and King, W. A. (1983). Occurrence of two different reciprocal translocations in the same litter of domestic pigs. *Hereditas* **99,** 257–267.

Hare, W. C. D., and Singh, E. L. (1979). "Cytogenetics in Animal Production." Commonw. Agric. Bur., Farnham Royal, Bucks, England.

Hare, W. C. D., Singh, E. L., Betteridge, K. J., Eaglesome, M. D., Randall, G. C. B., Mitchell, D., Bilton, R. J., and Trounson, A. O. (1980). Chromosomal analysis of 159 bovine embryos collected 12 to 18 days after estrus. *Can. J. Genet. Cytol.* **22,** 615–626.

Henricson, B., and Backström, L. (1964). Translocation heterozygosity in a boar. *Hereditas* **52,** 166–170.

Ilgren, E. B. (1981). On the control of the trophoblastic giant-cell transformation in the mouse: Homotypic cellular interactions and polyploidy. *J. Embryol. Exp. Morphol.* **62,** 183–202.

Iwasaki, S., Shioya, Y., Hanada, A., and Nakahara, T. (1988). Chromosome preparation from 2-cell bovine embryos derived from follicular oocytes fertilized *in vitro*. *Jpn. J. Anim. Reprod.* **34**(2), 79–82.

Iwasaki, S., Shioya, Y., Masuda, H., Hanada, A., and Nakahara, T. (1989). Incidence of chromosomal anomalies in early bovine embryos derived from *in vitro* fertilization. *Gamete Res.* **22,** 83–91.

Jacobs, P. A. (1982). Pregnancy loss and birth defects. *In* "Reproduction in Mammals" (C. R. Austin and R. V. Short, eds.), Vol. 2, pp. 142–158. Cambridge Univ. Press, London and New York.

Jagiello, G. M., Miller, W. A., Ducayen, M. B., and Lin, J. S. (1974). Chiasma frequency and disjunctional behavior of ewe and cow oocytes matured *in vitro. Biol. Reprod.* **10**, 354–363.

King, W. A. (1985). Intrinsic embryonic factors that may affect survival after transfer. *Theriogenology* **23**, 161–174.

King, W. A., and Picard, L. (1985). Haploidy in preattachment bovine embryos. *Can. J. Genet. Cytol.* **27**, 69–73.

King, W. A., Linares, T., and Gustavsson, I. (1981a). Cytogenetics of preimplantation embryos sired by bulls heterozygous for the 1/29 translocation. *Hereditas* **94**, 219–224.

King, W. A., Gustavsson, I., Popescu, C. P., and Linares, T. (1981b). Gametic products transmitted by rcp(13q$^-$; 14qt) translocation heterozygous pigs and resulting embryonic loss. *Hereditas* **95**, 239–246.

King, W. A., Bousquet, D., Greve, T., and Goff, A. K. (1986). Meiosis in bovine oocytes matured *in vitro* and *in vivo. Acta Vet. Scand.* **27**, 267–279.

King, W. A., Guay, P., and Picard, L. (1987). A cytogenetical study of 7-day-old bovine embryos of poor morphological quality. *Genome* **29**, 160–164.

King, W. A., Sirard, M.-A., and First, N. L. (1988). The influence of the time of insemination on fertilization in superovulated heifers. *Proc. Int. Congr. Anim. Reprod. Artif. Insemin.* **11**(3), 335–337.

King, W. A., Desjardin, M., Xu, K. P., and Bousquet, D. (1990). Chromosome analysis of horse oocytes cultured *in vitro. Genet. Sel. Evol.* **22**, 151–160.

Kovacs, A., and Csukly, S. (1980). Effects of the 1/29 translocation upon fertility in Hungarian Simmental cattle. *Proc. Eur. Colloq. Cytogenet. Domest. Anim., 4th,* Uppsala, pp. 35–43.

Kovacs, A., and Foote, F. H. (1989). Chromosome preparation from bovine spermatozoa. *Theriogenology* **31**, 213.

Logue, D. N. (1977). Meiosis in the domestic ruminants with particular reference to Robertsonian translocations. *Ann. Genet. Sel. Anim.* **9**, 493–507.

Logue, D. N., and Harvey, M. J. A. (1978). Meiosis and spermatogenesis in bulls heterozygous for a presumptive 1/29 Robertsonian translocation. *J. Reprod. Fertil.* **54**, 159–165.

Long, S. E. (1977). Cytogenetic examination of pre-implantation blastocysts of ewes mated to rams heterozygous for the Massey I (t$_1$) translocation. *Cytogenet. Cell Genet.* **18**, 82–89.

Long, S. E. (1978). Chiasma counts and non-disjunction frequencies in a normal ram and in rams carrying the Massey I (t$_1$) Robertsonian translocation. *J. Reprod. Fertil.* **53**, 353–356.

Long, S. E., and Williams, C. V. (1982). A comparison of the chromosome complement of inner cell mass and trophoblast cells in day-10 pig embryos. *J. Reprod. Fertil.* **66**, 645–648.

Ma, S., Kalousek, D. K., Zouves, C., Yuen, B. H., Gomel, V., and Moon, Y. S. (1989). Chromosome analysis of human oocytes failing to fertilize in vitro. *Fertil. Steril.* **51**(6), 992–997.

Makino, S., and Nishimura, I. (1952). Water pretreatment squash technique. *Stain Technol.* **27**, 1–7.

Martin, R. H. (1984). Comparison of chromosomal abnormalities in hamster egg and human sperm pronuclei. *Biol. Reprod.* **31**, 819–825.

Martin, R. H. (1989). Analysis of human sperm chromosome complements. *Proc. Serono Symp. Fertil. Mamm.,* Boston, Abstr., p. 30.

Maurer, R. R., and Chenault, J. R. (1983). Fertilization failure and embryonic mortality in parous and nonparous beef cattle. *J. Anim. Sci.* **56**, 1186–1189.
McFeely, R. A. (1966). A direct method for the display of chromosomes from early pig embryos. *J. Reprod. Fertil.* **11**, 161–163.
McFeely, R. A. (1967). Chromosome abnormalities in early embryos of the pig. *J. Reprod. Fertil.* **13**, 579–581.
McFeely, R. A., and Rajakoski, E. (1968). Chromosome studies on early embryos of the cow. *Proc. Int. Congr. Anim. Reprod. Artif. Insemin.* **6**, 905–907.
McGaughey, R. W., and Polge, C. (1971). Cytogenetic analysis of pig oocytes matured *in vitro*. *J. Exp. Zool.* **176**, 383–396.
Miller, B. G., and Armstrong, D. T. (1981). Effects of superovulatory dose of pregnant mare serum gonadotropin on ovarian function, serum estrodiol and progesterone levels and early embryo development in immature rats. *Biol. Reprod.* **25**, 161–171.
Miller, B. G., and Armstrong, D. T. (1982). Infertility in superovulated immature rats: Role of ovarian steroid hypersecretion. *Biol. Reprod.* **26**, 861–868.
Moon, R. G., Rashad, M. N., and Mi, M. P. (1975). An example of polyploidy in pig blastocysts. *J. Reprod. Fertil.* **45**, 147–149.
Moraes, J. C. F., and Mattevi, M. S. (1983). Chromosome study of embryos sired by a heterozygous bull for insertion 16. *Proc. Symp. Adv. Top. Anim. Reprod., 2nd,* pp. 205–212.
Murray, J. D., Moran, C., Boland, M. P., Doff, A. M., and Nancarow, C. D. (1985). Cytogenetic analysis of 34 early stage bovine embryos from superovulated Hereford donors. *Can. J. Genet. Cytol.* **27**, 483–486.
Murray, J. D., Moran, C., Boland, M. P., Nancarrow, C. D., Sutton, R., Hoskinson, R. M., and Scaramuzzi, R. J. (1986a). Polyploid cells in blastocysts and early fetuses from Australian Merino sheep. *J. Reprod. Fertil.* **78**, 439–446.
Murray, J. D., Boland, M. P., and Moran, C. (1986b). Frequency of chromosomal abnormalities in embryos from superovulated Merino ewes. *J. Reprod. Fertil.* **78**, 433–437.
Popescu, C. P. (1978). A study of meiotic chromosomes in bulls carrying the 1/29 translocation. *Ann. Biol. Anim. Biochim. Biophys.* **18**, 383–389.
Popescu, C. P. (1980). Cytogenetics study on embryos sired by a bull carrier of 1/29 translocation. *Proc. Eur. Colloq. Cytogenet. Domest. Anim., 4th,* Uppsala, pp. 182–186.
Popescu, C. P., and Boscher, J. (1982). Cytogenetics of preimplantation embryos produced by pigs heterozygous for the reciprocal translocation (4q +;14q −). *Cytogenet. Cell Genet.* **34**, 119–123.
Refsdal, A. O. (1976). Low fertility in daughters of bulls with 1/29 translocation. *Acta Vet. Scand.* **17**, 190–195.
Romagnano, A., Richer, C. L., King, W. A., and Betteridge, K. J. (1987). Analysis of X-chromosome inactivation in horse embryos. *J. Reprod. Fertil., Suppl.* **35**, 353–361.
Scofield, A. M. (1976). Embryonic mortality in the pig. *Vet. Annu.* **15**, 91–94.
Scott, I. S., and Long, S. E. (1980). An examination of chromosomes in the stallion *(Equus caballus)* during meiosis. *Cytogenet. Cell Genet.* **26**, 7–13.
Short, R. V. (1984). Species differences in reproductive mechanisms. In "Reproduction in Mammals" (C. R. Austin and R. V. Short, eds.), Vol. 4, pp. 24–61. Cambridge Univ. Press, London and New York.
Skinner, J. D., Van Zyl, J. H. M., and Oates, L. G. (1974). The effect of season on the breeding cycle of plains antelope of the Western Transvaal high veld. *J. S. Afr. Wildl. Manage. Assoc.* **4**, 15–23.
Snell, G. O., Bodemann, E., and Hollander, W. (1934). A translocation in the house mouse and its effect on development. *J. Exp. Zool.* **67**, 93–104.

Tateno, H., and Mikamo, K. (1987). A chromosomal method to distinguish between X- and Y-bearing spermatozoa of the bull in zona-free hamster ova. *J. Reprod. Fertil.* **81,** 119–125.

Tesarik, J. (1988). Developmental control of human preimplantation embryos: A comparative approach. *J. in Vitro Fertil. Embryo Transfer* **5,** 347–362.

Tripp, H. R. H. (1970). Repeoduction in the *Macroscelididae* with special reference to ovulation. Ph.D. Thesis, University of London.

van der Hoeven, F. A., Cuijpers, M. P., and de Boer, P. (1985). Karyotypes of 3- or 4-day-old pig embryos after short *in vitro* culture. *J. Reprod. Fertil.* **75,** 593–597.

Verini Supplizi, A., King, W. A., and Xu, K. P. (1988). The chromosomes of early cleavage stage bovine embryos. *Proc. Eur. Colloq. Cytogenet. Domest. Anim., 8th,* Bristol, Abstract.

Williams, C. V., and Long, S. E. (1980). The effect of superovulation on the chromosome complement of early sheep embryos. *Proc. Eur. Colloq. Cytogenet. Domest. Anim., 4th,* Uppsala, pp. 168–171.

Gene Mapping in the Cow

JAMES E. WOMACK

Department of Veterinary Pathology, College of Veterinary Medicine, Texas A&M University, College Station, Texas

I. Introduction
II. Methods of Bovine Gene Mapping
    A. Somatic Cell Genetics
    B. Pedigree Analysis
    C. *In Situ* Hybridization
III. Current Status of the Cow Map
IV. Comparative Maps
V. Considerations for the Future
    A. Multiple Mapping Methods
    B. Interspecific Hybrids
    C. The Cloning of DNA Probes
    D. Selection of Probes
References

I. Introduction

Mammalian genomic exploration has not only become experimentally feasible, but is now scientifically fashionable. It has not always been so. Gene mapping in mammals has historically been practiced by only a small group of hard-core mouse geneticists exploring the organization of the only mammalian genome accessible with the tools available to them. Twenty years ago, these tools consisted of a finite number of inbred strains and mutant stocks of mice that could be crossed, backcrossed, and intercrossed to sort Mendelian genes responsible for mutant phenotypes into linkage groups and to subsequently order those genes and assign map distances based on frequencies of recombination between parental combinations. Consequently, the mouse map contained only a few dozen genes. Mouse gene mapping flourished in the late 1970s with the discovery of extensive biochemical and immunological polymorphisms. Particularly valuable were the allozyme loci revealed by the discovery and implementation of isozyme technology (Markert, 1977; reviewed by Womack, 1982). The widespread availability of multiple-mutant stocks, congenic strains, recombinant–inbred strains, and genetically distant but interfertile subspecies of *Mus musculus* combined with this new wealth of variation generated a map of over 300 loci. Domestic animal geneticists, however, particularly those involved in the genetic improvement of livestock, still did not generally appreciate the potential practical application of gene mapping.

The current revolution in medical genetics also had its roots in the 1970s with the advent of somatic cell genetics and its application to human gene mapping (reviewed by Puck and Kao, 1982). This technology eliminated the need for extensive pedigrees or large breeding experiments, and therefore opened the door to gene mapping in virtually any mammalian species, including livestock. This surge in new genetic information also made extensive use of isozyme techniques. The somatic cell and isozyme mapping strategy is not without limitation, however, because it is applicable only to genes normally expressed in cell culture, primarily the housekeeping enzymes. Moreover, polymorphisms in these mapped loci were not found to be sufficiently abundant to provide markers for a large number of genetic diseases, and consequently the human gene map was not widely viewed as a valuable tool for genetic counseling or prenatal diagnosis. In retrospect, it is not surprising that most animal breeders still did not view gene maps of livestock as potentially valuable tools for marker-assisted selection of desirable phenotypes.

Human gene mapping came into its own as a practical medical endeavor with the recombinant DNA era of the 1980s. Polymorphic markers for a number of human diseases, including muscular dystrophy, cystic fibrosis, Huntington's disease, and Alzheimer's disease, have become available as diagnostic and counseling tools, thanks primarily to the development of DNA probes that identify ubiquitous restriction fragment length polymorphisms (RFLPs) and the mapping of these polymorphic loci through a combination of somatic cell genetics, *in situ* hybridization, and pedigree analysis in families segregating the inherited diseases. A new approach to genetic disease, so called "reverse genetics," has emerged from these technologies. The protein product of most disease genes is neither obvious nor predictable from even the most elaborate pathological investigations. Mapping a disease locus relative to a marker gene permits a search for concentrated polymorphisms in the region of the gene. Molecular walking and jumping technologies, beginning with very closely linked DNA markers, can lead to cloning and sequencing the gene, from which the primary structure of the protein product can be read directly from the DNA sequence. A gratifying example of the results from such a reverse genetics strategy is the identification and cloning of the cystic fibrosis gene (Rommens et al., 1989). The potential value of these new biotechnologies to animal genetics has now become obvious. It is now technically feasible to construct a foundation genetic map in cattle that will make it possible to map any simply inherited trait or even quantitative trait loci (Soller and Beckmann, 1983) relative to one or more polymorphic markers. Marker-assisted selection for disease resistance and meat and milk productivity is a reasonable goal now awaiting the development of gene maps in livestock species. Moreover, the development of a map sufficiently concentrated with polymorphic genes to use in reverse genetics is a not an unreasonable aspiration. The methodology, current status, and some future considerations for the gene map of domestic cattle will be discussed with the realization that the field is now moving at a pace that will render the "status" portion of this article obsolete before it is published.

II. Methods of Bovine Gene Mapping

A. Somatic Cell Genetics

The same hybrid somatic cell techniques that produced the human gene map of the 1970s have been used successfully to map bovine genes (Heuertz and Hors-Cayla, 1981; Dain et al., 1984; Womack and Moll, 1986). Briefly, bovine cells such as fresh leukocytes have been fused with hypoxanthine phosphoribosyltransferase (HPRT)-deficient Chinese hamster E36 cells in the presence of polyethylene glycol and subsequently grown in hypoxathine–aminopterin–thymidine (HAT) medium. Complementing hybrid cells can then be cloned and grown to quantities necessary for enzyme electrophoresis, DNA analysis, and karyotyping. Fusion and enzyme assay methods have been described in detail elsewhere (Womack and Moll, 1986). In our laboratory, we have also successfully fused bovine cells with thymidine kinase-deficient mouse LMTK cells and Chinese hamster lines auxotrophic for phosphoribosylglycinamide synthetase (PRGS), phosphoribosylaminoimidazole synthetase (PAIS), and thymidine kinase (TK) (McAvin et al., 1988). These rodent cell lines require different bovine chromosomes for complementation and can therefore be used to prefer-

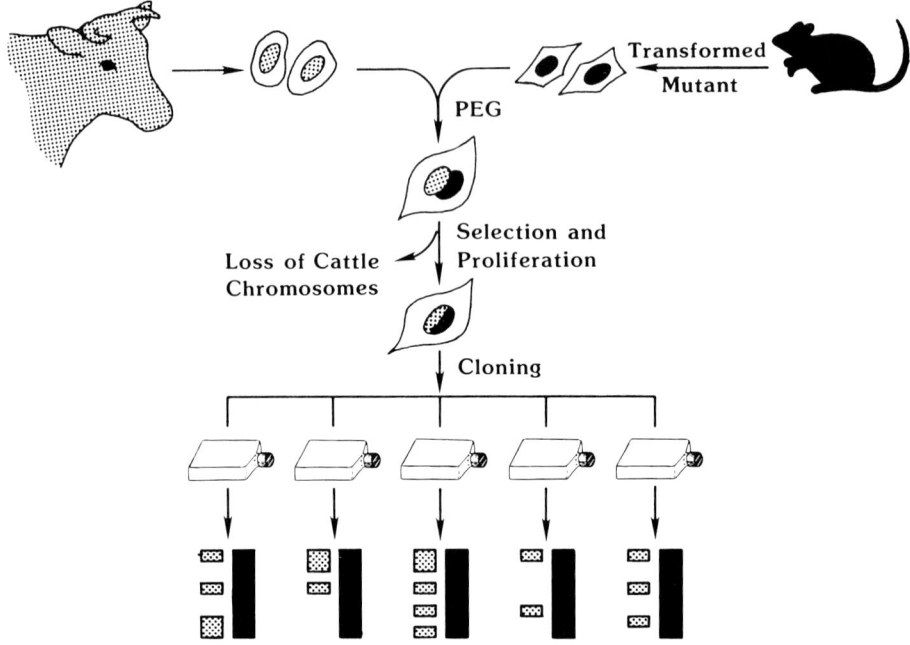

RELATIVE PROPORTIONS OF PARENTAL GENOMES RETAINED

FIG. 1. Schematic diagram of the construction of hybrid somatic cell clones. The cattle genome segregates under these conditions, resulting in a panel of clones, each with a different proportional representation of the cattle genome. (From Womack, 1988.)

entially retain selected bovine chromosomes. As a general rule in somatic cells genetics, chromosomes from a primary cell progenitor will be preferentially segregated when hybridized to a transformed cell line of another species. As expected, cow chromosomes were segregated in each of the panels of hybrid cells generated in our studies. Initially, enzyme electrophoresis was used to determine the presence or absence of several dozen bovine gene products. Using tables of concordancy, "syntenic" groups were then defined as groups of genes that were retained or segregated together. The assumption is made that genes of a common syntenic group are coded by the same chromosome (see Figs. 1 and 2).

The assignment of syntenic groups to chromosomes can be made by karyotypic analysis of the same panels of hybrid cells and the scoring of each clone for the presence or absence of each of the bovine chromo-

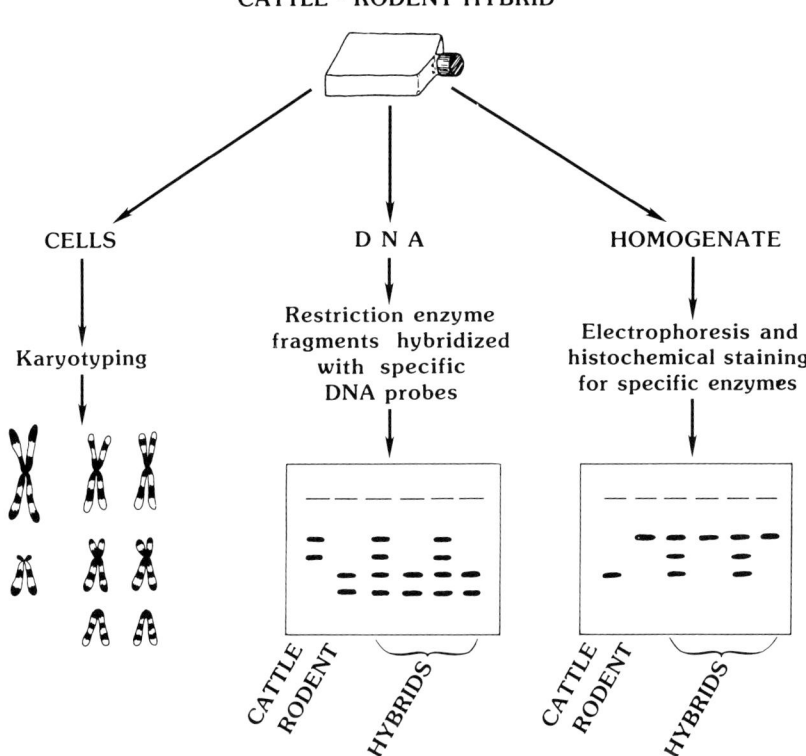

FIG. 2. Genetic analysis is performed on each hybrid cell clone. This analysis may include karyotyping, DNA blotting, enzyme electrophoresis, or other measures of phenotypes expressed in cultured cells. (From Womack, 1988.)

somes. Concordancy of retention of a gene or syntenic group with a particular chromosome is the basis for assignment of that gene or group to the respective chromosome. Also, rearranged chromosomes in these hybrid cells are potentially useful to regionally assign genes relative to breakpoints. The accurate karyotypic definition of hybrid cell panels, however, remains an enigma to somatic cell mapping of cattle. Many of the smaller cattle chromosomes are difficult to distinguish one from the other, especially in a partial bovine karyotype against a background of rodent chromosomes. Consequently, at this time, the assignment of genes to cattle chromosomes lags behind the definition of syntenic groups. It is not clear at this point whether the assignment of bovine syntenic groups to chromosomes will proceed more quickly from this approach or from the *in situ* approach discussed later. Ideally, one technique should be used to confirm the other.

The growing number of cloned DNA probes available to gene mappers gives an important new dimension to somatic cell genetics. Mapping is no longer restricted to genes whose products are expressed in cell culture, but any DNA sequence for which a cloned probe is available can now be mapped in a panel of hybrid cells. DNA can be prepared from the same hybrid cell clones that are analyzed for enzymes and chromosomes as described above. Hybrid cell DNA can then be cut with an appropriate restriction endonuclease, separated by agarose electrophoresis, and transferred to a nylon filter by the well-known method of Southern (1975). Hybridization with radiolabeled DNA probes, followed by autoradiography, identifies bands of genomic DNA homologous to the cloned probes. If the endonuclease cuts the hybridizing cow and rodent DNA into differently sized fragments, the presence or absence of bovine-specific fragments can be easily determined. The genetic distance between cattle and rodents makes fragment size differences highly probable regardless of the enzyme used. These fragments can be compared for concordancy with other genes and chromosomes analyzed in the same hybrid clones. Especially important to gene mapping for the purpose of identifying polymorphic markers of quantitative trait loci is the fact that the same probes used to identify RFLPs in breeding populations can be used for synteny analysis of hybrid cells (Adkison *et al.*, 1987, 1988). Consequently, two loci may first be determined to be syntenic, then the appropriate pedigrees segregating polymorphisms for the loci can be analyzed for linkage. This approach will prove to be much more efficient than the linkage analysis of random polymorphisms. Regional localization of genes to chromosomes, either by rearranged chromosomes in hybrid cells or by *in situ* hybridization, will facilitate the development of a linkage map, because some estimate of genetic spacing can be made from these physical maps.

B. Pedigree Analysis

The human gene map of the 1980s with markers for cystic fibrosis and other diseases is replete with DNA polymorphisms as a result of extensive pedigree analysis with cloned probes. Genomic DNA collected from members of reference pedigreed families can be probed repeatedly with different cloned probes in different laboratories, providing linkage analysis of numerous gene combinations from a single collection of samples. DNA, and even previously probed nylon filters, can be exchanged among laboratories for maximum efficiency of linkage testing. Such reference families of cattle are only now becoming available and consequently have not contributed significantly to the current map. It is certain, however, that the linkage map of the future will come from such reference families. Linkage relationships of markers to each other and to quantitative trait loci will necessarily come from this type of study, complemented by syntenic analysis of hybrid cells and by *in situ* hybridization.

C. *In Situ* Hybridization

Genes can be assigned to syntenic groups or chromosomes by somatic cell analysis and linkage relationships between polymorphic loci can be determined in pedigreed herds. Although regional chromosomal assignments can be made in hybrid clones carrying broken or translocated chromosomes, and gene order can be established from pedigree analysis, neither is a particularly efficient method for assigning genes to specific chromosomal loci. *In situ* hybridization of DNA probes directly to metaphase chromosomes has been used successfully for this purpose for a large number of human genes and recently by Fries and his colleagues to localize the bovine major histocompatibility complex (bovine leukocyte antigen; BoLA) and parathyroid hormone (Fries *et al.*, 1986, 1988b; Hediger *et al.*, 1987) genes. Our laboratory has successfully used the technique to map genes in both mice (Threadgill and Womack, 1988; Zneimer and Womack, 1988) and cattle (Zneimer and Womack, 1989). The bovine gene map of the future will undoubtedly benefit greatly from increased use of this valuable technique.

III. Current Status of the Cow Map

An updated version of the gene map of the cow, complete with references, is periodically published (Fries *et al.*, 1988a; Womack, 1987b). Briefly, the map now consists of 140 markers on all but one of the bovine syntenic groups (Table I). Two linkage groups remain unassigned to the syntenic map. Moreover, nine syntenic groups are now assigned to specific chromosomes. The alphabetical list of mapped genes (Table II) matches gene symbols from the map with names of gene loci. Complete references for this map appear in the latest issue of "Genetic Maps" (O'Brien, 1990).

The complementarity of various mapping methods may best be illus-

TABLE I

GENE MAP OF THE COW[a]

Syntenic group	Chromosome	Gene locus
U1		PGD, ENO1, AT3, ABLL
U2		SOD2, ME1, PGM3
U3	5	GAPD, LDHB, TPI1, PEPB, IFNG, A2M, INT1, HOX3, LALBA, KRAS2, GLI, PAH, NKNB, KRT2, GDH, LYS
U4	21	MPI, CYP11A, FES
U5		PKM2, NP, HEXA, FOS, KRT8L
U6		PGM1
U7		LDHA, TYR
U8		MDH2, ASL, PRM, GUSB, HBA
U9	18	GPI, DIA4
U10		SOD1, IFREC, PRGS, PAIS, CRYA1, SST, APP, ETS2, S100B, COL6A1, COL6A2, CBS, GAP43, PFKL, CD18, TF, CP
U11		ITPA, ADA, VIM
U12		ACY1, RHO
U13		HOX1, MET, COL1A2
U14		GSR, PLAT
U15	6	PGM2, PEPS, CASAS1, CASAS2, CASB, CASK
U16		ABL, ASS, GRP78, LGB, J
U17	8	IDH1, FN1, CRYG
U18		ACO1, IFNA, IFNB, GSN, GGTB2, ALDOB, ALDH1, C5, ITI, NEFM
U19	15	CAT, A, PTH, HBB, CRYA2, FSHB
U20	23	GLO1, CYP21, BoLA-A, BoLA-B, BoLA-D, PRL, TCP-1, M, HSPA1
U21	19	GH, HOX2, KRT1
U22		AMH, SPARC
U23		ALDH2, IL2, IGL
U24	14	TG, MOS, CA2, MYC, CYP11B
U25		PEPA
U26		GOT1, CYP17, ADRA2R
U27		POLR2
U28		MBP
U29		—
X	X	G6PD, HPRT, PGK1, GLA, F9, DMD
Y	Y	DYZB, DYZ1

[a]Linkage groups not assigned to syntenic groups or chromosomes: LG VI (ALB, GC), LG VII (S, PI2).

TABLE II

ALPHABETICAL LIST OF MAPPED BOVINE GENES

Gene symbol	Location	Description
A2M	Chr 5	α-2-Macroglobulin
A	Chr 15	Blood group A
ABL	U16	Abelson oncogene homologue
ABLL	U1	Abelson oncogene homologue-like
ACO1	U18	Aconitase 1, soluble
ACY1	U12	Aminoacylase 1
ADA	U11	Adenosine deaminase
ADRA2R	U26	Adrenergic, α-2-, receptor
ALB	LG VI	Albumin
ALDH1	U18	Aldehyde dehydrogenase 1, soluble
ALDH2	U23	Aldehyde dehydrogenase 2, mitochondrial
ALDOB	U18	Aldolase B
AMH	U22	Anti-Müllerian hormone
APP	U10	Amyloid β (A4) precursor protein
ASL	U8	Argininosuccinate lyase
ASS	U16	Argininosuccinate synthetase
AT3	U1	Antithrombin III
BoLA-A	Chr 23	Major histocompatibility complex, class I
BoLA-B	Chr 23	Major histocompatibility complex, class I
BoLA-D	Chr 23	Major histocompatibility complex, class II
C5	U18	Complement component 5
CA2	Chr 14	Carbonic anhydrase II
CASAS1	Chr 6	Casein, α-S1
CASAS2	Chr 6	Casein, α-S2
CASB	Chr 6	Casein, β
CASK	Chr 6	Casein, κ
CAT	Chr 15	Catalase
CBS	U10	Cystathionine-β-synthase
CD18	U10	Antigen CD18
COL1A2	U13	Collagen, type 1, α-2
COL6A1	U10	Collagen, type VI, α-1
COL6A2	U10	Collagen, type VI, α-2
CP	U10	Ceruloplasmin
CRYA1	U10	Crystallin, α, polypeptide 1
CRYA2	Chr 15	Crystallin, α, polypeptide 2
CRYG	Chr 8	Crystallin, γ
CYP11A	Chr 21	Cytochrome P450, subfamily XIA
CYP11B	Chr 14	Cytochrome P450, subfamily XIB
CYP17	U26	Cytochrome P40, family XVII
CYP21	Chr 23	Cytochrome P40, family XXI
DIA4	Chr 18	Diaphorase (NADH, NADPH)
DMD	X	Dystrophin
DYZB	Y	DNA segment
DYZ1	Y	DNA segment

(continued)

TABLE II *(Continued)*

Gene symbol	Location	Description
ENO1	U1	Enolase 1
ETS2	U10	Avian erythroblastosis virus E26 oncogene homologue
F9	X	Coagulation factor IX
FES	Chr 21	Feline sarcoma viral oncogene homologue
FN1	Chr 8	Fibronectin 1
FOS	U5	Murine FBJ osteosarcoma viral oncogene homologue
FSHB	Chr 15	Follicle-stimulating hormone, β peptide
GAP43	U10	Growth-associated protein (43 kDa)
GAPD	Chr 5	Glyceraldehyde-3-phosphate dehydrogenase
GC	LG VI	Vitamin D binding protein
GDH	Chr 5	Glucose dehydrogenase
GGTB2	U18	Glycoprotein-4-β-galactosyl transferase 2
GH	Chr 18	Growth hormone
GLA	X	Galactosidase, α
GLI	Chr 5	Glioma-associated oncogene homologue
GLO1	Chr 23	Glyoxalase 1
GOT1	U26	Glutamic-oxaloacetic transaminase 1, soluble
GPI	Chr 18	Glucose phosphate isomerase
GRP78	U16	Glucose-related protein (78 kDa)
GSN	U18	Gelsolin
GSR	U14	Glutathione reductase
GUSB	U8	Glucuronidase, β
G6PD	X	Glucose-6-phosphate dehydrogenase
HBA	U8	Hemoglobin, α
HBB	Chr 15	Hemoglobin, β
HEXA	U5	Hexosaminidase A
HOX1	U13	Homeo box region 1
HOX2	Chr 19	Homeo box region 2
HOX3	Chr 5	Homeo box region 3
HPRT	X	Hypoxanthine phosphoribosyltransferase
HSPA1	Chr 23	Heat-shock 70-kDa protein 1
IDH1	Chr 8	Isocitrate dehydrogenase 1, soluble
IFNA	U18	Interferon, α
IFNB	U18	Interferon, β
IFNG	Chr 5	Interferon, γ
IFREC	U10	Interferon receptor
IGLC	U23	Immunoglobulin λ polypeptide, constant region
IL2	U23	Interleukin 2
INT1	Chr 5	MMTV integration site oncogene homologue
ITI	U18	Inter-α-trypsin inhibitor, protein HC
ITPA	U11	Inosine triphosphatase
J	U16	Blood group J
KRAS2	Chr 5	Kirsten rat sarcoma 2 viral oncogene homologue
KRT1	Chr 19	Keratin (Type I)
KRT2	Chr 5	Keratin (Type II)
KRT8L	U5	Keratin 8-like
LALBA	Chr 5	Lactalbumin, α
LDHA	U7	Lactate dehydrogenase A

TABLE II *(Continued)*

Gene symbol	Location	Description
LDHB	Chr 5	Lactate dehydrogenase B
LGB	U16	Lactoglobulin, β
LYS	Chr 5	Lysozyme
M	Chr 23	Blood group M
MBP	U28	Myelin basic protein
MDH2	U8	Malate dehydrogenase, NAD, mitochondrial
ME1	U2	Malic enzyme 1, soluble
MET	U13	Met protooncogene
MOS	Chr 14	Moloney murine sarcoma viral oncogene homologue
MPI	Chr 21	Mannose phosphate isomerase
MYC	Chr 14	Avian myelocytomastis viral oncogene homologue
NEFM	U18	Neurofilament, medium peptide
NKNB	Chr 5	Neurokinin B
NP	U5	Nucleoside phosphorylase
PAH	Chr 5	Phenylalanine hydroxylase
PAIS	U10	Phosphoribosylaminoimidazole synthetase
PEPA	U25	Peptidase A
PEPB	Chr 5	Peptidase B
PEPS	Chr 6	Peptidase S
PFKL	U10	Phosphofructokinase, liver type
PGD	U1	Phosphogluconate dehydrogenase
PGK1	X	Phosphoglycerate kinase 1
PGM1	U6	Phosphoglucomutase 1
PGM2	Chr 6	Phosphoglucomutase 2
PGM3	U2	Phosphoglucomutase 3
PI2	LG VII	Protease inhibitor
PKM2	U5	Pyruvate kinase
PLAT	U14	Plasminogen activator, tissue
POLR2	U27	Polymerase (RNA) II (DNA directed) large polypeptide
PRGS	U10	Phosphoribosylglycinamide synthetase
PRL	Chr 23	Prolactin
PRM	U8	Protamine
PTH	Chr 15	Parathyroid hormone
RHO	U12	Rhodopsin
S	LG VII	Blood group S
S100B	U10	S100 protein, β-polypeptide
SOD1	U10	Superoxide dismutase 1, soluble
SOD2	U2	Superoxide dismutase 2, mitochondrial
SPARC	U22	Secreted protein, acidic, cystein rich
SST	U10	Somatostatin
TCP1	Chr 23	T complex protein
TF	U10	Transferrin
TG	Chr 14	Thyroglobulin
TPI1	Chr 5	Triosephosphate isomerase 1
TYR	U7	Tyrosinase
VIM	U11	Vimentin

trated by BoLA. The M blood group was initially found to be linked to BoLA genes by immunogenetic studies of pedigreed herds (Leveziel and Hines, 1984). Subsequently, BoLA RFLPs were identified with DNA probes and a family of linked BoLA genes were described (Andersson et al., 1986). Fries et al. (1986) then used a heterologous probe to localize BoLA on chromosome 23. The assignment of BoLA to a syntenic group completed (Skow et al., 1988) an important mapping story that includes linkage by meiotic recombination, chromosomal location by in situ hybridization, and, indirectly the assignment of other genes to that chromosome by synteny analysis in hybrid cells.

Auxotrophic mutants have also been useful for cattle gene mapping. Two Chinese hamster cell lines, one deficient for PRGS and the other for PAIS, two different enzymes of purine biosynthesis, were independently fused with cow leukocytes and maintained on medium selective for the complementing bovine enzymes. Segregation of cow chromosomes was extensive and only a few biochemical markers of cow chromosomes could be identified in each clone. Without exception, however, the bovine gene for cytoplasmic superoxide dismutase (SOD1) was retained. These experiments were interpreted to demonstrate synteny of the bovine genes for PRGS, PAIS, and SOD1 (McAvin et al., 1988). Clones from such panels may ultimately be recognized to have a single cow chromosome retained. These will be extremely valuable for the generation of single-chromosome libraries and the eventual fine-structure mapping of that chromosome.

IV. Comparative Maps

A large number of homologous genes have now been mapped in cattle, humans, and mice. A comparison of these maps reveals considerable conservation of syntenic groups in the three species (Womack and Moll, 1986). As the gene map of the cow grows, the comparative relationships become increasingly more complex and more interesting.

A sampling of the more interesting examples of interspecific chromosomal conservation are illustrated in Figs. 3–7. The major histocompatibility complex (MHC) has been mapped in a number of mammalian species. In humans, mice, and cattle, chromosomal conservation extends well beyond the limits of the MHC. Glyoxalase 1 (GLO1) and 21 steroid hydroxylase (21OH) are syntenic with the MHC in all three species (Fig. 3). Homologues of several genes on human (HSA) chromosome arm 6p also map to mouse (MMU) chromosome 17, whereas genes on the other arm, HSA 6q, are generally represented on another

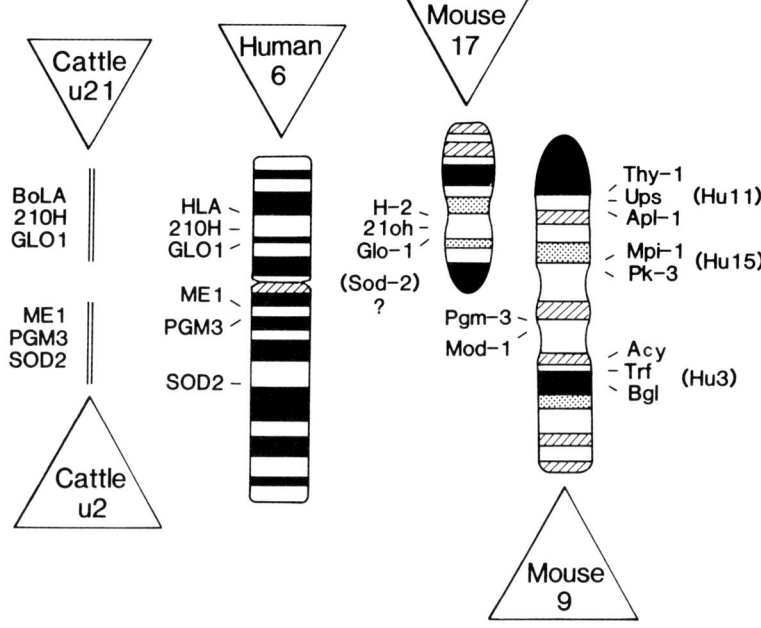

FIG. 3. Comparative cattle, human, and mouse maps of genes on human chromosome 6.

mouse chromosome, MMU 9. SOD2 is an exception to an exact arm conservation, however, in that it has been assigned to MMU 17 and appears to evidence an internal rearrangement involving a centromere in the ancestral lineage of HSA 6 and MMU 17. The gene for SOD2 in cattle, however, has remained with the chromosome carrying malic enzyme 1 (ME1) and phosphoglucomutase 3 (PGM3), which in cattle is different from chromosome 23, the chromosome carrying the bovine MHC (BoLA). There is no evidence to date to suggest that the evolution of HSA 6 and two corresponding bovine chromosomes was other than a simple centromeric fusion or fission.

A simple fusion or fission of chromosome arms may also explain the evolution of human and cattle chromosomes carrying the α and β interferons (IFNA and IFNB). These genes are syntenic with aconitase 1 (ACO1) on HSA 9p and also on cattle syntenic group U18. Whereas the same genes are syntenic on mouse chromosome 4 (Fig. 4), they are interrupted by the *Pgm-2* locus whose homologue maps to HSA 1 and to bovine syntenic group U6. Another HSA 1 gene, *Pgd*, maps more

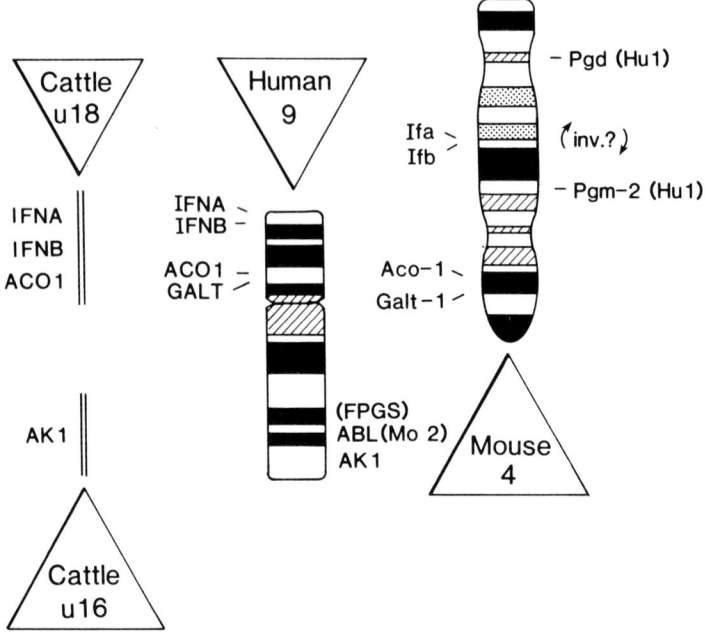

FIG. 4. Comparative cattle, human, and mouse maps of genes on human chromosome 9.

distal on MMU 4, suggesting an internal rearrangement in the evolutionary lineage of these mouse and human chromosomes. It is not possible to determine which lineage experienced the inversion, as the ancestral linkage arrangement in mammals is unknown. The suggestion of an inversion on the mouse chromosome in Fig. 4 is arbitrary. The human short arm, 9p, appears to be relatively intact as represented on cattle syntenic group U18.

Conservation across a human centromere is evidenced by the mapping in cattle of genes on HSA 12. Genes from both the p and q arms of HSA 12 are found on a single cattle chromosome (Fig. 5). Because all cattle autosomes are acrocentric, a pericentric inversion best accounts for the evolutionary history of these chromosomes. As with the other cases, it is premature to suggest which arrangement, if either, might be ancestral. Human chromosomal conservation is suggested in the mouse, wherein HSA 12p homologues map to MMU 6 and HSA 12q appears to be conserved on MMU 10. More extensive work in our laboratory suggests that the entirety of HSA 12 is located on only two cattle chromosomes (D. W. Threadgill, personal communication).

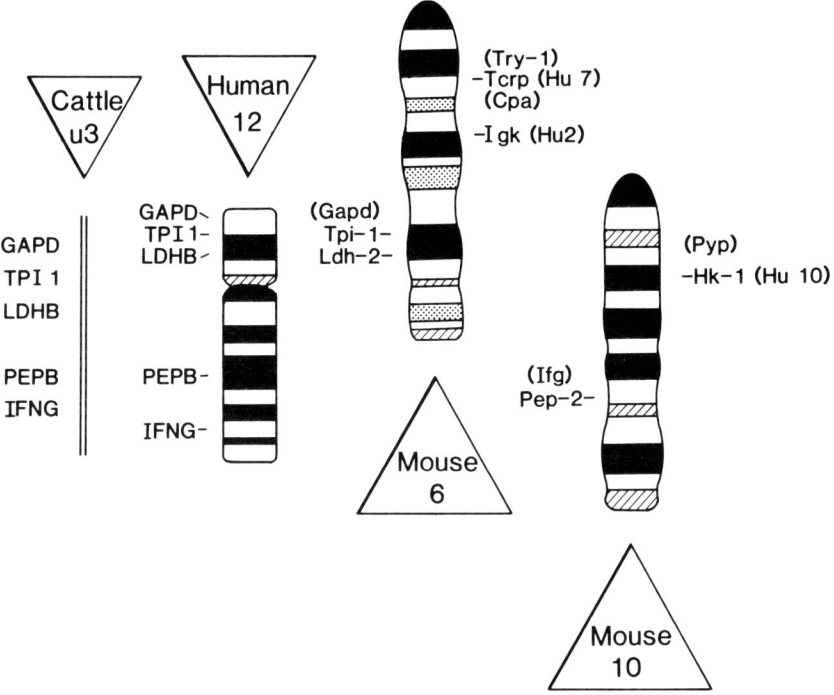

FIG. 5. Comparative cattle, human, and mouse maps of genes on human chromosome 12.

Human chromosome 21 has long been recognized as medically important because of its involvement in Down syndrome. Several of the genes on HSA 21 map to MMU 16, which is larger than HSA 21 and contains genes that map to human chromosomes other than 21 (Fig. 6). The bovine chromosome carrying syntenic group U10 contains the same genes found in MMU 16 but also contains α-crystallin (CRYA1) which maps to the *H-2* region of MMU 17. The identification of the chromosome carrying U10 is a high priority in bovine cytogenetics because it may provide an opportunity to study aneuploidy of a highly conserved region of human chromosome 21. As the map grows and more homologous genes are mapped, the extent of chromosomal conservation can be better appreciated and some of the "breakpoints" of disrupted groups will be defined. Gene mapping in cattle will then be able to benefit greatly from more generously funded human gene mapping studies. Hypotheses will be made regarding the chromosomal location of a cow gene based on the location of its homologue in the hu-

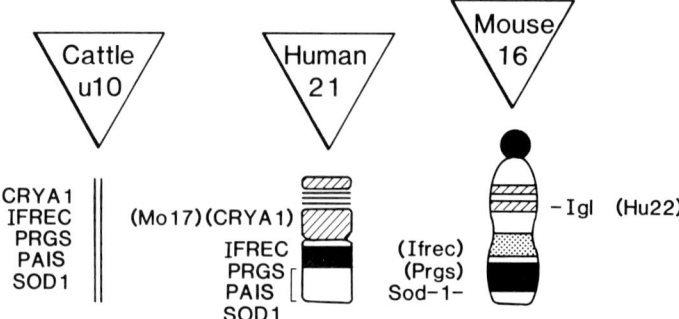

FIG. 6. Comparative cattle, human, and mouse maps of genes on human chromosome 21.

man map. Testing of such hypotheses is naturally much simpler and more efficient than random mapping. This is a very important consideration in light of the "human genome initiative," an international effort to map and sequence the human genome. Carefully planned comparative mapping in cattle will benefit directly from the enormous set of data likely to be generated from this superscience project.

As discussed previously by Kashi et al. (1986) and myself (Womack, 1987a), the number of randomly distributed markers required to saturate the bovine genome is much greater than the number required to simply dissect the genome into 30–40 centimorgan segments. The use of comparative mapping data, however, should allow us to identify markers with a high probability of the desired spacing. As an example, genes for γ-crystallin (CRYG) and fibronectin 1 (FN1) are syntenic on human chromosome 2q and mouse chromosome 1 (Skow et al., 1987; Zneimer and Womack, 1988). Somatic cell mapping in the cow also places the loci on a common bovine syntenic group (Adkison et al., 1988), which we now know to be bovine chromosome 8 (Zneimer and Womack, 1988). A reasonable hypothesis is that the physical distance between the two loci (and perhaps frequency of recombination, as well) has been conserved in cattle.

Comparative maps will ultimately prove to be extremely valuable in the improvement of cattle because they may be predictive of the location in the cattle genome of genes for production and health-related phenotypes. For example, a small region of mouse chromosome 1, probably the single locus, *Lsh*, is responsible for resistance or susceptibility to several intracellular bacterial and protozoan parasites, including *Leishmania, Mycobacterium bovis, Plasmodium,* and *Salmo-*

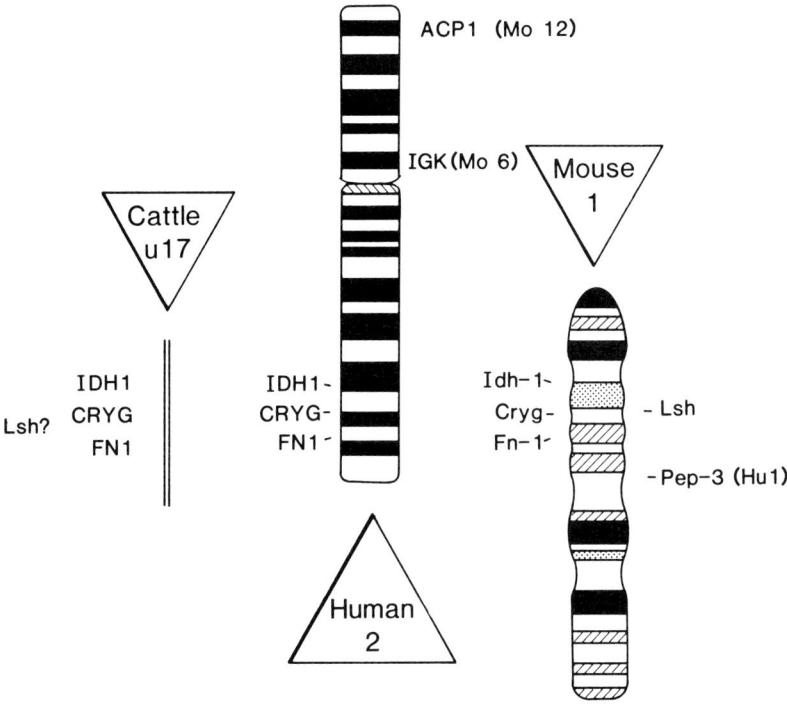

FIG. 7. Comparative cattle, human, and mouse maps of genes on human chromosome 2.

nella typhimurium. The gene is a part of the conserved segment marked by the fibronectin and γ-crystallin genes described above. Fibronectin or related proteins may mediate host cell attachment to a variety of bacterial and protozoan pathogens, including *Leishmania spp.* (Wyler *et al.*, (1985), *Treponema pallidum* (Thomas *et al.*, 1985), and *Trypanosoma cruzi* (Ouaissi *et al.*, 1986). A cluster of physically related proteins map to this general region in the mouse, one of which may be the product of the *Lsh* gene. Regardless of the specific gene product involved in host resistance, FN1 and CRYG are syntenic in cattle (Adkison *et al.*, 1988), and this conserved segment of cow chromosome 8 (Fig. 7) is now a prime target for genes in cattle that may be homologous to mouse *Lsh*. Moreover, these marker genes have now been precisely located on bovine chromosome 8 (Zneimer and Womack, 1989). The use of RFLPs for fibronectin and γ-crystallin to seek a cow homologue of the mouse *Lsh* locus will likely prove much more efficient than the use of random unmapped probes.

V. Considerations for the Future

A. MULTIPLE MAPPING METHODS

As previously discussed, each method of gene mapping produces a different type of information. A *physical map* is generated by somatic cell and *in situ* studies. This map localizes the position of genes on specific cow chromosomes. More precise physical maps may be generated by pulsed field electrophoresis of large DNA fragments to which multiple gene loci may be assigned. We have begun to apply this technique to multigene families in the cattle genome and have localized the entire casein gene family to a 400-kb segment on chromosome 6 (Threadgill and Womack, 1990). The ultimate physical map of a genome is its complete nucleotide sequence, now a realistic goal in human genetics. A *genetic map* is generated by analysis of meiotic recombination in pedigreed families. The complete map will be both a physical and genetic map, although it is the genetic map that will ultimately be utilized to identify and mark chromosomal regions that influence health and productivity.

B. INTERSPECIFIC HYBRIDS

The mouse map has gained a new surge of momentum from the use of interspecific backcrosses (Avner *et al.*, 1988). Heterozygosity is maximized in the F_1 hybrid between the subspecies *Mus spretus* and *M. musculus*. Because females of this cross are fertile, their meiotic products can be tested for linkage and recombination in a backcross generation. DNA from these backcross animals can be distributed to multiple laboratories to take full advantage of the wealth of heterozygosity in the F_1 parent. A comparable mapping resource is possible in the bovid species. Both the bison (*Bison bison*) and the gaur (*Bos gaurus*) interbreed with domestic cattle, to produce fertile female hybrid offspring. Only a few of these females as embryo donors could be used to produce a backcross generation of 100 or more offspring. DNA from these animals could be extremely important to the development of the bovine map, as the *Bos* and *Bison* hybrids appear to be every bit as heterozygous as are the invaluable *Mus* hybrids.

C. The Cloning of DNA Probes

DNA probes are extremely valuable mapping tools in that they can be used to identify RFLPs, to probe hybrid cell DNA, and also to hybridize to chromosomes *in situ*. Such a wealth of mapping information is not possible with any other type of genetic marker. Consequently, the development of the gene map of cattle stands to benefit greatly from the continued development of new DNA probes. Although heterologous probes often work well for RFLP and hybrid cell analysis, they are less likely to work for *in situ* hybridization. The continued construction of cattle cDNA and genomic libraries and the cloning of probes from these libraries are important steps in the future development of the gene map. The advent of the powerful new polymerase chain reaction (PCR) technology should facilitate the cloning of bovine genes by using primers from highly conserved regions of mouse and human homologues. An extremely valuable contribution to the bovine map would be the discovery of probes that reveal hypervariable loci, such as the variable number of tandem repeat (VNTR) loci in humans.

D. Selection of Probes

Ultimately, our goal is a map replete with highly polymorphic loci spaced at intervals no greater than 30 centimorgans, including the interval between both the centromeres and telomeres to the nearest marker. Such a map will ensure the linkage of quantitative trait loci for polymorphic markers with no greater than 15% recombination. As previously discussed, a reasonable approach to this goal is to select markers that are similarly spaced in conserved segments of genomes of other species. Another approach to a "practically useful" gene map is to seek and map polymorphisms of loci in chromosomal regions that have a sound physiological basis for involvement in the phenotype of interest. BoLA is one such target locus if the goal is to find a marker for disease resistance. Another target in this "candidate gene" approach might be the cluster of interferon genes on syntenic group U18 or the yet-unmapped immunoglobulin loci. We have been particularly interested in the region defined by FN1 and CRYG and the speculation that a bovine homologue of the mouse *Lsh* gene is located in this region. Here we have a candidate chromosomal region rather than a candidate gene to target, thanks to comparative mapping between cattle and mice.

For the next several years there will be "milepost" marker genes on the bovine map, with a gradual filling of the gaps in between. Ideally the use of comparative maps can help expedite the filling of gaps in an efficient manner. There is no reason, however, why the mileposts should not be loci with a reasonable expectation for involvement in the phenotypes we desire to mark.

REFERENCES

Adkison, L. R., Leung, D. W., and Womack, J. E. (1987). Somatic cell mapping and restriction fragment analysis of bovine alpha and beta interferon gene families. *Cytogenet. Cell Genet.* **47,** 62–65.

Adkison, L. R., Skow, L. C., Thomas, T. L., Petrash, M., and Womack, J. E. (1988). Somatic cell mapping and restriction fragment analysis of bovine genes for fibronectin and gamma crystallin. *Cytogenet. Cell Genet.* **47,** 155–159.

Andersson, L., Bohme, J., Rask, L., and Peterson, P. A. (1986.) Genomic hyrbidization of bovine class II major histocompatibility genes I. Extensive polymorphism of DQβ genes. *Anim. Genet.* **17,** 95–112.

Avner, P., Amar, L., Dandolo, L., and Guenet, J. L. (1988). Genetic analysis of the mouse using interspecific crosses. *Trends Genet.* **4,** 18–23.

Dain, A. R., Tucker, E. M., Donker, R. A., and Clarke, S. W. (1984). Chromosome mapping in cattle using mouse myeloma/calf lymph node hybridomas. *Biochem. Genet.* **22,** 429–439.

Fries, R., Hediger, R., and Stranzinger, G. (1986). Tentative chromosomal location of the bovine major histocompatibility complex by *in situ* hybridization. *Anim. Genet.* **17,** 287–294.

Fries, R., Beckmann, J. S., Georges, M., Soller, M., and Womack, J. E. (1988a). The bovine gene map. *Anim. Genet.* **20,** 3–29.

Fries, R., Hediger, R., and Stranzinger, G. (1988b). The loci for parathyroid hormone and beta-globin are closely linked and map to chromosome 15 in cattle. *Genomics* **3,** 302–307.

Hediger, R., Fries, R., and Stranzinger, G. (1987). Gene mapping in cattle: Two chromosomal assignments by *in situ* hybridization. *J. Dairy. Sci.* **70,** Suppl. 1, 240 (abstr.).

Heuertz, S., and Hors-Cayla, M.-C. (1981). Cattle gene mapping by somatic cell hybridization study of 17 enzyme markers. *Cytogenet. Cell Genet.* **30,** 137–145.

Kashi, Y., Soller, M., Hallerman, E., and Beckman, J. S. (1986). Restriction fragment length polymorphisms in dairy cattle improvement. *Proc. 3rd World Congr. Genet. Appl. Livest. Prod., 3rd,* Vol. 12, pp. 57–63.

Leveziel, H., and Hines, H. C. (1984). LInkage in cattle between major histocompatibility complex (BoLA) and the M blood group system. *Genet. Sel. Evol.* **16,** 405–416.

Markert, C. L. (1977). Isozymes: The development of a concept and its application. *Isozymes: Curr. Top. Biol. Med. Res.* **1,** 1–17.

McAvin, J. C., Patterson, D., and Womack, J. E. (1988). Mapping the bovine PRGS and PAIS genes in hybrid somatic cells: Syntenic conservation with human chromosome 21. *Biochem. Genet.* **26,** 9–18.

O'Brien, S. J., ed. (1990). "Genetic Maps." Cold Spring Harbor Lab., Cold Spring, New York.

Ouaissi, M. A., Cornette, J., Afchain, D., Carpon, A., Gras-Masse, H., and Tartar, A. (1986). *Trypanosoma cruzi* infection inhibited by peptides modeled from a fibronectin cell attachment domain. *Science* **234,** 603–606.

Puck, T. T., and Kao, F.-T. (1982). Somatic cell genetics and its applications to medicine. *Annu. Rev. Genet.* **16,** 225–271.
Rommens, J. M., Iannuzzi, M. C., Karem, B., Drumm, M. L., Melmer, G., Dean, M., Rozmahel, R., Cole, J. L., Kennedy, D., Hidaka, N., Zsiga, M., Buchwald, M., Riordan, J. R., Tsui, L. C., and Collins, F. S. (1989). Identification of the cystic fibrosis gene: Chromosome walking and jumping. *Science* **245,** 1059–1065.
Skow, L. C., Adkison, L., Womack, J. E., Beamer, W. G., and Taylor, B. A. (1987). Mapping of mouse fibronectin gene *(Fn-1)* to chromosome 1: Conservation of the *ldh-1–Cryg–Fn-1* synteny group in mammals. *Genomics* **1,** 283–286.
Skow, L. C., Womack, J. E., Petrash, J. M., and Miller, W. L. (1988). Synteny mapping of bovine genes for 21 steroid hydroxylase, alpha A-crystallin and class I bovine leucocyte antigen (BoLA) in cattle. *DNA* **7,** 143–149.
Soller, M., and Beckmann, J. S. (1983). Genetic polymorphism in varietal identification and genetic improvement. *Theor. Appl. Genet.* **67,** 25–33.
Southern, E. M. (1975). Detection of specific sequences among DNA fragments separated by gel electrophoresis. *J. Mol. Biol.* **98,** 503–517.
Thomas, D. D., Baseman, J. B., and Alderette, J. F. (1985). Fibronectin mediates *Treponema pallidum* cytoadherence through recognition of fibronectin cell-binding domain. *J. Exp. Med.* **161,** 514–525.
Threadgill, D. W., and Womack, J. E. (1988). Regional localization of mouse *Abl* and *Mos* protooncogenes by *in situ* hybridization. *Genomics* **3,** 82–86.
Threadgill, D. W., and Womack, J. E. (1990). Submitted for publication.
Womack, J. E. (1982). Linkage of mammalian isozyme loci: A comparative approach. *Isozymes: Curr. Top. Biol. Med. Res.* **6,** 207–246.
Womack, J. E. (1987a). Genetic engineering in agriculture: Animal genetics and development. *Trends Genet.* **3,** 65–68.
Womack, J. E. (1987b). A gene map of the cow. *Genet. Maps* **4,** 499–501.
Womack, J. E. (1988). Molecular cytogenetics of cattle: A genomic approach to disease resistance and productivity. *J. Dairy Sci.* **71,** 1116–1123.
Womack, J. E. (1989). A gene map of the cow. *Genet. Maps* **5** (in press).
Womack, J. E., and Moll, Y. D. (1986). A gene map of the cow: Conservation of linkage with mouse and man. *J. Hered.* **77,** 2–7.
Wyler, D. J., Sypek, J. P., and McDonald, J. A. (1985). *In vitro* parasite–monocyte interactions in human Leishmaniasis: Possible role of fibronectin in parasite attachment. *Infect. Immun.* **49,** 305–311.
Zneimer, S. M., and Womack, J. E. (1988). Regional localization of fibronectin and gamma crystallin genes to mouse chromosome 1 by *in situ* hybridization. *Cytogenet. Cell Genet.* **48,** 238–241.
Zneimer, S. M., and Womack, J. E. (1989). Chromosomal localization of the fibronectin and gamma crystallin genes to bovine chromosome 8. *Genomics* **5,** 215–220.

Gene Mapping in the Pig

R. FRIES, P. VÖGELI, AND G. STRANZINGER

Department of Animal Science, Swiss Federal Institute of Technology, ETH-Zentrum, Zürich, Switzerland

I. Gene Mapping and Animal Breeding
II. Methods Applied in Gene Mapping
   A. Physical and Genetic Maps
   B. Linkage Analysis
   C. Somatic Cell Genetics
   D. *In Situ* Hybridization
   E. Comparative Mapping
III. Status of the Map
IV. Conclusions
V. Appendix: Gene Loci in the Pig
   References

I. Gene Mapping and Animal Breeding

Most economically important traits of domestic species are quantitative traits, i.e., traits that exhibit continuous variation resulting from the action of multiple genes that is modified by the environment. The selection process of animal breeding is thought to act on the frequency of different versions of these genes; usually it results in an increased frequency of favorable versions in the population under selection. Determining the location and number of genes that condition quantitative traits and estimating the magnitude of individual gene effects have occupied quantitative geneticists since the beginning of this century. However, a preliminary dissection of the genetic factors affecting quantitative characters was achieved only in experimental organisms such as *Drosophila melanogaster* (Thoday, 1961; Shrimpton and Robertson, 1988a,b) and very recently in some plant species such as tomato (Paterson *et al.*, 1988). Despite the fact that genetic factors affecting quantitative characters in domestic species have not been systematically identified, impressive breeding success has been achieved for many characters during the last three decades.

The breeding success for a trait depends on its heritability (the proportion of the variance of the breeding value to the nongenetic variance). Traits such as fertility, disease resistance, and disease susceptibility exhibit low heritability. However, these traits play an important role in animal agriculture. Identification of single genes with a certain action could be the first step toward a more successful handling of such traits by animal breeding. The identification of the so-called halothane gene responsible for the malignant hyperthermia syndrome in pigs, as well as the Booroola gene responsible for an increased ovulation rate in sheep, are good examples for this approach. A more systematic dissection of the genome (i.e., the gene complement of an organism) with respect to loci affecting traits of economic importance may be achieved by gene mapping. McKusick (1980) has proposed considering the genome as part of the anatomy of an organism. The anatomy of the genome offers the most powerful view of an organism, because the genes are the blueprint not only for the structure but also for the functioning of an animal.

The first step in genome dissection could consist of establishing a map of genes. Mapping a gene means to determine its chromosomal position on a chromosome and/or its position relative to other genes. This mapping information can be applied, e.g., for marker-based selection (Geldermann, 1975, 1976; Soller and Beckmann, 1982, 1983, 1985; Geldermann *et al.*, 1985; Smith and Simpson, 1986; Beckmann and Soller, 1987). The indirect selection for genotypes determining the halothane reaction based on closely linked marker loci is presently the main application of this approach in swine (Vögeli *et al.*, 1988 Vögeli, 1989a). Mapping information will also be the basis of map-based molecular cloning of unknown but mapped genes. This approach, often referred to as reverse genetics (Orkin, 1986; Fries and Ruddle, 1986), uses tightly linked DNA markers as entry points to "walk" along the chromosome to the gene of interest. Reverse genetics has already been used to clone several genes involved in hereditary diseases of humans (Royer-Pokora *et al.*, 1986; Monaco *et al.*, 1986). Map-based cloning will certainly be the method of choice to clone the halothane gene in swine (Davies *et al.*, 1988). Ultimately, reverse genetics will lead to a better understanding of the processes modifying animal performances.

This article provides a review of the methods applied to study the "genomic anatomy" of the pig and other species and presents the status of the porcine gene map in order to define the starting point for future efforts.

II. Methods Applied in Gene Mapping

A. PHYSICAL AND GENETIC MAPS

There are two different but complementary types of gene maps, the *physical* and the *genetic* maps, that are established by the synthesis of data derived by several different methods. Studying the meiotic linkage relationships of gene loci (linkage analysis) is the basis of the genetic maps. Physical maps are arrived at by methods that make use of gene transfer among mammalian somatic cells from different species (somatic cell hybridization), by methods that involve the direct assignment of genes by hybridization of DNA of specific type to fixed chromosomes (*in situ* hybridization), and by comparative investigations that allow provisional mapping based on the evolutionarily conserved location of genes.

B. LINKAGE ANALYSIS

Genetic maps provide information on the distance between gene loci, given as the function of the frequency of meiotic crossing-over occurring between the gene loci. Each meiotic crossing-over can be counted as a recombination event between alleles at the two loci in informative families, i.e., families in which at least one parent is heterozygous at both loci. If the recombination frequency (θ) is less than 0.50 and if the assumption of random segregation at the loci is correct, one can conclude that the two loci are on the same chromosome, at a distance from each other that is proportional to the frequency of recombination. As a statistical test to determine whether the hypothesis of linkage can be accepted or must be rejected the logarithm of the odds (lod) score test (Wald, 1947; Morton, 1955) is now widely used. Lod scores of $+3.0$ or more, meaning that the likelihood of linkage is at least 1,000 times greater than the likelihood of nonlinkage, are considered as sufficient evidence for linkage, whereas lod scores of -2.0 are sufficient for the rejection of linkage. The map distance measured in cross-over units, or centimorgans (cM), can be estimated based on θ and an appropriate mapping function (e.g., Kosambi, 1944). Several computer programs were developed to facilitate lod score calculation in complex pedigrees and to determine the likelihood of the order of several linked genes (Lathrop, 1984; Ott, 1976).

For genetic mapping, one would want to have all points of the genome within not much more than 20 cM of a mapped marker locus, in order to enable linkage relationships to be established with a reasonable number of animals.

It has now become generally accepted that the most efficient way to obtain the required number and distribution of polymorphic markers is to make use of DNA restriction fragment length polymorphisms (RFLPs) (Botstein et al., 1980; Beckmann and Soller, 1983). These have been detected at high frequencies in man (White et al., 1985). A linkage map of the human genome, based on the pattern of inheritance of about 400 marker loci, mostly RFLPs, has recently been established (Donis-Keller et al., 1987). Complete marker maps are also available for some plant species and are already being applied in breeding programs (Helentjaris, 1987; Tanksley et al., 1989).

A complete and efficient marker map should consist of highly polymorphic marker loci that are not more than 40 cM apart from each other. This maximum distance between marker loci is given by the requirement that any locus should be within 20 cM of the next marker locus to enable efficient linkage analysis. The porcine genome can be assumed to span 3,000 cM (Fries and Ruddle, 1986). Thus, on an average porcine chromosome of 160 cM, one would need four well-spaced markers per chromosome—two about 20 cM from the centromere and the telomere, respectively, and two 40 cM apart in the center. That is, less than 80 marker loci, well spaced along the chromosomes, would initially be sufficient for complete coverage of the 19 different porcine chromosomes. In fact, because the markers will be selected at random from a given DNA library, the number of markers required to achieve the desired goal is considerably more than 80. The number of markers required to cover the genome may depend on the strategy employed to find RFLPs. One strategy involves the use of a genomic library whereas the second, more efficient approach uses libraries from single chromosomes or even parts of chromosomes. From this second type of library, markers can be selected to avoid choosing new probes for a chromosome that already carries sufficient markers.

C. Somatic Cell Genetics

Mapping data obtained with methods based on somatic cell genetics are part of the physical gene map. Gene mapping by somatic cell genetics is based on parasexual events that allow the transfer of genetic material between cells. The delivery of genes in a random fashion into recipient cells is possible through somatic cell hybridization (Yerganian and Nell, 1966; Pontecorvo, 1975). The use of mutant cell lines allows the efficient selection of hybrid cells from parental cells (Littlefield, 1964; Baker *et al.*, 1974). If mouse and hamster cells are combined with cells from another species, such as human or pig, there is progressive and preferential loss of the chromosomes of the nonmouse or nonhamster species (Weiss and Green, 1967). Panels of hybrid cells are generated, each retaining a partial complement of the genome of the segregating progenitor species. It is possible to draw conclusions about synteny (location of genes on the same chromosome) or to assigne gene loci to particular chromosomes after the investigation of the chromosomal complement and the determination of the presence or absence of gene products or specific cellular phenotypes in a panel of about 20–30 hybrid clones. When a gene probe is available, the presence of a gene can be directly determined by restriction fragment analyses (Ruddle, 1981).

Karyotypic analysis of hybrid cells is often difficult, because single chromosomes of the segregating progenitor species need to be distinguished from the hamster or mouse chromosomes. A special staining technique has been developed to facilitate distinction between the chromosomes of different species (Bobrow and Cross, 1974). *In situ* hybridization (see below) of total labeled DNA from a species is also used to mark the chromosomes in hybrid cells. We routinely apply a sequential procedure, whereby the chromosomes of the pig–hamster hybrids are first stained with quinacrine to induce Q-bands. Suitable metaphase spreads are photographed and subsequently hybridized *in situ* with total porcine DNA. After autoradiography, heavy labeling of the pig chromosomes can be observed, whereas there are only few grains associated with the hamster chromosomes. The chromosomes identified as porcine chromosomes can then be unequivocally typed using the photographs taken before.

D. *In Situ* Hybridization

Hybridization of suitable probes with fixed preparations of metaphase chromosomes is now routinely applied to map single-copy genes in man and other species. Harper and Saunders (1981) improved a technique that was first developed by Gall and Pardue (1969) and John *et al.* (1969). The original method allowed only the localization of highly reiterated or amplified genes. Improvement in the hybridization procedure, including the use of dextran sulfate in the reaction mixture, made possible the routine mapping of single-copy genes by *in situ* hybridization. The probes are labeled to high specific activities by nick translation with ^{3}H-labeled nucleotides. ^{125}I- and ^{35}S-labeled nucleotides are also used to label probes for *in situ* hybridization (Rabin et al., 1985; Geffrotin et al., 1984). However, ^{3}H-labeled nucleotides are frequently used now. For radioactive *in situ* hybridization, a 10-fold increase of the specific radioactivity of the probes (over that by nick translation) was recently achieved by "oligolabeling" (Feinberg and Vogelstein, 1983, 1984) with three ^{3}H-labeled nucleotides (Lin et al., 1985; Fries et al., 1986). This enables the mapping of genes by *in situ* hybridization even when using relatively short cDNA or heterologous sequences as probes. Detection of the radioactive signal is by autoradiography, a procedure that may take up to 4 weeks. The distribution of silver grains along the chromosomes is evaluated and a significant accumulation of grains over a specific chromosome region is considered as a signal of specific hybridization of the probe.

Procedures based on nonradioactive labeling allow for a more precise localization of the probe signal on the chromosomes and therefore for an increased mapping resolution. Moreover, with nonisotopic methods, a signal may be generated within hours, rather than within days, a distinct advantage over autoradiography. Yet nonradioactive methods are not sufficiently sensitive to routinely map single-copy genes. However, Landegent et al. (1987) demonstrated that the use of cosmid clones as probes in nonradioactive *in situ* hybridization resulted in an improved detection limit. Cherif et al. (1989) have recently been able to chromosomally locate unique DNA sequences of less than 2 kb in length using biotinylated probes generated by oligolabeling and an improved immunofluorescence detection technique including signal amplification. A faint signal may also be detected using a camera sensitive to low light levels, digital storing of images, and time averaging of images for noise reduction (Albertson et al., 1988).

An essential step in gene mapping by *in situ* hybridization is the unambiguous identification of chromosomes. Our approach to solving this problem consists of photographing, prior to the hybridization, quinacrine (Q)-banded chromosomes (Caspersson et al., 1969) and scoring of silver grain distribution in the prephotographed spreads after autoradiography. This procedure guarantees an unbiased selection of spreads. This is of special importance when mapping genes in the pig, because most gene assignments are first assignments in this species.

In combination with somatic cell genetics, *in situ* hybridization will be indispensable in establishing the physical gene map. Newly developed marker loci should be chromosomally assigned by *in situ* hybridization, in order to allow marker spacing to be monitored during the development of the marker map.

The resolution of mapping by *in situ* hybridization, like the maximum resolution by subchromosomal panel mapping, depends on the band resolution of the chromosomes and is, therefore, in the range of 5–10 cM (Ruddle, 1981). This level of resolution is not sufficient to bridge the gap between physical chromosome mapping and mapping on the molecular level, even when using novel molecular techniques such as pulsed-field gradient electrophoresis (Barlow and Lehrach, 1987), cloning in yeast (Cooke, 1987), or jumping and linking libraries (Poustka and Lehrach, 1986). Only genetic mapping allows for a resolution in the range of 1 cM, a distance that is amenable to the new molecular techniques.

E. Comparative Mapping

Comparative mapping is based on the observation that the location of genes on specific chromosome regions is conserved in different species. The chromosomal distribution of homologous genes among different species can be characterized in three ways, depending on the number and order of genes in each segment. *Homology segments* are marked by a single gene that is considered homologous in different species based on the 10 criteria established by Lalley *et al.* (1987). Two or more pairs of homologous genes located on the same chromosome compose a *conserved synteny group*. The term conserved synteny is used regardless of whether the gene order is conserved. In a *conserved linkage segment* both synteny and gene order must be conserved.

Synteny conservation (not linkage conservation) is most complete for the X chromosome. All 14 genes of the mouse and three porcine genes that have been assigned to the X chromosomes in these species have homologous counterparts in man that map to the human X chromosome (Nadeau, 1989). This conservation of the gene content of the X chromosomes supports Ohno's law (Ohno, 1973) that chromosomal rearrangements involving the X chromosome and autosomes are strongly selected against, presumably due to selective constraints of the release of X-linked genes from the dosage compensation mechanism.

The mapping of homologous genes to the autosomes has also revealed synteny and linkage conservation of autosomal segments, although to a lesser degree than the complete chromosomal conservation of the X chromosome. Comparative mapping data are presently available for more than 25 species of mammals. However, the number of genes mapped in more than one species is less than 20 for most pairs and an estimation of the degree of evolutionary conservation of chromosome segments is presently only possible for mice and humans, based on more than 250 homologous gene assignments in these species. More than 40 conserved synteny segments are known for humans and mice. The average length of conserved autosomal linkages is 8–12 cM (Nadeau, 1989). In other pairs of species, conservation of chromosome segments may be even more extensive, e.g., in cattle and humans (Womack and Moll, 1986). The number genes that have been mapped in humans *and* in the pig is too small to provide comment on the degree of linkage conservation in these two species.

Comparative mapping makes use of the knowledge about chromosome segment conservation in different species to predict the position of homologous genes in a species in which the genes have not been mapped. The application of this strategy to map porcine genes may be illustrated with the following example. The porcine gene for glucose phosphate isomerase (GPI) has been assigned by *in situ* hybridization close to the centromere of chromosome 6. This assignment is of special interest in the pig, because GPI is closely linked to the locus controlling the so-called halothane sensitivity gene (HAL). Because the region around HAL and GPI is deplete of DNA marker loci, a saturation with this type of marker loci will be the first step toward the cloning of the HAL gene. A direct approach to the cloning of marker loci could consist of microdissecting (Lüdecke *et al.*, 1989) the chromosome region to which GPI has been assigned. Genomic libraries constructed from the DNA obtained by microdissection could then be used as a source for probes specific for this region. An alternative approach, based on comparative gene mapping, consists of selecting genes that map close to GPI in humans and/or mice as probes to screen a porcine genomic library. Positive clones will be immediately mapped by *in situ* hybridization to determine whether they belong to the region of GPI. If they do, they will be used as probes to detect RFLPs useful as landmarks in walking toward the HAL gene.

Comparative mapping will allow the construction of a preliminary but extensive porcine gene map fairly rapidly. Only relatively few well-chosen mapping experiments will be necessary. Based on conserved synteny between humans and mice (or other species), one will select genes from the boundaries of the conserved segments to be mapped in the pig. If they actually map to the same porcine chromosome, it can be assumed that all genes that are flanked by the two genes map also to that porcine chromosome region. Thus, a provisional map can be drawn using the well advanced human gene map with over 3,500 gene assignments (McAlpine et al., 1988) as a guide.

III. Status of the Map

The gene map of the porcine chromosomes shows only a few specific assignments (Fig. 1), similar to the human gene map as presented more than 10 years ago by McKusick and Ruddle (1977). A total of 107 loci have been described in swine (see Section V). The nomenclature follows the guidelines for human gene nomenclature (Shows et al., 1987). Whenever a homologous gene has been mapped in humans, the same symbol was chosen to designate the porcine locus. Such a nomenclature will facilitate comparative mapping. When chosing a symbol for a locus without a presently known homologous human counterpart, care has been taken to use a symbol not used for a human gene. Most of the loci listed in Section V exhibit multiple alleles. At a few loci, variation has also been detected at the DNA level (RFLPs). For some combinations of loci, linkage analysis has been carried out. Table I summarizes the known linkage groups. The synteny groups established by the analysis of hybrid panels are also listed in Table I.

IV. Conclusions

The porcine gene map is not as far advanced as is the human gene map. However, powerful methods used to map the human genome can also be applied in pig gene mapping. Mapping the porcine genome clearly can profit technically from the human gene mapping. Conservation of the gene order among mammalian species will allow gene mapping in the pig to draw directly on the success in human and murine gene mapping. A major effort should therefore be made to map porcine genes with homologous counterparts in other mammalian species. Comparative mapping along with the development of a DNA marker system will serve as an essential first step toward the ultimate

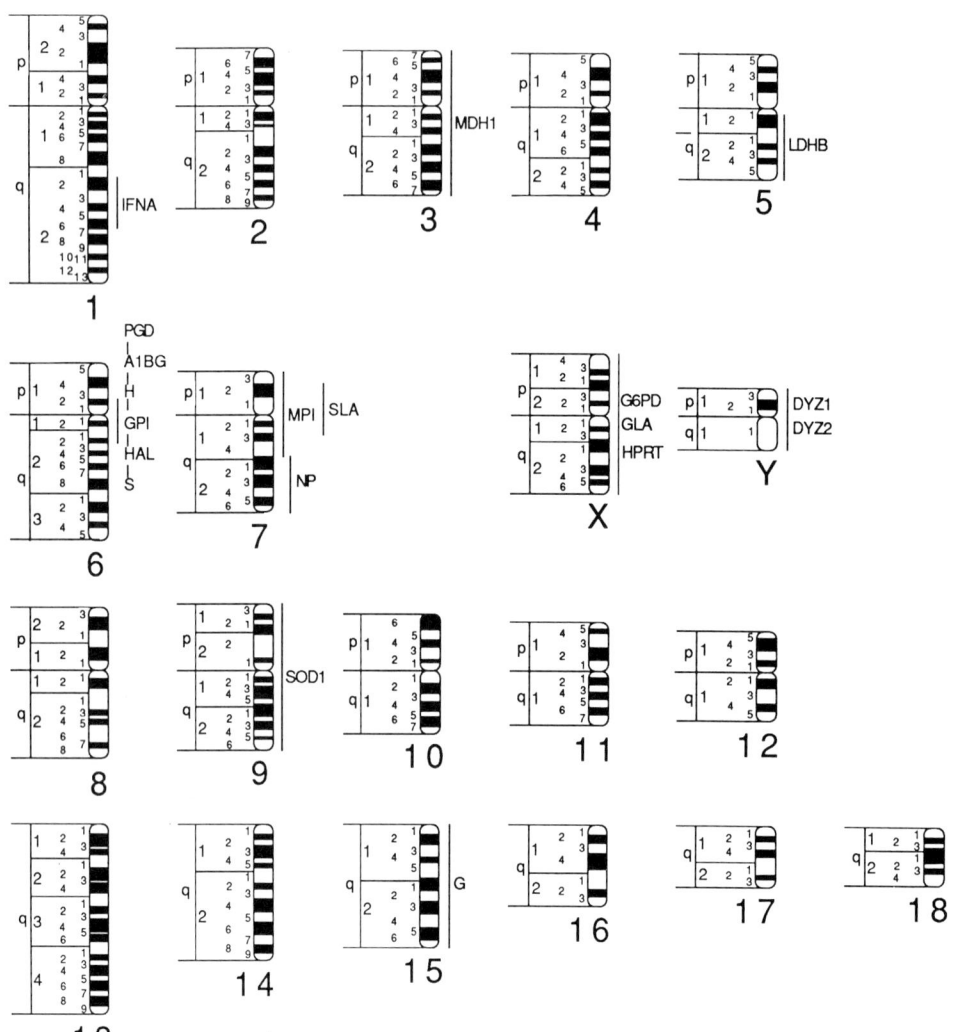

FIG. 1. Pictorial representation of the chromosomal gene assignments in swine. Inconsistent assignments are not included. The idiogram represents the international standard of swine chromosomes (Gustavsson, 1988). The explanation of the locus symbols is given in Section V. SLA comprises SLA-DQA, SLA-DQB, SLA-DRA, SLA-DRB, SLA-B, SLA-C, SLA-A, and C4 (see Table I).

TABLE I

Synteny and Linkage of Gene Loci in the Pig[a]

Assigned linkage and synteny groups	
Chromosome	Linked/*syntenic* loci
6	PGD-A1BG-H-GPI-HAL-S *(PGM1?)*
7	C-J-DQA-DQB-DRA-DRB-B-C-A, *C4,* *MPI, NP (PKM2?)*
X	*G6PD, HPRT, GLA*
Y	*DYZ1, DYZ2*
Unassigned linkage groups	
Linkage group	Linked loci
LGI	K-HPX
LGII	I-AM
LGIII	ELF-TF-CP
LGIV	L-SLB
LGV	APOB, APOT, APOU
LGVI	PI1-PI4-PI5-PI2, IGHG1, IGHG2, IGHG3, IGHG4

[a]Gene symbols are defined in Section V. Loci for which the order is known are separated by a hyphen; loci for which the order is not known are separated by commas. Syntenic loci are indicated in italics. The underlined loci belong to the SLA complex.

goal of dissecting the genetic variation of important traits in the pig to its Mendelian components, and of manipulating them at a genomic rather than a phenotypic level.

V. Appendix: Gene Loci in the Pig

In the following alphabetical tabulation of gene loci in the pig, the position of a locus is given as assignment to a chromosome or a chromosome region (see also Fig. 1) or to a linkage group (LG). The methods used for mapping and the status of assignments are symbolized as follows (McAlpine et al., 1988): A, *in situ* hybridization; L, linkage/family studies; R, recombinant DNA methodology; S, somatic cell hybrids; C, confirmed (results of two independent laboratories or from several families); P, provisional (results from only one laboratory or one family); I, inconsistent (results inconsistent between laboratories). The presence of a RFLP is denoted by the plus sign.

Symbol	Component	Location	Method	Status	RFLP	References
A	Blood group A	—	L	C		Rasmusen (1964); Hojný and Hála (1965); Vögeli et al. (1983)
A1BG	α-1-B-glycoprotein (postalbumin-2; Po2)	6	L	C		Juneja et al. (1983); Gahne (1987); Van Zeveren et al. (1988); Vögeli et al. (1988); Vögeli (1989a)
A2M	α-2-macroglobulin (S-α-2)	—	L	P		Schröffel (1965)
ACP	Acid phosphatase	—	L	P		Meyer and Verhorst (1973)
ADA	Adenosine deaminase (Ada)	—	L	C		Widar et al. (1974); Widar and Ansay (1975); Hyldgaard-Jensen and Wegger (1977)
ALB	Albumin (Alb-1)	—	L	P		Kristjansson (1966)
ALP	Alkaline phosphatase (Akp)	—	L	C		Dinklage (1970); Verhorst (1973b); Kierek-Jaszcuk et al. (1978)
AMY	Amylase (Am)	LGII	L	C		Ashton (1960); Andresen (1966b); Hesselholt (1970); Kurosawa et al. (1987)
AMY2	Amylase-2 (Am-2)	—	L	P		Jumkov and Nikonchik (1977)
AMY3	Amylase-3 (Am-3)	—	L	P		Rozhkov (1983)
APOB	Apolipoprotein B (Lpb)	LGV	L	C	+	Rapacz (1982); Wysshaar (1988); Maeda et al. (1988)
AFOR	Apolipoprotein R (Lpr)	—	L	C		Rapacz (1982); Wysshaar (1988)
APOS	Apolipoprotein S (Lps)	—	L	P		Rapacz (1982)
AP?T	Apolipoprotein T (Lpt)	LGV	L	P		Rapacz (1982)
APOU	Apolipoprotein U (Lpu)	LGV	L	P		Rapacz (1982)
B	Blood group B	—	L	C		Andresen (1962); Baker and Andresen (1964)
C	Blood group C	7	L	C		Andresen and Baker (1964); Rasmusen (1965a); Andresen (1966a); Hradecký et al. (1982)

C4	Complement component 4	7	L	P	Vaiman et al. (1986)
CA	Carbonic anhydrase	—	L	C	Kloster et al. (1970); Verhorst (1973b)
CASB1	Casein, β-1 (β-1-Cn)	—	L	C	Glasnák (1966); Kemmer et al. (1972)
CASB2	Casein, β-2 (β-2-Cn)	—	L	C	Glasnák (1966); Kemmer et al. (1972)
CASZ	Casein-Z (Z-protein; Z-Cn)	—	L	P	Glasnák (1968)
CAT	Catalase	—	L	P	Baranov (1970)
CP	Ceruloplasmin	LGIII	L	C	Imlah (1964); Oishi et al. (1980); Juneja et al. (1989)
D	Blood group D	—	L	C	Saison et al. (1967); Hradecký and Linhart (1970)
DIA1	Diaphorase-1	—	L	P	Makaveev (1979)
DIA2	Diaphorase-2	—	L	P	Makaveev (1979)
DYZ1	DNA segment, repetitive, 3.8-kb probe	Y	R	P	McGraw et al. (1988)
DYZ2	DNA segment, repetitive, 3.8-kb probe	Y	R	P	Mileham et al. (1988)
E	Blood group E	—	L	C	Andresen (1957) (1962) (1963) (1965); Andresen and Wroblewski (1959); Rasmusen (1965b); Dinklage and Major (1968); Dinklage et al. (1969); Baker (1971); Hojný and Hradecký (1972a) (1973) (1974); Hradecký and Hojný (1972); Linhart (1974); Linhart and Romanov (1975); Hojný (1989)
ECK88	Escherichia coli K88 small intestinal receptors	—	L	C	Sellwood et al. (1975); Bijelsma et al. (1982); Rapacz and Hasler-Rapacz (1986)
ELF	Early lethal factor	LGIII	L	C	Imlah (1970); Juneja et al. (1989)
ES	Esterase	—	L	P	Kúbek (1970)
ESAR	Esterase, aryl (Ar)	—	L	C	Augustinsson and Olsson (1961); Gahne (1970); Gahne et al. (1972)
ESB	Esterase II (Es II)	—	L	P	Grunder and Kristjansson (1974)
ESD	Esterase D	—	L	C	Tanaka et al. (1980); Hyldgaard-Jensen and Thorup (1981)

(continued)

Symbol	Component	Location	Method	Status	RFLP	References
F	Blood group F	—	L	C		Andresen (1957); Hdradecký and Hojný (1970); Voron and Sokolenko (1971); Hojný et al. (1984)
G	Blood group G	15	L	C		Andresen (1957); Andresen and Wroblewski (1961); Tikhonov et al. (1979); Fries et al. (1983), (1984)
G6PD	Glucose-6-phosphate dehydrogenase	X	S	C		Verhorst (1973a); Förster et al. (1980); Leong et al. (1983b)
GC	Group-specific component (vitamin D binding protein)	—	L	P		Ljungqvist and Hyldgaard-Jensen (1983)
GLA	Galactosidase, α	X	S	P		Leong et al. (1983b)
GP	Globulin	—	L	P		Janik et al. (1983)
GPI	Glucose phosphate isomerase (phosphohexose isomerase; Phi)	6p12–q22	L, A	C	+	Kúbek and Dinklage (1971); Saison and O'Reilly (1971); Rasmusen (1981); Juneja et al. (1983); Hojný et al. (1985); Davies et al. (1987), (1988); Van de Weghe et al. (1988); Van Zeveren et al. (1988); Vögeli et al. (1988); Vögeli (1989a)
GPX	Glutathione peroxidase	—	L	P		Agar and Board (1984)
H	Blood group H	6	L	C		Andresen (1957), (1964a); Andresen and Wroblewski (1961); Nielsen (1962); Hojný and Hradecký (1972b); Hojný (1973); Rasmusen (1981); Juneja et al. (1983); Hojný et al. (1985); Van Zeveren et al. (1988); Vögeli et al. (1988); Vögeli (1989a)
HAL	Halothane sensitivity (malignant hyperthermia)	6	L	C		Smith and Bampton (1977); Rasmusen (1981); Juneja et al. (1983); Gahne and Juneja (1985); Hojný et al. (1985); Van Zeveren et al. (1988); Vögeli et al. (1988); Vögeli (1989a)

			L	P	+	
HBB	Hemoglobin, β	—				Rando and Masina (1985)
HP	Haptoglobin (Hp)	—	L	C		Hesselholt (1963); Kristjansson (1961)
HPRT	Hypoxanthine phosphoribosyltransferase	X	S	C		Förster et al. (1980); Leong et al. (1983b)
HPX	Hemopexin	LGI	L	C		Kristjansson (1961); Brummerstedt-Hansen and Hesselholt (1962); Imlah (1965); Schröffel (1966); Hesselholt and Hristić (1966); Baker (1967); Tanaka et al. (1979); Oishi et al. (1980)
I	Blood group I	LGII	L	C		Andresen (1957), (1964b), (1966b)
IFNA	Interferon, α (leukocyte)	1q22–q26	A	C		Yerle et al. (1986); Grunwald et al. (1986)
IGHG1	Immunoglobulin heavy chain gamma 1 polypetide (Igh1)	LGVI	L	C		Rapacz and Hasler-Rapacz (1982); Juneja et al. (1986); Vögeli et al. (1987)
IGHG2	Immunoglobulin heavy chain gamma 2 polypetide (Igh2)	LGVI	L	P		Rapacz and Hasler-Rapacz (1982)
IGHG3	Immunoglobulin heavy chain gamma 3 polypetide (Igh3)	LGVI	L	P		Rapacz and Hasler-Rapacz (1982)
IGHG4	Immunoglobulin heavy chain gamma 4 polypetide (Igh4)	LGVI	L	P		Rapacz and Hasler-Rapacz (1982)
J	Blood group J	7	L	C		Andresen (1957), (1966a); Rasmusen (1965a); Hojný and Hradecký (1972b); Hradrecký et al. (1982)
K	Blood group K	LGI	L	C		Andresen (1957), (1962), (1963); Andresen and Irwin (1959); Imlah (1965); Brucks (1966); Hojný et al. (1979b); Nielsen and Vögeli (1982)

(continued)

Symbol	Component	Location	Method	Status	RFLP	References
K1	Protein K1	—	L	P		Dostál (1968)
K2	Protein K2	—	L	P		Dostál (1968)
L	Blood group L	LGIV	L	C		Andresen (1962); Brucks (1964); Hojný et al. (1966); Linhart (1971); Hruban et al. (1978)
LALBA	Lactalbumin, α (α-La)	—	L	C		Schmidt and Ebner (1972); Bell et al. (1981)
LDHA	Lactate dehydrogenase A	2, 5	S	I		Förster and Hecht (1986); Ryttman et al. (1986)
LDHB	Lactate dehydrogenase B	5q12–qter	S	C		Förster and Hecht (1986); Ryttman et al. (1986)
LDHC	Lactate dehydrogenase C	—	L	P		Valenta et al. (1967)
LGB	Lactoglobulin, β (β-Lg)	—	L	C		Kemmer (1969); Erhardt and Senft (1987)
M	Blood group M		L	C		Nielsen (1961); Dinklage and Major (1969); Hojný and Hradecký (1972b); Hojný et al. (1979a); Hojný and Van Zeveren (1985)
MDH1	Malate dehydrogenase, NAD (soluble)	3	S	P		Förster and Hecht (1984)
ME1	Malic enzyme 1	1 or 17	S	P		Förster and Hecht (1984)
MPI	Mannose phosphate isomerase	7q21–pter	S	C		Gellin et al. (1980), (1981); Echard et al. (1984); Kaufmann et al. (1985a); Förster and Hecht (1985); Dolf and Stranzinger (1986); Ryttman et al. (1986), (1988)
N	Blood group N	—	L	C		Hojný et al. (1966); Saison (1967)
NF	Nucleoside phosphorylase	7q21–qter	S	C		Gellin et al. (1981); Echard et al. (1984); Kaufmann et al. (1985a); Förster and Hecht (1985); Dolf and Stranzinger (1986); Ryttman et al. (1988)

O	Blood group O	—	L	C	Hojný et al. (1966); Vögeli (1989b)
PEPB	Peptidase B	5, 11	S	I	Förster and Hecht (1984); Ryttman et al. (1986)
PEPC	Peptidase C	—	L	P	Saison (1973)
PEPE	Peptidase E (leucine amino-peptidase; Lap)	—	L	P	Randi et al. (1986)
PGD	Phosphogluconate dehydrogenase	6	L	C	Saison and Giblett (1969); Rasmusen (1981); Juneja et al. (1983); Hojný et al. (1985); Archibald and McTeir (1988); Van Zeveren et al. (1988); Vögeli et al. (1988): Vögeli (1989a)
PGM1	Phosphogluco-mutase-1	6, 10	S	I	Förster and Hecht (1984); Ryttman et al. (1986)
PGM2	Phosphogluco-mutase-2	—	L	C	Safarova et al. (1972); Vögeli et al. (1982)
PGM3	Phosphogluco-mutase-3	—	L	P	Pretorius et al. (1977)
PI1	Protease inhibitor-1 (α-1-antitrypsin)	LGVI	L	C	Kristjansson (1963); Juneja and Gahne (1981); Juneja et al. (1986); Gahne and Juneja (1987); Vögeli et al. (1987)
PI2	Protease inhibitor-2 (α-1-antichymotrypsin)	LGVI	L	C	Gahne and Juneja (1986), (1987); Juneja et al. (1986); Vögeli et al. (1987); Kühne et al. (1989)
PI3	Protease inhibitor-3 (Pi3; α-cysteine protease inhibitor?)	—	L	P	Stratil and Gábrišová (1989)
PI4	Protease inhibitor-4 (Po1A; α-cysteine protease inhibitor?)	LGVI	L	C	Gahne and Juneja (1986); Juneja et al. (1986); Vögeli et al. (1987); Kühne et al. (1989)
PI5	Protease inhibitor-5 (Po1B)	LGVI	L	C	Gahne and Juneja (1986); Juneja et al. (1986); Vögeli et al. (1987); Kühne et al. (1989)

(continued)

Symbol	Component	Location	Method	Status	RFLP	References
PKLR	Pyruvate kinase, red blood cells (Pk)	—	L	P		Imamura and Tanaka (1972)
PKM2	Pyruvate kinase, muscle	7, 13–18	S	I		Gellin et al. (1980), (1981); Echard et al. (1984); Kaufmann et al. (1985b)
PLG	Plasminogen	—	L	P		Rapacz et al. (1988)
PPR	Pancreatic proteinase	—	L	P		Takahashi et al. (1974)
S	Blood group S	6	L	C		Rasmusen (1964); Hojný and Hála (1965); Vögeli et al. (1983), (1988); Hojný et al. (1985); Rasmusen (1981); Van Zeveren et al. (1988); Vögeli (1989a)
SLA-A	Swine leukocyte alloantigen (major histocompatibility complex, class I)	7p12–q12	L, A	C	+	Hradecký et al. (1982); Singer et al. (1982), (1987); Geffrotin et al. (1984); Chardon et al. (1985); Rabin et al. (1985); Kirszenbaum et al. (1985); Renard et al. (1988)
SLA-B	Swine leukocyte alloantigen (major histocompatibility complex, class I)	7	L	C	+	Singer et al. (1982), (1987); Chardon et al. (1985); Kirszenbaum et al. (1985); Renard et al. (1988)
SLA-C	Swine leukocyte alloantigen (major histocompatibility complex, class I)	7	L	C	+	Singer et al. (1982), (1987); Chardon et al. (1985); Kirszenbaum et al. (1985); Renard et al. (1988)
SLA-DQA	Swine leukocyte alloantigen (major histocompatibility complex, class II, α)	7	L	C	+	Chardon et al. (1985); Kirszenbaum et al. (1985); Vaiman et al. (1986); Vaiman (1987); Renard et al. (1988)
SLA-DQB	Swine leukocyte alloantigen (major histocompatibility complex, class II, β)	7	L	C	+	Chardon et al. (1985); Kirszenbaum et al. (1985); Vaiman et al. (1986); Vaiman (1987); Renard et al. (1988)
SLA-DRA	Swine leukocyte alloantigen (major histocompatibility complex, class II, α)	7	L	C	+	Chardon et al. (1985); Kirszenbaum et al. (1985); Vaiman et al. (1986); Vaiman (1987); Renard et al. (1988)

SLA-DRB	Swine leukocyte alloantigen (major histocompatibility complex, class II, β)	7	L	C	Chardon et al. (1985); Kirszenbaum et al. (1985); Vaiman et al. (1986); Vaiman (1987); Renard et al. (1988)
SLB	Swine leukocyte alloantigen B (non-MHC)	LGIV	L	C	Hruban et al. (1978), (1988)
SLC	Swine leukocyte alloantigen C (non-MHC)	—	L	P	Hruban et al. (1983)
SLD	Swine leukocyte alloantigen D (non-MHC)	—	L	P	Philipsen et al. (1985)
SOD1	Superoxide dismutase 1, soluble	9	S	C	Leong et al. (1983a); Förster and Hecht (1985)
SORD	Sorbitol dehydrogenase (Sdh)	—	L	P	Op't Hof et al. (1972)
SPL	Splay leg	X	L	P	Lax (1971)
TAIII	Tremor AIII, congenital	—	L	P	Harding et al. (1973)
TF	Transferrin	LGIII	L	C	Kristjansson (1960); Imlah (1965); Schröffel (1966); Baker (1968); Imlah (1970); Glasnák et al. (1976); Kurosawa et al. (1987); Kurosawa and Tanaka (1988); Juneja et al. (1989)
W2P	Whey-2 protein (κ-caseinlike protein)	—	L	C	Kraeling and Gerrits (1967); Althen and Gerrits (1972)
XB	X-protein	—	L	P	Glasnák (1968)

Acknowledgments

We thank J. Hojný and A. Stratil for their help in compiling the list of gene loci.

References

Agar, N. S., and Board, P. G. (1984). Phenotypic variation of erythrocyte glutathione peroxidase in the pig. *Anim. Blood Groups Biochem. Genet.* **15,** 63–66.
Albertson, D. G., Fishpool, R., Sherrington, P., Nacheva, E., and Milstein, C. (1988). Sensitive and high resolution *in situ* hybridization to human chromosomes using biotin labelled probes: Assignment of the human thymocyte CD1 antigen genes to chromosome 1. *EMBO J.* **7,** 2801–2805.
Althen, T. G., and Gerrits, R. J. (1972). Polymorphism of whey 2 protein of sow's milk. *J. Dairy Sci.* **55,** 331–332.
Andresen, E. (1957). Investigations on blood groups of the pig. *Nord. Veterinaermed.* **9,** 274–284.
Andresen, E. (1962). Blood groups in pigs. *Ann. N.Y. Acad. Sci.* **97,** 205–225.
Andresen, E. (1963). A study of blood groups in pigs. Thesis, Munksgaard, Copenhagen.
Andresen, E. (1964a). Further studies on the H blood group system in pigs with special reference to a new red cell antigen Hc. *Acta Genet.* **14,** 319–326.
Andresen, E. (1964b). The inheritance of the blood factors Ia and Ib in pigs of the Duroc and Hampshire breeds. *Vox Sang.* **9,** 617–621.
Andresen, E. (1965). Minus ($-/-$) Ea Ed phenotypes and new allele Eeg (= E7) in pigs of the Hampshire breed. *Vox Sang.* **10,** 738–741.
Andresen, E. (1966a). Additional linkage data involving the C and J blood group loci in pigs. *Vox Sang.* **11,** 120–123.
Andresen, E. (1966b). Blood groups of the I system in pigs: Association with variants of serum amylase. *Science* **153,** 1660–1661.
Andresen, E., and Baker, L. N. (1964). The C blood group system in pigs and the detection and estimation of linkage between the C and J systems. *Genetics* **49,** 379–386.
Andresen, E., and Irwin, M. R. (1959). The K blood group system of the pig. *Acta Agric. Scand.* **9,** 253–260.
Andresen, E., and Wroblewski, A. (1959). The E blood group system of the pig. *Nord. Veterinaermed.* **11,** 548–558.
Andresen, E., and Wroblewski, A. (1961). The G and H blood group systems of the pig. *Acta Vet. Scand.* **2,** 267–280.
Archibald, A. L., and McTeir, B. L. (1988). A new allele at the Pgd locus in pigs. *Anim. Genet.* **19,** 189–191.
Ashton, G. C. (1960). Thread protein and β-globulin polymorphism in the serum proteins of pigs. *Nature (London)* **186,** 991–992.
Augustinsson, K. B., and Olsson, B. (1961). Genetic control of arylesterase in the pig. *Hereditas* **47,** 1–22.
Baker, L. N. (1967). A new allele, Hp4, in the hemopexin system in pigs. *Vox Sang.* **12,** 397–400.
Baker, L. N. (1968). New allele in the transferrin system of pigs, TfE Ames, an apparent mutation. *Vox Sang.* **14,** 446–451.
Baker, L. N. (1971). E red cell system in pigs: Irregular genetic transmission. *Vox Sang.* **21,** 57–64.
Baker, L. N., and Andresen, E. (1964). The Bb blood factor in pigs. *Vox Sang.* **9,** 359–362.

Baker, R. M., Brunette, D. M., Mankovitz, R., Thompson, L. H., Whitmore, G. F., Siminovitch, L., and Till, J. E. (1974). Ouabain-resistant mutants of mouse and hamster cells in culture. *Cell (Cambridge, Mass.)* **1,** 9–21.

Baranov, O. K. (1970). An immunoelectrophoretic study of protein polymorphism in hemolysates of pigs and cattle. *Biochem. Genet.* **4,** 549–564.

Barlow, D. P., and Lehrach, H. (1987). Genetics by gel electrophoresis: The impact of pulsed field gel electrophoresis on mammalian genetics. *Trends Genet.* **3,** 167–171.

Beckmann, J. S., and Soller, M. (1983). Restriction fragment length polymorphisms in genetic improvement: Methodologies, mapping and costs. *Theor. Appl. Genet.* **67,** 35–43.

Beckmann, J. S., and Soller, M. (1987). Molecular markers in genetic improvement of farm animals. *Bio/Technology* **5,** 573–576.

Bell, K., McKenzie, H. A., and Shaw, D. C. (1981). Porcine alpha-lactalbumin A and B. *Mol. Cell. Biochem.* **35,** 113–119.

Bijelsma, I. G. W., Ne Nijs, A., Von der Meer, C., and Frik, J. F. (1982). Different pig phenotypes affect adherence of *Escherichia coli* to jejuna brush borders by K88ab, K88ac or K88ad antigen. *Infect. Immun.* **37,** 891–894.

Bobrow, M., and Cross, J. (1974). Differential staining of human and mouse chromosomes in interspecific cell hybrids. *Nature (London)* **251,** 77–79.

Botstein, D., White, R. L., Skolnick, M., and Davis, R. W. (1980). Construction of a genetic linkage map in man using restriction fragment length polymorphisms. *Am. J. Hum. Genet.* **32,** 314–331.

Brucks, R. (1964). Die Blutgruppensysteme des Schweines unter besonderer Berücksichtigung des L-Systems. *Z. Tierzuecht. Zuechtungsbiologie* **80,** 66–80.

Brucks, R. (1966). A study of the K blood group system of swine. *In* "Polymorphismes Biochimiques des Animaux," pp. 167–170. INRA, Paris.

Brummerstedt-Hansen, E., and Hesselholt, M. (1962). Haptoglobin polymorphism in sera from pigs of Danish Landrace. *Arsberet.—K. Vet.- Landbohoejsk., Inst. Sterilitetsforsk.* **5,** 211–219.

Caspersson, T., Zech, L., Modest, E. J., Foley, G. E., Wagh, U., and Simonsson, E. (1969). Chemical differentiation with fluorescence alkalyting agents in *Vicia faba* metaphase chromosomes. *Exp. Cell Res.* **58,** 128–140.

Chardon, P., Vaiman, M., Kirszenbaum, M., Geffrotin, C., Renard, C., and Cohen, C. (1985). Restriction fragment length polymorphism of the major histocompatibility complex of the pig. *Immunogenetics* **21,** 161–171.

Cherif, D., Bernard, O., and Berger, R. (1989). Detection of single-copy genes by nonisotopic *in situ* hybridization on human chromosomes. *Hum. Genet.* **81,** 358–362.

Cooke, H. (1987). Cloning in yeast: An appropriate scale for mammalian genomes. *Trends Genet.* **3,** 173–174.

Davies, W., Harbitz, I., and Hauge, J. G. (1987). A partial cDNA clone for porcine glucosephosphate isomerase: Isolation, characterization and use in detection of restriction fragment length polymorphisms. *Anim. Genet.* **18,** 233–240.

Davies, W., Harbitz, I., Fries, R., Stranzinger, G., and Hauge, J. G. (1988). Porcine malignant hyperthermia carrier detection and chromosomal assignment using a linked probe. *Anim. Genet.* **19,** 203–212.

Dinklage, H. (1970). The alkaline phosphatase system in the pig. *Eur. Conf. Anim. Blood Groups Biochem. Polymorphism, Proc., 11th,* Warsaw, *1968,* pp. 359–361.

Dinklage, H, and Major, F. (1968). Eaegi (= E8), a new allele in the E blood-group system of the pig. *Vox Sang.* **14,** 315–317.

Dinklage, H., and Major, G. (1969). New factors and alleles in the M blood-group system of the pig. *Vox Sang.* **17,** 316–319.

Dinklage, H., Schahmirzadi, H., Hradecky, J., and Hojny, J. (1969). Eedghj (= E9), a new allele in the E blood-group system of the pig. *Vox Sang.* **17,** 129–133.

Dolf, G., and Stranzinger, G. (1986). Pig gene mapping: Assignment of the genes for mannosephosphate isomerase (MPI) and nucleoside phosphorylase (NP) to chromosome no. 7. *Génét. Sél. Evol.* **18,** 375–384.

Donis-Keller, H., Green, P., Helms, C., Cartinhour, S., Weiffenbach, B., Stephens, K., Keith, T. P., Bowden, D. W., Smith, D. R., Lander, E. S., Botstein, D., Akots, G., Rediker, K. S., Gravius, T., Brown, V. A., Rising, M. B., Parker, C., Powers, J. A., Watt, D. E., Kauffman, E. R., Bricker, A., Phipps, P., Muller-Kahle, H., Fulton, T. R., Ng, S., Schumm, J. W., Braman, J. C., Crooks, S. M., Lincoln, S. E., Daly, M. J., and Abrahamson, J. (1987). A genetic linkage map of the human genome. *Cell (Cambridge, Mass.)* **51,** 319–337.

Dostál, J. (1968). A study on polymorphic proteins of seminal vesicle fluid and seminal plasma in boars. *Immunogenet. Lett.* **5,** 117–119.

Echard, G., Gellin, J., Benne, F., and Gillois, M. (1984). Progress in gene mapping of cattle and pigs using somatic cell hybridization. *Cytogenet. Cell Genet.* **37,** 458–459.

Erhardt, G., and Senft, B. (1987). Protein polymorphisms in porcine milk. *Anim. Genet.* **18,** Suppl. 1, 56–57.

Feinberg, A. P., and Vogelstein, B. (1983). A technique for radiolabeling DNA restriction endonuclease fragments to high specific activity. *Anal. Biochem.* **132,** 6–13.

Feinberg, A. P., and Vogelstein, B. (1984). A technique for radiolabeling DNA restriction endonuclease fragments to high specific activity (addendum). *Anal. Biochem.* **137,** 266–267.

Förster, M., and Hecht, W. (1984). Some provisional gene assignments in pig. *Proc. Eur. Colloq. Cytogenet. Domest. Anim., 6th,* Zurich, pp. 351–355.

Förster, M., and Hecht, W. (1985). Genlokalisierungen für die Superoxid Dismutase (SOD-1), Nukleosid Phospho-Isomerase (NP) und Mannose Phospho-Isomerase (MPI) beim Schwein. *Zuechtungskunde* **54,** 249–255.

Förster, M., and Hecht, W. (1986). Assignment of the genes for lactate dehydrogenase A and B in the pig to chromosome no. 4 and no. 5 by somatic cell hybrids. *J. Anim. Breed. Genet.* **103,** 46–50.

Förster, M., Stranzinger, G., and Hellkuhl, B. (1980). X-chromosome gene assignment of swine and cattle. *Naturwissenschaften* **67,** 48.

Fries, R., and Ruddle, F. H. (1986). Gene mapping in domestic animals. *Beltsville Symp. Agric. Res.* **10,** 19–37.

Fries, R., Stranzinger, G., and Vögeli, P. (1983). Provisional assignment of the G blood group locus to chromosome 15 in swine. *J. Hered.* **74,** 426–430.

Fries, R., Rasmusen, B. A., Jarrell, V. L., and Maurer, R. R. (1984). Mapping of the gene for G blood group antigens to chromosome 15 in swine. *Anim. Blood Groups Biochem. Genet.* **15,** 251–258.

Fries, R., Hediger, R., and Stranzinger, G. (1986). Tentative chromosomal localization of the bovine major histocompatibility complex by *in situ* hybridization. *Anim. Genet.* **17,** 287–294.

Gahne, B. (1970). The genetic control of arylesterase activity in pig serum. *Anim. Blood Groups Biochem. Genet.* **1,** 33–42.

Gahne, B. (1987). Pig Blood Group and Polymorphic Protein Workshop, Pawlowice (Poland). Personal communication.

Gahne, B., and Juneja, R. K. (1985). Prediction of the halothane (Hal) genotypes of pigs by deducing Hal, Phi, Po2, Pgd haplotypes of parents and offspring: Results from a large scale-practice in Swedish breeds. *Anim. Blood Groups Biochem. Genet.* **16,** 265–283.

Gahne, B., and Juneja, R. K. (1986). Extensive genetic polymorphism of four plasma alpha-protease inhibitors in pigs and evidence for tight linkage between the structural loci of these inhibitors. *Anim. Genet.* **17**, 135–157.

Gahne, B., and Juneja, R. K. (1987). Genetic polymorphism of plasma protease inhibitors in pig and some other species of domestic animals. *Anim. Genet.* **18**, Suppl.1, 46–50.

Gahne, B., Bengtsson, S., and Kleppenes, O. (1972). At least eight alleles controlling the arylesterase activity in pig serum. *Eur. Conf. Anim. Blood Groups Biochem. Polymorphism* Budapest, 1970, pp. 379–382.

Gall, J. G., and Pardue, M. L. (1969). Formation and detection of RNA-DNA hybrid molecules in cytological preparations. *Proc. Natl. Acad. Sci. U.S.A.* **63**, 378–383.

Geffrotin, C., Popescu, C. P., Cribiu, E. P., Boscher, J., Renard, C., Chardon, P., and Vaiman, M. (1984). Assignment of MHC in swine to chromosome 7 by *in situ* hybridization and serological typing. *Ann. Génét.* **27**, 213–219.

Geldermann, H. (1975). Investigations on inheritance of quantitative characters in animals by gene markers. I. Methods. *Theor. Appl. Genet.* **46**, 319–330.

Geldermann, H. (1976). Investigations on inheritance of quantitative characters in animals by gene markers. II. Expected effects. *Theor. Appl. Genet.* **47**, 1–4.

Geldermann, H., Pieper, U., and Roth, B. (1985). Effects of marked chromosome sections on milk performance in cattle. *Theor. Appl. Genet.* **70**, 138–146.

Gellin, J., Benne, F., Hors-Cayla, M. C., and Gillois, M. (1980). Carte génique du porc (Sus scrofa L.) I. Etude de deux groups synténiques G6PD, PGK, HPRT et PKM2, MPI. *Ann. Génét.* **23**, 15–21.

Gellin, J., Echard, G., Benne, F., and Gillois, M. (1981). Pig gene mapping: PKM2–MPI–NP synteny. *Cytogenet. Cell Genet.* **30**, 56–62.

Glasnák, V. (1966). Protein polymorphism in sow's milk. *In* "Polymorphismes Biochimiques des Animaux," pp. 433–435. INRA, Paris.

Glasnák, V. (1968). Inter- and intraspecific differences in milk proteins of cattle and swine. *Comp. Biochem. Physiol.* **25**, 355–357.

Glasnák, V., Stratil, A., and Schleger, W. (1976). A transferrin variant TfI in crosses of the wild and domestic pigs. *Anim. Blood Groups Biochem. Genet.* **7**, 59–64.

Grunder, A. A., and Kristjansson, F. K. (1974). Genetic control of serum esterases in day-old pigs. *Anim. Blood Groups Biochem. Genet.* **5**, 143–151.

Grunwald, D., Geffrotin, C., Chardon, P., Frelat, G., and Vaiman, M. (1986). Swine chromosomes: Flow sorting and spot blot hybridization. *Cytometry* **7**, 582–588.

Harding, J. D. J., Done, J. T., Harbourne, J. F., Randall, C. J., and Gilbert, F. R. (1973). Congenital tremor type AIII in pigs: An hereditary sex-linked cerebrospinal hypomyelinogenesis. *Vet. Rec.* **92**, 527–529.

Harper, M. E., and Saunders, G. F. (1981). Localization of single copy DNA sequences on G-banded human chromosomes by *in situ* hybridization. *Chromosoma* **83**, 431–439.

Helentjaris, T. (1987). A genetic linkage map for maize based on RFLPs. *Trends Genet.* **3**, 217–221.

Hesselholt, M. (1963). Haptoglobin polymorphism in pigs. *Acta Vet. Scand.* **4**, 238–246.

Hesselholt, M. (1970). Additional studies into serum amylase in swine. *Eur. Conf. Anim. Blood Groups Biochem. Polymorphism, Proc, 11th,* Warsaw, 1968, pp. 347–353.

Hesselholt, M., and Hristić, V. (1966). Haemopexin polymorphism in pigs. *Acta Vet. Scand.* **7**, 187–188.

Hojný, J. (1973). Further contribution to the H system in pigs. *Anim. Blood Groups Biochem. Genet.* **4**, 161–168.

Hojný, J. (1989). Blood groups in pigs. *Rep.: Pig Blood Group Polymorphic Protein Workshop,* Stara Zagora, Bulgaria, pp 1–9.

Hojný, J., and Hála, K. (1965) A contribution to the study of the blood group system A in pigs. *In* "Blood Groups of Animals" (J. Matoušek, ed.), pp. 155–161. Pub. House Czech. Acad. Sci., Prague.

Hojný, J., and Hradecký, J. (1972a). El-Em, the fourth closed E subsystem of blood groups in pigs. *Anim. Blood Groups Biochem. Genet.* **3**, 51–57.

Hojný, J., and Hradecký, J. (1972b). A contribution to the study on H, J and M blood group systems in pigs. *Eur. Conf. Anim. Blood Groups Biochem. Polymorphism [Proc.], 12th,* Budapest, *1970,* pp. 299–303.

Hojný, J., and Hradecký, J. (1973). En-Eo—Further new factors in the complex E blood group system of the pig. *Anim. Blood Groups Biochem. Genet.* **4**, 27–34.

Hojný, J., and Hradecký, J. (1974). Factor Er and allele Edeghjmnr in blood groups of the pig. *Anim. Blood Groups Biochem. Genet.* **5**, 189–191.

Hojný, J., and Van Zeveren, A. (1985). Ml, a new factor in the porcine M blood group system. *Anim. Blood Groups Biochem. Genet.* **16**, 69–72.

Hojný, J., Gavalier, M., Hradecký, J., Linhart, J. (1966). New blood factors in pigs. *In* "Polymorphismes Biochimiques des Animaux" pp. 151–158. INRA, Paris.

Hojný, J., Hradecký, J., and Camacho, A. (1979a). Further factors and alleles of the M blood group system in pigs. *Proc. Int. Conf. Anim. Blood Groups Biochem. Polymorphism, 16th,* Leningrad, *1978,* Vol. 3, pp. 114–119.

Hojný, J., Hradecký, J., and Pazdera, J. (1979b). The blood group factor Kf and allele Kae in the pig. *Anim. Blood Groups Biochem. Genet.* **10**, 175–180.

Hojný, J., Hradecký, J., and Linhart, J. (1984). New blood group allele (Fad) in the pig. *Anim. Blood Groups Biochem. Genet.* **15**, 227–228.

Hojný, J., Čepica, S., and Hradecký, J. (1985). Gene order and recombination rates in the linkage group S-Phi-Hal-H-(Po2)-Pgd in pigs. *Anim. Blood Groups Biochem. Genet.* **16**, 307–318.

Hradecký, J., and Hojný, J. (1970). Blood factor Fb in pigs. *Anim. Blood Groups Biochem. Genet.* **1**, 125–126

Hradecký, J., and Hojný, J. (1972). E blood group system in miniature pigs. *Conf. Anim. Blood Groups Biochem. Polymorphism [Proc.], 12th, 1970,* pp. 293–297.

Hradecký, J., and Linhart, J. (1970). Db—Next blood group factor of the D system in pigs. *Anim. Blood Groups Biochem. Genet.* **1**, 65–66.

Hradecký, J., Hruban, V., Pazdera, J., and Klaudy, J. (1982). Map arrangement of the SLA chromosomal region and the J and C blood group loci in the pig. *Anim. Blood Groups Biochem. Genet.* **13**, 223–224.

Hruban, V., Hradecký, J., Pazdera, J., Simon, M., and Veselský, L. (1978). SLB, a new alloantigenic system of the pig. *J. Immunogenet.* **5**, 173–178.

Hruban, V., Dvořák, P., Hradecký, J., Pazdera, J., and Müller, J. (1983). Non-MHC alloantigenic system in pigs (SLC) detected by leucoagglutination. *Anim. Blood Groups Biochem. Genet.* **14**, 299–304.

Hruban, V., Hradecký, J., and Dvořák, P. (1988). Polymorphism of the SLB serologically defined (non-MHC) alloantigenic system in pigs. *Anim. Genet.* **19**, 285–290.

Hyldgaard-Jensen, J., and Thorup, I. (1981). Esterase D polymorphism in Danish Landrace pigs (in Danish). *Arsberet—K. Vet.- Landbohoejsk., Inst. Sterilitetsforsk.,* **24**, 110–117.

Hyldgaard-Jensen, J., and Wegger, I. (1977). Adenosine deaminase in pigs. II. Qualitative and quantitative genetic variation (in Danish). *Arsberet.—K. Vet.- Landbohoejsk., Inst. Sterilitetsforsk.* **20**, 131–139.

Imamura, K., and Tanaka, T. (1972). Multimolecular forms of pyruvate kinase from rat and other mammalian tissue. *J. Biochem. (Tokyo)* **71**, 1043–1051.

Imlah, P. (1964). Inherited variants in serum ceruloplasmins of the pig. *Nature (London)* **203**, 658–659.

Imlah P. (1965). A study of blood groups in pigs. In "Blood Groups of Animals" (J. Matoušek, ed.). pp. 109–122. Pub. House Czeck. Acad. Sci., Prague.

Imlah, P. (1970). Evidence for the Tf locus being associated with an early lethal factor in a strain of pigs. *Anim. Blood Groups Biochem. Genet.* **1**, 5–13.

Janik, A., Hojný, J., and Duniec, M. (1983). Allotype polymorphism of serum globulins (Gp system) in pigs. *Anim. Blood Groups Biochem. Genet.* **14**, 63–70.

John, H. A., Birnstiel, M. L., and Jones, K. W. (1969). RNA–DNA hybrids at the cytological level. *Nature (London)* **223**, 582–587.

Jumkov, V. A., and Nikonchik, L. I. (1977). Serum amylase-2 polymorphism in pigs. *Anim. Blood Groups Biochem. Genet.* **8**, 247–250.

Juneja, R. K., and Gahne, B. (1981). Polymorphic serum prealbumin (Pa) of pig, identified as an alpha-1-protease inhibitor. *Anim. Blood Groups Biochem. Genet.* **12**, 47–51.

Juneja, R. K., Gahne, B., Edfors-Lilja, I., and Andresen, E. (1983). Genetic variation at a pig serum protein locus, Po-2 and its assignment to the Phi, Hal, S, H, Pgd linkage group. *Anim. Blood Groups Biochem. Genet.* **14**, 27–36.

Juneja, R. K., Gahne, B., Rapacz, J., and Hasler-Rapacz, J. (1986). Linkage between the porcine genes encoding immunoglobulin heavy-chain allotypes and some serum alpha-protease inhibitors: A conserved linkage in pig, mouse and human. *Anim. Genet.* **17**, 225–233.

Juneja, R. K., Kuryl, J., Gahne, B., and Zurkowski, M. (1989). Linkage between the loci for transferrin and ceruloplasmin in pigs. *Anim. Genet.* **20**, 307–311.

Kaufmann, U., Avery, B., and Christensen, K. (1985a). Chromosome mapping in domestic pigs *(Sus scrofa):* MPI and NP located to chromosome 7. *Hereditas* **102**, 231–235.

Kaufmann, U., Avery, B., and Christensen, K. (1985b). Chromosome mapping in domestic pigs *(Sus scrofa):* PK is not linked to the syntenic group MPI-NP on chromosome no. 7. *Hereditas* **102**, 305–306.

Kemmer, B. (1969). Beta-Laktoglobulin-Typen in der Sauenmilch. *Zuechtungskunde* **41**, 331–334.

Kemmer, B., Gruhn, R., and Dinklage, H. (1972). Studies on protein polymorphism in sow's milk. *Con. Anim. Blood Groups Biochem. Polymorphism [Proc.] 12th,* Budapest, *1970,* pp. 393–396.

Kierek-Jaszcuk, D., Zurkowski, M., Skladanowska-Krzyzanowska, E., and Tomaszewska-Guszkiewicz, K. (1978). Serum alkaline phosphatase polymorphism in pigs. *Anim. Blood Groups Biochem. Genet.* **9**, 15–18.

Kirszenbaum, M., Renard, C., Geffrotin, C., Chardon, P., and Vaiman, M. (1985). Evidence for mapping pig C4 gene(s) within the pig major histocompatibility complex (SLA). *Anim. Blood Groups Biochem. Genet.* **16**, 65–68.

Kloster, G., Larsen, B., and Nielsen, P. B. (1970). Carbonic anhydrase polymorphism in cattle and swine. *Acta Vet. Scand.* **11**, 318–321.

Kosambi, D. D. (1944). The estimation of map distances from recombination values. *Ann. Eugen.* **12**, 172–175.

Kraeling, R. R., and Gerritis, R. J. (1967). Polymorphism of a crystalline protein in sow's whey. *J. Anim. Sci.* **26**, 877 (abstr.).

Kristjansson, F. K. (1960). Genetic control of two blood serum proteins in swine. *Can. J. Genet. Cytol.* **2**, 295–300.

Kristjansson, F. K. (1961). Genetic control of three haptoglobins in pigs. *Genetics* **46**, 907–910.

Kristjansson, F. K. (1963). Genetic control of two pre-albumins in pigs. *Genetics* **48**, 1059–1063.

Kristjansson, F. K. (1966). Fractionation of serum albumin and genetic control of two albumin fractions in pigs. *Genetics* **53**, 675–679.

Kúbek, A. (1970). Electrophoretical study of the esterases in pig serum. *Eur. Conf. Anim. Blood Groups Biochem. Polymorphism, Proc., 11th,* Warsaw, *1968,* pp. 355–358.

Kúbek, A., and Dinklage, H. (1971). Phosphohexose isomerase polymorphism of pigs. *Anim. Blood Groups Biochem. Genet.* **2,** 35–38.

Kühne, R., Vögeli, P., Kuhn, B., Kaufmann, A., and Stranzinger, G. (1989). Four new alpha-protease inhibitor variants PO1A-A', PO1A-I*, PO1Bt* and P12-Y* in pigs detected by horizontal 2D electrophoresis. *Anim. Genet.* **20,** Suppl. 1, 70–71.

Kurosawa, Y., and Tanaka, K. (1988). Electophoretic variants of serum transferrin in wild pig populations of Japan. *Anim. Genet.* **19,** 31–35.

Kurosawa, Y., Amano, T., Okada, I., Ota, K., Namikawa, T., Maeda, Y., Hasnath, M. A., Mostafa, K. G., Faruque, M. O., and Majid, M. A. (1987). Blood groups and biochemical polymorphisms in the native pig populations of Bangladesh. *In* "Genetic Studies on Breed Differentiation of the Native Domestic Animals in Bangladesh, Part II," pp. 59–74. Faculty of Applied Biological Science, Hiroshima University.

Lalley, P. A., and McKusick, V. A. (1985). Report of the committee on comparative mapping. Human Gene Mapping 8. *Cytogenet. Cell Genet.* **40,** 536–566.

Lalley, P. A., O'Brien, S. J., Créau-Goldberg, N., Davisson, M. T., Roderick, T. H., Echard, G., Womack, J. E., Graves, J. M., Doolittle, D. P., and Guidi, J. N. (1987). Report of the committe on comparative mapping. *Cytogenet. Cell Genet.* **46,** 367–389.

Landegent, J. E., Jansen in de Wal, N., Dirks, R. W., Baas, F., and Van der Ploeg, M. (1987). Use of whole cosmid cloned genomic sequences for chromosomal localization by non-radioactive *in situ* hybridization. *Hum. Genet.* **77,** 366–370.

Lathrop, G. M. (1984). Easy calculation of lod scores and genetic risks on small computers. *Am. J. Hum. Genet.* **36,** 460–465.

Lax, T. (1971). Hereditary splayleg in pigs. *J. Hered.* **62,** 250–251.

Leong, M. M. L., Lin, C. C., and Ruth, R. F. (1983a). Assignment of superoxide dismutase (SOD-1) gene to chromosome no. 9 of domestic pig. *Can. J. Genet. Cytol.* **25,** 233–238.

Leong, M. M. L., Lin, C. C., and Ruth, R. F. (1983b). The localization of genes for HPRT, G6PD, and alpha-GAL onto the X-chromosome of domestic pig (Sus scrofa domesticus). *Can. J. Genet. Cytol.* **25,** 239–245.

Lin, C. C., Draper, P. N., and De Braekeleer, M. (1985). High-resolution chromosomal localization of the β-gene of the human beta-globin gene complex by *in situ* hybridization. *Cytogenet. Cell Genet.* **39,** 269–274.

Linhart, J. (1971). Lm, a new blood group factor of the L sysem in pigs. *Anim. Blood Groups Biochem. Genet.* **2,** 243–245.

Linhart, J. (1974). Further studies on the E blood group system in pigs. *Anim. Blood Groups Biochem. Genet.* **5,** 129–132.

Linhart, J., and Romanov, J. D. (1975). Eabgmnop (=E15), a new allele in the E bloodgroup system of the pig. *Anim. Blood Groups Biochem. Genet.* **6,** 57–59.

Littlefield, J. W. (1964). Selection of hybrids from matings of fibroblasts *in vitro* and their presumed recombinants. *Nature (London)* **256,** 495–497.

Ljungqvist, L., and Hyldgaard-Jensen, J. (1983). Genetic poymorphism of the vitamin D binding protein (Gc protein) in pig plasma determined by agarose isoelectrofocusing. *Anim. Blood Groups Biochem. Genet.* **14,** 293–297.

Lüdecke, H.-J., Senger, G., Claussen U., and Horsthemke, B. (1989). Cloning defined regions of the human genome by microdissection of banded chromosomes and enzymatic amplification. *Nature (London)* **338:** 348–350.

Maeda, N., Ebert, D. L., Doers, T. M., Newman, M., Hasler-Rapacz, J., Attie, A. D., Rapacz, J., and Smithies, O. (1988). Molecular genetics of the apolipoprotein B gene in pigs in relation to artheriosclerosis. *Gene* **70,** 213–229.

Makaveev, T. (1979). On the genetic polymorphism of NAD H_2 methemoglobin reductase in the erythrocytes of sheep, cattle and swine. *Proc: Conf. Anim. Blood Groups Biochem. Polymorphism, 16th,* Leningrad, *1978* Vol. 3, pp. 91–97.

McAlpine, P. J., Boucheix, C., Pakstis, Stranc, L. C., Berent, T. G., and Shows, T. B. (1988). The 1988 catalog of mapped genes and report of the nomenclature committee. *Cytogenet. Cell Genet.* **49,** 4–38.

McGraw, R. A., Jacobson, R. J., and Akamatsu, M. (1988). A male-specific repeated DNA sequence in the domestic pig. *Nucleic Acids Res.* **16,** 10389.

McKusick, V. A. (1980). The anatomy of the human genome. *J. Hered.* **71,** 370–391.

McKusick, V. A., and Ruddle, F. H. (1977). The status of the gene map of the human chromosomes. *Science* **196,** 390–405.

Meyer, J. N., and Verhorst, D. (1973). The evidence of erythrocyte acid phosphatase by starch gel electrophoresis in the pig. *Anim. Blood Groups Biochem. Genet.* **4,** 129–131.

Mileham, A. J., Siggens, K. W., and Plastow, G. S. (1988). Isolation of a porcine male specific DNA sequence. *Nucleic Acids Res.* **16,** 11842.

Monaco, A. P., Neve, R. L., Coletti-Feener, C., Bertelson, C. J., Kurnit D. M., Kunkel, L. M. (1986). Isolation of candidate cDNAs for portions of the Duchenne muscular dystrophy gene. *Nature (London)* **323,** 646–650.

Morton, N. E. (1955). Sequential tests for the detection of linkage. *Am. J. Hum. Genet.* **7,** 277–318.

Nadeau, J. H. (1989). Maps of linkage and synteny homologies between mouse and man. *Trends Genet.* **5,** 82–86.

Nielsen, P. B. (1961). The M blood group system of the pig. *Acta Vet. Scand.* **2,** 246–253.

Nielsen, P. B. (1962). A new allele in the H blood group system in pigs. *Arsberet.—K. Vet.- Landbohoejsk., Inst. Sterilitetsforsk.* **5,** 201–204.

Nielsen, P. B., and Vögeli, P. (1982). A new Kd subgroup designated Kg in the porcine K blood group system. *Anim. Blood Groups Biochem. Genet.* **13,** 65–66.

Ohno, S. (1973). Ancient linkage groups and frozen accidents. *Nature (London)* **244,** 259–262.

Oishi, T., Tomita, T., and Komatsu, M. (1980). New genetic variants detected in the haemopexin and ceruloplasmin systems of Ohmini miniature pigs. *Anim. Blood Groups Biochem. Genet.* **11,** 59–62.

Op't Hof, J., Osterhoff, D. R., and de Beer, G. (1972). Polymorphism of sorbitol dehydrogenase and 6-phosphgluconate dehydrogenase in swine. (Sus Scrofa). *Anim. Blood Groups Biochem. Genet.* **3,** 237–239.

Orkin, S. H. (1986). Reverse genetics and human disease. *Cell (Cambridge, Mass.)* **47,** 845–850.

Ott, J. (1976). A computer program for linkage analysis of general human pedigrees. *Am. J. Hum. Genet.* **28,** 528–529.

Paterson, A. H., Lander, E. S., Hewitt, J. D., Peterson, S., Lincoln, S. E., and Tanksley, S. D. (1988). Resolution of quantitative traits into Mendelian factors by using a complete linkage map of restriction fragment length polymorphisms. *Nature (London)* **335,** 721–726.

Philipsen, M., Hruban, V., and Hradecký, J. (1985). Detection of a new non-MHC alloantigenic system (SLD) in pigs. *Anim. Blood Groups Biochem. Genet.* **16,** 175–182.

Pontecorvo, G. (1975). Production of mammalian somatic cell hybrids by means of polyethylene glycol (PEG) treatment. *Somatic Cell Genet.* **1,** 397–400.

Poustka, A., and Lehrach, H. (1986). Jumping libraries and linking libraries: The next generation of molecular tools in mammalian genetics. *Trends Genet.* **2,** 174–179.

Pretorius, A. M. G., Schmid, D. O., Cwik S., Meyer, J., and Albert, E. D. (1977). PGM3 locus and its genetic polymorphism in lymphocytes of the pig. *J. Immunogenet.* **4,** 363–365.

Rabin, M., Fries, R., Singer, D., and Ruddle, F. H. (1985). Assignment of the porcine major histocompatibility complex to chromosome 7 by *in-situ* hybridisation. *Cytogenet. Cell Genet.* **39,** 206–209.

Randi, E., Apollonio, M., and Toso, S. (1986). Electrophoretic polymorphism of erythrocyte leucine aminopeptidase in the wild boar, Sus scrofa. *Anim. Genet.* **17,** 359–362.

Rando, A., and Masina, P. (1985). Restriction site polymorphisms in the pig β-globin gene cluster. *Anim. Blood Groups Biochem. Genet.* **16,** 35–40.

Rapacz, J. (1982). Current status of lipoprotein genetics applied to livestock production in swine and other domestic species. *Proc. World Congr. Genet. Appl. Livest. Prod., 2nd,* Madrid, *1982,* Vol. 6, pp. 365–374.

Rapacz, J., and Hasler-Rapacz, J. (1982). Immunogenetic studies on polymorphism, postnatal passive acquisition and development of immunoglobulin gamma (IgG) in swine. *Proc. World Congr. Genet. Appli. Livest. Prod., 2nd,* Madrid, *1982,* Vol. 8, pp. 601–606.

Rapacz, J., and Hasler-Rapacz, J. (1986). Polymorphism and inheritance of swine small intestinal receptors mediating adhesion of three serological variants of *Escherichia coli*-producing K88 pilus antigen. *Anim. Genet.* **17,** 305–321.

Rapacz, J., Jr., Reiner, Z., Ye, S.-Q., Hasler-Rapacz, J., Rapacz, J., and McConathy, W. J. (1988). Detection of plasminogen polymorphism in swine. *In* "Fibrinogen 3. Biochemistry, Biological Functions, Gene Regulation and Expression" (Mosesson *et al.,* eds.), pp. 351–354. Elsevier Science Publishers, New York.

Rasmusen, B. A. (1964). Gene interaction and the A-O blood group system in pigs. *Genetics* **50,** 191–198.

Rasmusen, B. A. (1965a). Linkage between the loci for C and J blood groups in pigs. *Vox Sang.* **10,** 239–241.

Rasmusen, B. A. (1965b). Eaef (= E6), a sixth allele at the E blood-group locus in Yorkshire pigs. *Vox Sang.* **10,** 242–245.

Rasmusen, B. A. (1981). Linkage of genes for PHI, halothane sensitivity, A-O inhibition, H red blood cell antigens and 6-PGD variants in pigs. *Anim. Blood Groups Biochem. Genet.* **12,** 207–209.

Renard C., Kristensen, B., Gautschi, C., Hruban, V., Fredholm, M., and Vaiman, M. (1988). Joint report of the first International Comparison Test on Swine Lymphocyte Alloantigens (SLA). *Anim. Genet.* **19,** 63–72.

Royer-Pokora, B., Kunkel, L. M., Monaco, A. P., Goff, S. C., Newburger, P. E., Baehner, R. L., Cole, F. S., Curnutte, J. T., and Orkin, S. H. (1986). Cloning the gene for an inherited human disorder—chronic granulomatous disease—on the basis of its chromosomal location. *Nature (London)* **322,** 32–38.

Rozhkov, Y. I. (1983). Genetic polymorphism of amylases revealed by polyacrylamide gel electrophoresis in some species of artiodactyla. *Genetica* **19,** 488–497.

Ruddle, F. H. (1981). A new era in mammalian gene mapping: Somatic cell genetics and recombinant DNA methodologies. *Nature (London)* **294,** 115–120.

Ryttman, H., Thebo, P., Gustavsson, I., Gahne, B., and Juneja, R. K. (1986). Further data on chromosomal assignments of pig enzyme loci LDHA, LDHB, MPI, PEPB and PGM1, using somatic cell hybrids. *Anim. Genet.* **17,** 323–333.

Ryttman, H., Thebo, P., and Gustavsson, I. (1988). Regional assignments of NP and MPI on chromosome 7 in pig, Sus scrofa. *Anim. Genet.* **19,** 197–200.

Safarova, P., Karadjole, I., Hyldgaard-Jensen, J., Nielsen, P. B., and Lycik, G. (1972). Phosphoglucomutase polymorphism in porcine red cells. *Acta Vet. Scand.* **13,** 134–136.

Saison, R. (1967). Two new antibodies, anti-Nb and anti-Nc in the N blood-group system in pigs. *Vox Sang.* **12**, 215–220.

Saison, R. (1973). Red cell peptidase polymorphism in pigs, cattle, dogs, and mink. *Vox Sang.* **25**, 173–181.

Saison, R., and Giblett, E. R. (1969). 6-Phosphogluconate dehydrogenase polymorphism in the pig. *Vox Sang.* **16**, 514–516.

Saison, and R., O'Reilly, M. (1971). Phosphohexose isomerase variants in pigs. *Vox Sang.* **20**, 274–276.

Saison, R., Rasmusen, B. A., and Hradecký, J. (1967). Da, a factor in a new blood-group system in pigs. *Can. J. Genet. Cytol.* **9**, 794–798.

Schmidt, D. V., and Ebner, K. E. (1972). Multiple forms of pig, sheep and goat alpha-lactalbumin. *Biochim. Biophys. Acta* **263**, 714–720.

Schröffel, J. (1965). Genetic determination of the serum "thread proteins" and the slow alpha-2 globulin polymorphism in pigs. *In* "Blood Groups of Animals" J. Matoušek, (ed.), pp. 321–329. Publ. House Czech. Acad. Sci., Prague.

Schröffel, J. (1966). New genetic variants of transferrins and haptoglobins in pigs. *Nature (London)* **210**, 1274–1275.

Sellwood, R., Gibbons, R. A., Jones, G. W., and Rutter, J. M. (1975). Adhesion of enteropathogenic *Escherichia coli* to pig intestinal brush borders: The existence of two pig phenotypes. *J. Med. Microbiol.* **8**, 405–411.

Shows, T. B., McAlpine, P. J., Boucheix, C., Collins, F. S., Conneally, P. M., Frezal, J., Gershowitz, H., Goodfellow, P. N., Hall, J. G., Issit, P., Jones, C. A., Knowles, B. B. Lewis, M., McKusick, V. A., Meisler, M., Morton, N. E., Rubinstein, P., Schanfield, M. S., Schmickel, R. D., Skolnick, M. H., Spence, M. A., Sutherland, G. R., Traver, M., Van Cong, N., and Willard, H. F. (1987). An international system for human gene nomenclature (ISGN, 1987). *Cytogenet. Cell Genet.* **46**, 11–28.

Shrimpton, A. E., and Robertson, A. (1988a). The isolation of polygenic factors controlling bristle score in *Drosophila melanogaster*. I. Allocation of third chromosome sternopleural bristle effects to chromosome sections. *Genetics* **118**, 437–443.

Shrimpton, A. E., and Robertson, A. (1988b). The isolation of polygenic factors controlling bristle score in *Drosophila melanogaster*. II. Distribution of third chromosome sternopleural bristle effects within chromosome sections. *Genetics* **118**, 445–459.

Singer, D. S., Camerini-Otero, D., Satz, M. C., Osborne, B., Sachs, D., and Rudikoff, S. (1982). Characterization of a porcine genomic clone encoding a major histocompatibility antigen: Expression in mouse L cells. *Proc. Natl. Acad. Sci. U.S.A.* **79**, 1403–1407.

Singer, D. S., Ehrlich, R., Satz, L., Frels, W., Bluestone, J., Hodes, R., and Rudikoff, S. (1987). Structure and expression of class I MHC genes in the miniature swine. *Vet. Immunol. Immunopathol.* **17**, 211–221.

Smith, C., and Bampton, P. R. (1977). Inheritance of reaction to halothane anaesthesia in pigs. *Genet. Res.* **29**, 287–292.

Smith, C., and Simpson, S. P. (1986). The use of genetic polymorphisms in livestock improvement. *J. Anim. Breed. Genet.* **103**, 205–217.

Soller, M., Beckmann, J. S. (1982). Restriction fragment length polymorphisms and genetic improvement. *Proc. World Congr. Genet. Appl. Livest. Prod., 2nd,* Madrid, *1982*, Vol. 6, pp. 396–404.

Soller, M., Beckmann, J. S. (1983). Genetic polymorphism in varietal identification and genetic improvement. *Theor. appl. Genet.* **67**, 25–33.

Soller, M., and Beckmann, J. S. (1985). Restriction fragment length polymorphisms and animal genetic improvement. *Rev. Rural Sci.* **6**, 10–18.

Stratil, A., Gábrišová, E. (1989). Polymorphic proteins of the pig *(Sus scrofa). Rep.: Pig Blood Group Polymorphic Protein Workshop,* Stara Zagora, Bulgaria, 1–6.

Takahashi, A., Tanaka, H., Tamada, S., Shibata, H., and Inagaki, J. (1974). Genetic variations of pancreatic proteinase in pigs (in Japanese). *Res. Bull. Aichi-Ken Agric. Res. Center., Ser. E* **4**, 27–32.

Tanaka, K., Oishi, T., and Kurosawa, Y. (1979). Genetic studies on the native pigs in Taiwan. I. Blood groups and electrophoretic variants of serum proteins in Taoyan breed. *Jpn. J. Swine Sci.* **16**, 37–44.

Tanaka, K., Kurosawa, Y., Kurosawa, K., and Oishi, T. (1980). Genetic polymorphism of erythrocyte esterase-D in pigs. *Anim. Blood Groups Biochem. Genet.* **11**, 193–197.

Tanksley, S. D., Young, N. D., Paterson, A. H., and Bonierbale, M. W. (1989). RFLP mapping in plant breeding: New tools for an old science. *Biotechnology* **7**, 257–264.

Thoday, J. M. (1961). Location of polygenes. *Nature (London)* **191**, 368–370.

Tikhonov, Y. N., Borovich, Y. E., and Gorelov, I. G. (1979). A new notion of the genetical structure of the blood group locus G in pigs according to the finding of the alleles Gbc, Gbd, Gad. *Proc. Int. Conf. Anim. Blood Groups Biochem. Polymorphism, 16th,* Leningrad, *1978*, Vol. 3, pp. 110–113.

Vaiman, M. (1987). MHC in farm animals. *Anim. Genet.* **18**, Suppl, 7–10.

Vaiman, M., Chardon, P., and Cohen, D. (1986). DNA polymorphism in the major histocompatibility complex of man and various farm animals. *Anim. Genet.* **17**, 113–133.

Valenta, M., Hyldgaard-Jensen, J., and Moustgaard, J. (1967). Three lactic-dehydrogenase isoenzyme systems in pig spermatozoa and the polymorphism of subunits controlled by a third locus C. *Nature (London)* **216**, 506–507.

Van de Weghe, A., Yablanski, T., and Van Zeveren, A. (1988). A third variant of glucose phosphate isomerase in pigs. *Anim. Genet.* **19**, 55–58.

Van Zeveren, A., Van de Weghe, A., Bouquet, Y., and Varewyck, H. (1988). The porcine stress linkage group. II. The position of the Halothane locus and the accuracy of the Halothane test diagnosis in Belgian Landrace pigs. *J. Anim. Breed. Genet.* **105**, 187–194.

Verhorst, D. (1973a). Polymorphism in glucose-6-phosphate dehydrogenase in the German Large White. *Anim. Blood. Groups Biochem. Genet.* **4**, 65–68.

Verhorst, D. (1973b). Enzym- und Serumproteinpolymorphismen in Schweinezuchtlinien. Thesis, University of Göttingen.

Vögeli, P. (1989a). Position of the Phi and Po2 loci in the Hal linkage group in pigs. *Génét. Sél. Evol.* **21**, 119–125.

Vögeli, P. (1989b). Blood groups of pigs, serological and genetical studies (in German). Habilitation Thesis, ETH Zurich.

Vögeli, P., Gerwig, C., Schneebeli, H., and Wäfler, P. (1982). Gene frequencies of important polymorphic systems of two divergent lines of Landrace pigs using index selection procedures (in German). *Schweiz. Landwirtsch. Monatsh.* **60**, 234–240.

Vögeli, P., Gerwig, C., and Schneebeli, H. (1983). The A-O and H blood group systems, some enzyme systems and halothane sensitivity of two divergent lines of Landrace pigs using index selection procedures. *Livest. Prod. Sci.* **10**, 159–169.

Vögeli, P., Kühne, R., Wysshaar, M., and Stranzinger, G. (1987). Recombination rates and gene order for some serum alpha-protease inhibitors and immunoglobulin heavy-chain allotypes in pigs. *Anim. Genet.* **18**, 351–360.

Vögeli, P., Kühne, R., Gerwig, C., Kaufmann, A., Wysshaar, M., and Stranzinger, G. (1988). Prediction of the halothane genotypes with the aid of the S, Phi, Hal, H, Po2, Pgd haplotypes of parents and offspring in Swiss Landrace pigs. *Zuechtungskunde* **60**, 24–37.

Voron, F. P., and Sokolenko, N. T. (1971). Dalneishie -izuchenie sistemy F grupy krovi sviney. *Genetika*, **7**, 58–61.

Wald, A. (1947). "Sequential Analysis." Dover, New York.

Weiss, M. C., and Green, H. (1967). Human–mouse hybrid cell lines containing partial complements of human chromosomes and functioning human genes. *Proc. Natl. Acad. Sci. U.S.A.* **58,** 1104–1111.

White, R., Leppert, M., Bishop, D. T., Barker, D., Berkowitz, J., Brown, C., Callahan, P., Holm, T., and Jerominski, L. (1985). Construction of linkage maps with DNA markers for human chromosomes. *Nature (London)* **313,** 101–105.

Widar, J., and Ansay, M. (1975). Adenosine deaminase in the pig: Tissue specific patterns and expression of the silent ADA O allele in nucleated cells. *Anim. Blood Groups Biochem. Genet.* **6,** 109–116.

Widar, J., Ansay, M., and Hanset R. (1974). Polymorphism of adenosine deaminase in the pig: Allelic variation in erythrocytes. *Anim. Blood Groups Biochem. Genet.* **5,** 115–124.

Womack, J. E., and Moll, Y. D. (1986). Gene map of the cow: Conservation of linkage with mouse and man. *J. Hered.* **77,** 2–7.

Wysshaar, M. (1988). Polymorphic lipoprotein systems and their relationships to economical traits in pigs. Thesis 8534, ETH Zürich.

Yerganian, G., and Nell, M. B. (1966). Hybridization of dwarf hamster cells by UV-inactivated Sendai virus. *Proc. Natl. Acad. Sci. U.S.A.* **55,** 1066–1073.

Yerle, M., Gellin, J., Echard, G., Lefevre, F., and Gillois, M. (1986). Chromosomal localization of leukocyte interferon gene in pig (*Sus scrofa domestica* L.) by *in situ* hybridization. *Cytogenet. Cell Genet.* **42,** 129–132.

GLOSSARY OF COMMONLY USED TERMS[1]

Androgenetic	Having origin from the male parent only, with no contribution of the female parent.
Aneuploidy	Chromosome number that is not an exact multiple of the characteristic number for the species.
Autosome	Any chromosome that is not a sex chromosome.
C-band	Regions of chromosomes having special staining properties and containing large blocks of heterochromatin.
Centric fusion	A type of translocation whereby two single armed chromosomes are joined at their centric ends to form a single bi-armed chromosome.
Centromere	The localized region of a chromosome to which spindle fibers are attached at mitosis and meiosis.
Chimera	An embryo or an animal having cells with genetically different components. The component cell lines are derived from genetically different gametes.
Chromosome lag	Delayed migration of a chromosome from the equatorial plate of metaphase to the poles, resulting in its exclusion from either of the daughter cells.
Deletion	Loss of a segment of a chromosome.
Dispermy	Penetration of an ovum by two spermatozoa.
Digyny	Presence of two maternal pronuclei in an ovum.
Diploid	The chromosome number characteristic of a species ($2n$).
Euploidy	A chromosome number that is an exact mul-

[1] Adapted from N. S. Fechheimer (1990), The Domestic Chicken (*Gallus domestica*) as an Organism for the Study of Chromosome Aberrations. *In* "Farm Animals in Biomedical Research" (V. Pliska and G. Stranzinger, eds.), pp. 43–54. Verlag Paul Perry, Hamburg and Berlin.

tiple of the characteristic number for the species.

G-banding Differentiation of segments of a chromosome into darkly and lightly staining regions by treatment with trypsin or other agents, followed by staining with Giemsa stain.

Gonosomes Sex chromosomes (X and Y in most mammals and Z and W in birds).

Haploid Cell or organism containing the chromosome number characteristic of gametes of that species (n).

Heteroploid Cell or organism with a chromosome number that is different from that which its characteristic for the species.

Heterochromatin Genetically inactive region of chromosome that has staining properties different than those of the remainder of the chromosome.

Hyperdiploid Chromosome complement differing from the normal diploid ($2n$) by the addition of one or more chromosomes.

Hypodiploid Chromosome complement differing from the normal diploid ($2n$) by the absence of one or more chromosomes.

Inversion Rotation through 180° of an interstitial chromosome segment so that the sequence of genes it contains has a new position relative to the other genes of the chromosome.

Marker chromosome A chromosome with markedly altered morphology by which it is readily identified and distinguished from other chromosomes.

Meiosis The process of cell division of germ cells that requires two successive divisions, i.e., meiosis I and meisois II.

Mitosis The process of cell division of somatic cells.

Monosomy Chromosome complement differing from the diploid number by having one chromosome missing ($2n - 1$).

Mosaic Embryo or organism composed of a mixture of genetically different cells that were derived from a single fertilized egg.

Multivalent Configuration of more than two chromosomes in paired association at prophase and metaphase of the first meiotic division.

n Gametic chromosome number characteristic for the species; the haploid chromosome number.

Nondisjunction	Failure of chromatids (or homologous chromosomes in the first meiotic division) to separate at anaphase and move in opposite directions. The result is one daughter cell that is trisomic and one that is monosomic.
NOR	Nucleolar organizing region of particular chromosomes identified by a silver stain procedure.
p arm	The short arm of a bi-armed chromosome.
Parthenogenesis	The production of an embryo from a female gamete without the participation of a male gamete.
Pentaploid	Chromosome number that is five times the gametic number characteristic for the species ($5n$).
Pericentric inversion	An inversion that includes the centromere.
Polyploid	Chromosome number that is an exact multiple, of three or greater, of the gametic number of the species ($3n$, $4n$, $5n$, etc.).
q arm	The long arm of a chromosome.
Q-banding	Differentiation of chromosomal segments into brightly and dully fluorescing regions following staining with quinacrine stain.
R-bands	Differentiated segments of chromosomes that are darkly and lightly stained (the reverse of the staining properties of G-bands), i.e., darkly stained G-bands are lightly stained R-bands and vice versa.
Synaptonemal complex	Proteinaceous structure that enables pairing of homologous chromosomes at prophase of the first meiotic division.
Telomere	The terminal end of a chromosome arm.
Tetraploid	Chromosome number four times that of the gametic number characteristic of the species ($4n$).
Translocation	Exchange of segments between nonhomologous chromosomes.
Triploid	Chromosome number three times that of the gametic number characteristic of the species ($3n$).
Trisomy	Chromosome complement differing from the number characteristic for the species by having one additional chromosome ($2n + 1$).

INDEX

A

Acid/saline/Giemsa technique, 33
Acrocentric chromosomes, 10
  Zebu cattle, 62–64
Amino acids, codons coding for, 15
Amniotic cell cultures (horse), 133
Amniotic fluid, chromosome preparations from, 27–28
Anaphase, mitotic, 6
Anaphase I, 28
Aneuploidy
  characterization, 10
  in chickens
    autosomal, 190, 195–196
    sex chromosomes, 190, 195
  embryonic
    effects of, 243
    incidence of, 237—239
  in fish, 210
  occurrence, 10–11
Autoradiography, chromosome identification with, 31–32
Autosomal trisomy
  development to term and, 243
  in horses, 150–151
Azoospermia, XXY-associated (cattle), 58

B

Barr body, see Sex chromatin body
Bone marrow cells, chromosome preparations from, 27
Bone marrow cultures (horse), 134
Brachygnathia, trisomy 18-associated, 57–58
Breeding, gene mapping and, 273—275
5-Bromodeoxyuridine, for R-band staining, 33
Bull twins, 11–12

C

Cattle chromosomes
  abnormalities
    autosomal heteroploidies, 57–58
    distribution of abnormal embryos, 240
    freemartinism, see Freemartins
    intersexuality, see Intersexuality
    monosomies, 57
    numerical, 56–59
    1/29 Robertsonian translocation, 47–48
      effects of, 50–55
      eradication of, 55–56
      origin of, 48–50
      transmission of, 53–55
    sex chromosomes, see Sex chromosomes
    structural, 46–56
    trisomy 18-associated, 57–58
  aneuploid and diploid secondary spermatocytes and oocytes, 232–233
  frequency of embryos producing heterozygotes for structural alterations, 236
  karyotype, 41–46
    bull heterozygous for 1/29 translocation, 48
    bull homozygous for 1/29 translocation, 49
    normal bull, 42
    C-band
    RBA, 45
    normal cow, RBG, 45
C-banding
  cattle chromosomes, 43
  chicken chromosomes, 176, 180–182
  differential staining, 33–34
  fish chromosomes, 220
  goat chromosomes, 111
  horse chromosomes, 138, 141

309

Cell division, blockage at mitotic metaphase, 24–25
Cell lines
  Chinese hamster auxotrophic mutants, 253, 262
  mouse LMTK cells, 253
  pig
    C23, 96
    C26, 96
    ENS 122, 97
    NADL, 96–97
    PK-2a, 95–97
    PK(13), 95
    PK(14), 95–96
    PK(15), 95–97
    PTF, 97
    R206, 96
    R208, 96
    R338, 95
    R344, 95
Cellular origin theory, of freemartinism, 61–62
Centric fusion, 11, see also Robertsonian translocation
  trisomy with, 58
Centric fusion translocations
  fish, 211
  goats, 120–121
  horses, 149–150
  pigs, 75–76, 89
  sheep, 113–115
Centromere position, chromosome morphology and, 10, 23
Centromeric indexes, for chicken chromosomes, 179
Centromeric staining, 34
Chiasmata, 8, 28
  counts at diakinesis/metaphase (chicken), 189
  counts at diplotene and diakinesis, 28
Chicken chromosomes
  abnormalities
    aneuploid/aneuploid mosaicism, 196
    autosomal aneuploidy, 190, 195–196
    diploid/aneuploid mosaicism, 196
    diploid/diploid chimeras, 194–195
    diploid/tetraploid mosaicism, 194
  diploid/triploid chimeras, 194–195
  in embryos, 191–193
  euploidy, 189–190
  experimentally produced, 197–198
  pentaploidy, 194
  pericentric inversions, 197–199
  reciprocal translocations, 197, 199–201
  sex chromosome aneuploidy, 190, 195
  spontaneously occurring, 196–197
  tetraploidy, 194
  triploidy, 193–194
  banding procedures, 176
  centromeric indexes of, 179
  DNA content of nuclei, 170–171
  heterochromatin, 171
  karyotype, 171
    meiotic, 183–189
    mitotic, 177–173
  knowledge of, 201–202
  lengths of, 179
  microchromosomes, 171
  types of, 171
  W chromosome, 177
  Z chromosome, 177
    C-banding, 180–182
    description, 177
    length and centromeric index for, 179
    morphology, 180
Chimerism
  characterization, 11
  in chickens
    diploid/diploid, 194–195
    diploid/triploid, 194–195
    in embryos, 191–192
    euploid, 190
    origins and etiology, 192–193
  freemartins, see Freemartins
  XX/XXY, in pigs, 92
  XX/XY
    in cattle, 61–62
    in goats, 123
    in pigs, 92
  XX/YY, in pigs, 92
Chromomycin A_3 staining, fish nucleolar organizer regions, 220

Chromosomal analyses, 3
    germ cells during first meiotic division, 231
    sexing of bovine embryos, 65
Chromosome 2 (human), comparative maps of genes on (cattle, human, mouse), 267–268
Chromosome 6 (human), comparative maps of genes on (cattle, human, mouse), 262–263
Chromosome 8 (cattle), genes homologous to mouse *Lsh*, 267
Chromosome 9 (human), comparative maps of genes on (cattle, human, mouse), 263–264
Chromosome 12 (human), comparative maps of genes on (cattle, human, mouse), 264–265
Chromosome 21 (human), comparative maps of genes on (cattle, human, mouse), 265–266
Chromosome abnormalities, *see also* specific abnormality
    distribution of abnormal embryos, 240
    frequencies
        in chick embryos, 191
        of embryos producing heterozygotes for structural alterations, 236
        in the general population (porcine), 92–93
    heteroploidies
        aneuploid (pigs), 82–84
        autosomal (cattle), 57–58
        euploid (pigs), 81–82
    incidence of (chickens), 196–197
    in vivo induction in pigs, 93–95
    numerical, 10–11
        cattle, 56–59
        chickens, 189–196
        fish, 210, 221
        goats, 121
        pigs, 81–84
        sheep, 113
    structural, 11–12
        cattle, 46–56
        chick embryos, 191–192
        chickens, 196–201
        fish, 210
        goats, 120–123
        pigs, 84–89
        sheep, 113–120
        undefined (porcine), 89–90
Chromosome banding
    cattle, 42–43
    C-bands, 33–34
    centromeric staining, 34
    G-bands, 32–33
    nomenclature for, 36–37
    Q-bands, 32
    R-bands, 32–33
    T-bands, 34
Chromosome deletions, 11
    in chickens, 197
    in fish, 211
    in pigs, 89
    in sheep, 117
    X chromosome, in cattle, 56
    Xp, in horses, 150
Chromosome duplications
    in fish, 89
    in pigs, 89
Chromosome identification
    autoradiography, 31–32
    differential staining
        C-bands, 33–34
        centromeric, 34
        G-bands, 32–33
        high-resolution banding, 35–37
        nomenclature for, 36–37
        nucleolar organizer regions, 34
        Q-bands, 32
        R-bands, 33
        sister chromatids, 34–35
        T-bands, 34
    markers, 31
    morphology, 31
Chromosomes
    display of, 8–10
    elongated, production, 35–37
    meiotic, 6–9
    in metaphase, morphology, 10
    mitotic, 4–6
    mitotic stimulators, 9–10
    p arm, 10
    q arm, 10
Codons
    coding for amino acid sequences, 15
    control sequences, 15

312 INDEX

Colchicine, blockage of cell division at mitotic metaphase with, 24
Committee for Standardized Karyotype of *Ovis aries*, 113
Concanavalin A, for lymphocyte cultures, 24
Crossbreeding, Zebu × European cattle, 64
Crossing-over process, meiotic, 6, 28
Cytogenetics
  bovine embryos, methods for sexing, 65
  chicken
    applicability to mammals, 202–203
    as model organism, 202
  fish
    in situ DNA hybridization, 222
    as model organisms, 213–215
  germ cells and embryos, 230–231
  history of, 1–4
  horse, clinical applications, 146–147

D

Deacetylmethylcolchicine, blockage of cell division at mitotic metaphase with, 24
Deletions, *see* Chromosome deletions
Diakinesis, 8, 28
  chiasmata counts at, 28
  crossing-over frequencies, 28
Differential staining
  C-bands, 33–34
  centromeric, 34
  G-bands, 32–33
  high-resolution banding, 35–37
  nucleolar organizer regions, 34
  Q-bands, 32
  R-bands, 33
  sister chromatids, 34–35
  T-bands, 34
Diploid/polyploid mixoploid embryos, 241
  effects of, 244
Diplotene stage, in meiosis, 8, 28
  chiasmata counts at, 28
  crossing-over frequencies, 28
Disease resistance genes, *Lsh* locus in cattle and mice, 266–267
Disjunctions, pig chromosomes, 86–88
DNA
  cloning, 16
  composition, 12–13
  fish
    chromosome numbers and, 210–211
    flow cytometry, 221–222
  nucleotide strands, 13
  replication, 13
DNA probes
  for gene mapping (cattle), 256, 269–270
  Y chromosome identification by hybridization with (cattle), 65
Drumstick appendages, 21–22
Duplications, *see* Chromosome duplications
Dysgenesis, gonadal (cattle), 60

E

Eggs (chicken)
  handling, 173
  incubation, 173
  processing of embryonic tissue, 173–174
Electron microscopy, chromosome banding with (horse), 143
Elongated chromosomes, production, 35–37
Embryos
  abnormal, effect on fertility and litter size, 235–243
  chicken
    handling and incubation of eggs, 173
    with haploid component, 192–193
    structural abnormalities, 191–192
    tissue processing, 173–174
  cultures of (horse), 133–134
  cytogenetic study of, 230–231
  diploid/polyploid mixoploids, 241
  haploid/diploid, 241
  haploid/diploid mixoploids, 240
  haploidy, 240
  hyperdiploidy, 237–239
  hypodiploidy, 237–239
  in vitro maturation of oocytes, 241–243
  mortality, 244–245
  producing heterozygotes for structural alterations, 236
  sexing (cattle), 64–65
  tetraploid, 241
  triploid, 11, 240–241
Endoreduplication, 11

ENS 122 cell line, 97
Environmental toxicology, fish as *in vivo* models, 213–214
Ethidium bromide, for high-resolution banding, 36
Euploidy, in chickens
  chimeras, 190
  polyploidy, 189

F

Fertility
  centric fusion translocation effects (sheep), 115
  effects of heterozygosity for structural alterations, 233
  pericentric inversion effects (chicken), 198
  reciprocal translocation effects (chicken), 199
  reduction, Y chromosome effects (cattle), 64
  1/29 translocation effects (cattle), 50–51
Fetal loss, incidence of, 244–245
Fibroblast cultures
  chicken, 175
  chopping of tissue, 26
  fish, long-term, 219–220
  harvesting, 27
  horse, 133
  plasma clot method, 26
  subculturing, 27
  trypsinization, 26
First International Conference for the Standardization of Domestic Animal Karyotypes, 4, 113, 143–144
Fish chromosomes
  banding, 220–221
  karyotype, 210–213
  ploidy levels, 221–222
  ploidy manipulation, 217–218
  sex determination, 215–217
  transgenic fish, 222
Fixation, lymphocytes cultures, 26
Flow cytometry, fish DNA quantities, 221–222
Fluorescent-plus-Giemsa technique
  for R-band staining, 33
  for sister chromatid exchanges, 34–35

Fluorochromes, for Q-band staining, 32
Freemartins, 11–12
  cattle
    cellular origin theory, 60–61
    characterization, 61
    chimerism, 61
    hormonal theory of, 61
    occurrence, 60–61
    role of H-Y antigen, 60–61
  goats, 123
  sheep, 118

G

G1 period, of mitosis, 6
G2 period, of mitosis, 6
Gametogenesis, 1/29 translocation effects, 51–53
G-banding
  cattle chromosomes, 42–43
  chicken chromosomes, 176, 180
  differential staining, 32–33
  fish chromosomes, 220
  goat chromosomes, 111
  horse chromosomes, 135, 144
  pig chromosomes, 77
  sheep chromosomes, 111, 113
Gene cloning, 15–16
Gene dosage compensation, in cattle, 58
Gene mapping, 3–4
  bovine, 42, 46
    comparative maps of homologous genes (cattle, humans, mice), 262–268
    current status, 257–262
    DNA probes, 269
    in situ hybridization, 257
    interspecific hybrids, 268
    list of mapped genes, 259–261
    pedigree analysis, 256–257
    somatic cell genetics, 253–256
  breeding and, 273–275
  conserved linkage segments, 279
  conserved synteny groups, 279
  genetic maps, 268, 275
  homology segments, 279
  physical maps, 268, 275
  porcine
    comparative mapping, 279–281

Gene mapping (continued)
    current status, 281
    gene assignments, 282
    in situ hybridization, 277–279
    linkage analysis, 275–276
    list of gene loci, 284–291
    somatic cell genetics, 276–277
    synteny and linkage of gene loci, 283
Genes, 12–15
    codons, 15
    DNA composition, 12–13
    inborn errors of metabolism, 12
    introduction into germs lines of fish, 218
    linear arrangement, 12
    mapped, bovine, 259–261
    traits, 12
Gene therapy, 3
Genetic manipulation (fish), 217–218
Gene transfer (fish), 218
Germ cells
    cytogenetic study of, 230–231
    meiosis
        in females, 231–232
        in males, 231
Giemsa bands, see G-banding
Giemsa staining, for R-bands, 33
Goat chromosomes
    abnormalities
        centric fusion translocations, 120–121
        freemartins, 123
        goat–sheep hybrids, 124–125
        intersexuality, 121–123
        true hermaphrodites, 123–124
        X chromosome polyploidy, 121
        Y chromosome polyploidy, 121
    banding patterns, 111
    karyotype, female, 110
    normal complement, 109–111
    X chromosome, 109
    Y chromosome, 109
Goat–sheep hybrids, 124–125
Gonadal dysgenesis, in cattle, 60
Growth hormone, fusion gene constructs
    (fish), 218

H

Haploid/diploid mixoploid embryos, 240–241
    effects of, 243–244

Haploidy, embryonic, 240
Harvesting, fibroblast cultures, 27
Hatchability
    pericentric inversion effects (chicken), 198
    reciprocal translocation effects (chicken), 199
Hermaphroditism
    in fish, 215–217
    pseudohermaphroditism
        cattle, 60
        horses, 155
        pigs, 91
        sheep, 120
    true
        cattle, 59–60
        goats, 123–124
        pigs, 90–91
Heterochromatin
    chicken chromosomes, 171
    goat chromosomes, 113
    pig chromosomes
        centromeric, polymorphism for, 80–81
        groups of, 78
Heteroploidies
    aneuploid
        in chickens
            autosomal, 190
            sex chromosome, 190
        in pigs, 82–84
    autosomal, in cattle, 57–58
    euploid
        in chickens, 189–190
        in pigs, 81–82
High-resolution banding, 35–37
Hinnies, 159
Histones, in metaphase chromosomes, 13
Hormonal theory, of freemartinism, 61
Horse chromosomes
    abnormalities
        autosomal trisomy, 150–151
        centric fusion translocation, 149
        clinical studies on, 148
        intersexuality, 155
        isochromosomes, 149
        Turner's syndrome, 152–153
        types of, 149
        X/autosome translocation, 148
        Xp deletion, 150

XXX condition, 154–155
X/XX mosaics, 153–154
XX/XXX mosaics, 154–155
X/XY mosaics, 154
XY sex reversal, 156
aneuploid and diploid secondary spermatocytes and oocytes, 232–233
banding techniques, 135–143
comparative studies, 158–159
karyotype
 idiograms of G-banded chromosomes, 144
 measurements of unbanded chromosomes, 144
 morphology, 143
 normal, 143–145
 Paris Conference, 144–145
 Reading Conference, 143–144
 variants, 145
meiotic, 134–135
 conventional, 134
 synaptonemal complex analysis, 134–135
mitotic
 amniotic cell cultures, 133
 bone marrow cultures, 134
 embryo cultures, 133–134
 fibroblast cultures, 133
 lymphocyte cultures, 132–133
Horses, domestic
 breeds, 157–158
 evolution of, 157
 hybrids, 159–160
Hot spots, in pig karyotype, 84
H-Y antigen
 monoclonal antibody, bovine embryo sexing with, 65
 role in freemartinism, 61–62
 60,XX intersex goats, 123
Hybridization with DNA probes, sexing of bovine embryos with, 65
Hybrids
 Equidae, 159–160
 goat–sheep, 124–125
 interspecific, use for gene mapping (bovine), 268
Hyperdiploid embryos, 237–239
Hypodiploid embryos, 237–239
Hypotonic treatment
 history of, 2
 for lymphocyte cultures, 25–26

I

Idiograms, G- and R-banded horse chromosomes, 144
Inborn errors of metabolism, 12
In situ hybridization
 fish, 222
 for gene mapping
  bovine, 257
  porcine, 277–279
Interphase cells, 5–6
 preparation, 20–22
  drumstick appendages, 21–22
  Lyon hypothesis of X inactivation, 20–21
  sex chromatin body, 20–21
Intersexuality
 cattle, 59–60
  gonadal dysgenesis, 60
  pseudohermaphroditism, 60
  testicular feminization syndrome, 60
  true hermaphroditism, 59–60
 chickens, 189–190
 goats, 121–124
 horses, 155
 pigs, 82, 90–92
  causes of, 91–92
  pseudohermaphroditism, 91
  true hermaphroditism, 90–91
 sheep, 118–120
  freemartins, 118
  pseudohermaphroditism, 120
  testicular feminization, 119–120
Interspecific hybrids, for gene mapping (bovine), 268
Inverions, chromosomal, 11
 pericentric, *see* Pericentric inversions
Isochromosomes (horse), 149

K

Karyotypes
 cattle, 41–46
  bull heterozygous for 1/29 translocation, 48
  bull homozygous for 1/29 translocation, 49
  cow carrying the X/autosome translocation, RBA, 57
  definition of hybrid cell panels, 255

316 INDEX

Karyotypes (continued)
  with monosomy 1 from embryo sired by bull carrying 1/29 translocations, 54
  normal bull
    C-band, 45
    Giemsa stained, 42
    RBA, 45
  normal cow, RBG, 45
  Zebu bull, 63
chicken
  meiotic
    primary spermatocytes, 183–186
    secondary spermatocytes, 187
    synaptonemal complexes, 187–189
  mitotic
    C-bands, 180–182
    G-bands, 180
    morphometry, 177–180
    Q-bands, 180
    R-bands, 180
  normal, 171–172
display of, 8–10
fish, 210–213
  salmonid, evolution of, 212
goat, female, 110
horse, 136–140
  C-band variants, 145
  chromosome 12 and 13 variants, 145
  comparative studies, 158–159
  idiograms, 144
  measurement of unbanded chromosomes, 144
  morphology, 143
  NOR-band variants, 145
  normal, 143–145
  normal female, 139
  normal male, 138
  Paris Conference, 144–145
  Reading Conference, 143–144
  X chromosome variants, 145
  Y chromosome length variation, 145
pig
  centric fusion, 75–76
  diagrammatic representation, GTG-banded, 79
  evolutionary aspects, 74–76
  normal boar, GTG-banded, 76
sheep
  ram, 112
  ram heterozygous for 1p−;20q+ reciprocal translocation, 116
  standardization
    Committee for Standardized Karyotype of *Ovis aries,* 113
    First International Conference, 4, 143–144
    Second International Conference, 4, 144–145
Klinefelter syndrome, in sheep, 118

L

Leptotene stage, in meiosis, 8, 28
Linkage analysis, 275–276
Linkage segments, conserved, 279
Litter size
  effects of heterozygosity for structural alterations, 233
  reciprocal translocation effects (pig), 85
Lymphocyte cultures, 23–24
  blockage of cell division, 24–25
  chicken, 174–175
  fish, 219
  fixation, 26
  horse, 132–133
  hypotonic treatment, 25–26
  mitogens, 24
Lyon hypothesis of X inactivation, 20–21

M

Major histocompatibility complex, complementarity of mapping methods (bovine), 259, 262
Markers, for chromosome identification, 31
Meiosis
  female, 231–232
    abnormal, 233–235
  male, 231
  nondisjunction rates, 232
Meiosis I, 6–8
  anaphase I, 8
  cell divisions in, 6
  chiasmata, 8
  crossing over, 6
  diakinesis, 8
  diploidtene stage, 8

equational division in, 6
leptotene stage, 8
metaphase I, 8
pachytene stage, 8
prophase I, 8
reductional division in, 6
synapsis, 8
telophase I, 8
tetrads, 8
zygotene stage, 8
Meiosis II
 completion of, 8
 incidence of chromosomally abnormal embryos, 237–243, 246
 metaphase II, 8
Meiotic chromosomes
 chicken, 172, 175
 horse
  conventional, 134
  synaptonemal complex analysis, 134–135
 pig, 80
  effects on litter size, 85–88
  preparation, 28–29
   female, 29
   male, 29
Messenger RNA, 15
Metabolism, inborn errors of, 12
Metacentric chromosomes, 10
Metaphase chromosomes, 6
 chick embryos, 173–174
 fibroblast culture technique, 26–28
  chicken, 175
  horse, 133
  histones, 13
 lymphocyte culture technique, 23–26
  blockage of cell division, 24–25
  fixation, 26
  hypotonic treatment, 25–26
  mitogens, 24
 preparation, 23–28
 shapes, 10
Metaphase I, 8, 28
Metaphase II, 8
 nondisjunction assessment at, 28–29
Methotrexate, for high-resolution banding, 36
Microchromosomes, 171–172
Mitogens, for lymphocyte cultures, 24

Mitosis
 anaphase, 6
 cell division phase, 5–6
 G1 period, 6
 G2 period, 6
 interphase, 5–6
 metaphase, 6
 prophase, 6
 S period, 6
 telophase, 6
Mitotic chromosomes
 autosomes, 4
 characterization, 4–5
 chicken
  embryo cultures, 173–174
  fibroblast cultures, 175
  lymphocyte cultures, 174–175
 horse
  amniotic cell cultures, 133
  bone marrow cultures, 134
  embryo cultures, 134
  fibroblast cultures, 133
  lymphocyte cultures, 132–133
 pig, 76–79
Mitotic stimulators, 9
Mixoploid embryos, effects of, 243–244
Molecular genetics, 15–16
Monoclonal antibodies, for H-Y antigen, bovine embryo sexing with, 65
Monosomic cells, 10
Monosomies
 cattle, 57
 chicken, 195–196
 horse, X chromosome, 152–153
 pig, 83
 tertiary, 89–90
Morphology, chromosome
 centromere position and, 10, 23
 identification of chromosomes by, 31
 in metaphase, 10
Mosaics, 11
 chicken
  aneuploid/aneuploid, 196
  diploid/aneuploid, 196
  diploid/tetraploid, 194
  embryos, 192
 horse
  X/XX, 153–154
  XX/XXX, 154–155
Mules, 159

Mutation research, fish as models for, 214–215

N

NADL cell line, 96–97
Nomenclature, chromosome banding, 36–37
Nondisjunction
  rates during male and female meiosis, 232
  at second metaphase, 28–29
Nucleolar organizer regions
  bovine chromosomes, silver nitrate staining, 46
  chicken chromosomes
    characterization, 182
    silver nitrate staining, 177
  differential staining, 34
  fish chromosomes
    chromomycin A_3 staining, 220
    ploidy determination by, 222
    silver nitrate staining, 46
  horse chromosomes, silver nitrate staining, 141–143
  pig chromosomes
    polymorphism for, 81
    silver nitrate staining, 78
  silver nitrate staining, 34
Nucleolar satellites, 2, 20
Nucleotide strands, in DNA, 13

O

Oligospermia, XXY-associated (cattle), 58
Oncological research, fish as models for, 214
Oocytes
  chromosome loss during fixation and preparation, 233
  in vitro maturation, 241

P

Pachytene stage, in meiosis, 8, 28
Pairing
  pericentric inversion effects (chicken), 198–199
  reciprocal translocation effects (chicken), 200
Paris Conference, for standardization of banded karyotypes, 4, 144–145
Pedigree analysis, bovine, 256–257
Pentaploidy, chick embryos, 194
Pericentric inversions, 11
  chicken, 172
  effects on
    fertility and hatchability, 199
    pairing and segregation, 199–200
  fish, 211
  horse, 158–159
  Y chromosome of European cattle, 63–64
Phages, 16
Phytohemagglutinin, 9
  for lymphocyte cultures, 24
Pig chromosomes
  abnormalities
    aneuploid heteroploidy, 82–84
    autosomes, 83–84
    centric fusion translocations, 89
    deletions, 89
    distribution of abnormal embryos, 240
    duplications, 89
    euploid heteroploidy, 81–82
    in general population, 92–93
    in vivo induction of aberrations, 93–95
    numerical aberrations, 81–84
    reciprocal translocations, 84–89
    sex chromosomes, 82–83
    structural aberrations, 84–89
    triploidy, 81–82
  aneuploid and diploid secondary spermatocytes and oocytes, 232–233
  centric fusion, 75
  karyotype, 74–79
    hot spots in, 84
  meiosis, 80
  mitosis, 76–79
  polymorphisms
    heterochromatin, 80–81
    nucleolar organizer regions, 81
  synaptonemal complex analyses, 80
PK-2A cell line, clonal lines derived from, 95–97
Plasma clot method, 26
Plasmids, 16
Ploidy manipulation (fish), 217–218

Pokeweed mitogen, 9
  for lymphocyte cultures, 24
Polling gene, in goats, 122–123
Polymorphisms, pig chromosomes
  for centromeric heterochromatin, 81–81
  for nucleolar organizer regions, 81
Polyploidy
  characterization, 10
  in chickens, 189–190
  in fish, 210–211, 221–222
  in goats, 121
  mechanisms, 11
Prophase, mitotic, 6
Prophase I, 8, 28
  completion of, 8
  stages in, 8
Proteins, in eukaryotic chromosomes, 13
Protein synthesis, RNA types in, 15
Pseudohermaphroditism
  in cattle
    female, 60
    male, 60
  in horses, 155
  in pigs, 91
  in sheep, 120
PTF cell line, 97

Q

Q-banding
  chicken chromosomes, 176, 180
  differential staining, 32
  fish chromosomes, 220
  goat chromosomes, 111
  horse chromosomes, 135, 144
  pig chromosomes, 77
  sheep chromosomes, 111
Quinacrine, for Q-band staining, 32

R

R-banding
  cattle chromosomes, 43
  chicken chromosomes, 176, 180
  differential staining, 33
  goat chromosomes, 111
  horse chromosomes, 135, 138, 144
  pig chromosomes, 77

Reading Conference, for standardization of banded karyotypes, 4, 143–144
Reciprocal translocations, 11
  chickens
    effects on fertility and hatchability, 199
    experimentally produced, 197
    pairing and segregation, 200
    spontaneously occurring, 197
    transmission of translocated chromosomes, 200–201
  pigs, 84–89
  sheep, 115–117
Recombination nodules, chicken synaptonemal complexes, 187
Replication, 13
Restriction fragment length polymorphisms, 252, 256, 276
Reverse genetics, 252–253
Ribosomal RNA, 15
Robertsonian translocation, 11, *see also* Centric fusion
  in fish, 210–211
1/29 Robertsonian translocation
  common origin hypothesis, 49–50
  effects on
    fertility, 50–51
    gametogenesis, 51–53
  eradication of, 55–56
  frequency, 49
  occurrence, 47
  recurrent mutation hypothesis, 48–49
  transmission of, 53–55

S

Satellites, markers for chromosome identification, 31
Secondary constrictions, markers for chromosome identification, 31
Second International Conference for the Standardization of Domestic Animal Karyotypes, 4, 144–145
Segregation
  pericentric inversion effects (chicken), 198–199
  reciprocal translocation effects, 200
Sex chromatin body, 2, 20–21
Sex chromosomes, 4–5
  aneuploidy effects, 243

320   INDEX

Sex chromosomes (*continued*)
  birds
    ZW (female), 6
    ZZ (male), 6
  cattle, 41
    X/autosome translocations, 56
    X chromosome deletions, 56
    XXX condition, 59
    XXY condition, 58
    XYY condition, 59
  chickens, aneuploidy, 190, 195
  fish, 215–217
  freemartinism, *see* Freemartins
  goats, anomalies, 121
  intersexuality, *see* Intersexuality
  monosomy effects, 243
  pigs, 77, 82–083
  sheep, anomalies, 117–120
Sex determination
  bovine embryos, 64–65
  fish, 215–217
Sex reversal
  gene for (goat, mouse), 122–123
  phenotypic (fish), 217
Sheep chromosomes
  abnormalities
    centric fusion translocations, 113–115
    chromosome 20-associated, 117
    deletions, 117
    distribution of abnormal embryos, 240
    freemartins, 118
    intersexuality, 118–120
    pseudohermaphroditism, 120
    reciprocal translocations, 115–117
    testicular feminization, 119–120
  aneuploid and diploid secondary spermatocytes and oocytes, 232–233
  banding patterns, 111–113
  karyotype (ram), 112
  normal complement, 111–113
Sheep–goat hybrids, 124–125
Silver nitrate staining, for nucleolar organizer regions
  bovine chromosomes, 46
  chicken chromosomes, 177
  fish chromosomes, 220
  horse chromosomes, 141–143
  pig chromosomes, 78
Sister chromatid exchanges, identification, 34–35

Sister chromatids, differential staining, 34–35
Somatic cell genetics, for gene mapping, 252
  bovine, 253–256
  porcine, 276–277
S period, of mitosis, 6
Spermatocytes
  chromosome loss during fixation and preparation, 233
  primary, meiotic chromosomes (chicken), 183–186
  secondary
    chromosome preparation from, 233
    meiotic chromosomes (chicken), 187
Staining, differential, *see* Differential staining
Subculturing, fibroblast cultures, 27
Submetacentric chromosomes, 10
Synapsis, 8
Synaptonemal complex analyses
  chicken chromosomes, 175–176
  chicken oocytes in microspread preparations, 187–189
  horse chromosomes, 134–135
  pig chromosomes (male), 80
Syntenic groups, 254–255
  conserved, 279

T

T-banding
  differential staining, 34
  pig chromosomes, 78
Telocentric chromosomes, 10
Telophase, mitotic, 6
Testicular feminization
  in cattle, 60
  in sheep, 119–120
Testicular hypoplasia, XXY-associated
  in cattle, 58
  in pigs, 58
Tetraploidy, 10
  cellular, 11
  chicken, origins and etiology, 194
  embryonic, 241
Thymidine, chromosome identification with, 31–32
Tissue cultures, for fish chromosomes, 219–220

T-lymphocyte stimulator, see Concanavalin A
Toxicology, environmental, see Environmental toxicology
Traits, genetic, 12
  dominant, 12
  recessive, 12
Transcription, 15
Transfer RNA, 15
Transgenic fish, 218, 222
Translocations, 11
  1/29, see 1/29 Robertsonian translocation
  centric fusion
    fish, 211
    goats, 120-121
    horses, 149–150
    pigs, 75–76, 89
    sheep, 113–115
  chicken, 172
  fish, 211
  reciprocal, 11
    chickens, 197–201
    pigs, 84–89
    sheep, 115–117
  Robertsonian (fish), 211
  X/autosome
    cattle, 56
    horses, 148
Triploid/diploid mixoploid embryos, effects of, 244
Triploid embryos, mechanism, 11
Triploidy, 10
  chicken, origins and etiology, 193–194
  chicken embryos, 189, 191
  effects of, 244
  embryonic, 240–241
  fish, 210
  pigs, 81–82
Trisomies, 10
  autosomal
    development to term and, 243
    in horses, 150–151
  cattle, 57–58
  with centric fusion, 58
  chick embryos, 192
  chickens, 190, 195–196
  pigs, tertiary, 89–90
Trisomy 17 (pig), 83

Trisomy 18
  cattle, 57–58
  pig, 83
Trisomy 23 (horse), 151
Trisomy 26 (horse), 151
Trisomy 28 (horse), 136, 151–152
Trisomy 30 (horse), 152–153
Trisomy X (horse), 154–155
Trypsin G-band technique, 33
Trypsinization, fibroblast cultures, 26
Turner's syndrome
  in horses, 152–153
  in sheep, 117–118

W

W chromosomes (chicken), 117
  ZW teleomeres, 187–189

X

X/autosome translocations
  in cattle, 56
  in horses, 148
X chromosomes
  cattle, 41
    C-banding, 43
    deletions, 56
    R-banding, 43
    X/autosome translocations, 56
  goats, 109
    polyploidy, 121
  horses
    C-band staining for, 33
    monosomy, 152–153
    variants, 145
  inactivated, autoradiographic identification, 32
  pigs, 77
    synteny conservation, 279–280
X irradiation
  chicken semen, 197
  in vivo induction of pig chromosome aberrations by, 94–95
  PK(14) clonal lines derived from, 95–96
XO (Turner) syndrome
  in horses, 152–153
  in sheep, 117–118

Xp deletion (horse), 150
XXX condition
  in cattle, 59
  in horses, 154–155
X/XX mosaics (horse), 153–154
XX/XXX mosaics (horse), 154–155
XX/XY chimeras
  cattle, 61–62
  goats, 123
  horses, 155
  pigs, 92
XX/XY mosaics (horse), 155
XX/XY system (fish), 215–216
XXY condition
  cattle, 58
  sheep, 118
X/XY mosaics (horse), 154
XY sex reversal syndrome, in horses, 156
XYY condition
  cattle, 59
  sheep, 118

Y

Y chromosomes
  cattle, 41
  C-banding, 43
  effects on fertility, 64
  embryonic, identification by hybridization with DNA probes, 65
  pericentric inversion, 63–64
  polymorphism of, 62, 64
  R-banding, 43
  Zebu cattle, 62–64
  Zebu × European crosses, 64
  goats, 109
  anomaly in, 121
  horses, length variation, 145
  pigs, 77

Z

Z chromosomes (chicken)
  C-banding, 180–182
  description, 177
  length and centromeric index, 179
  morphology, 180
  ZW teleomeres, 187–189
Zygotene stage, in meiosis, 8, 28

NOV 2 7 1990